Budgeting and Financial Management in the Federal Government

Volume 1 in the Series
Research in Public Management

Series Editors: Lawrence R. Jones and Nancy C. Roberts
Naval Postgraduate School, Monterey, CA

Budgeting and Financial Management in the Federal Government

Jerry L. McCaffery

Professor of Public Budgeting
Graduate School of Business and Public Policy
Naval Postgraduate School

and

L. R. Jones

Wagner Professor of Public Management
Graduate School of Business and Public Policy
Naval Postgraduate School

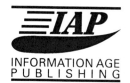

INFORMATION AGE
PUBLISHING

80 Mason Street • Greenwich, Connecticut 06830 • www.infoagepub.com

ISBN: 1-931576-12-2 (paper); 1-931576-13-0 (cloth)

Printed in the United States of America

CONTENTS

LIST OF TABLES, FIGURES, GRAPHS, AND EXHIBITS

INTRODUCTION

This book is more ambitious in its scope than originally intended. In the beginning we were simply attempting to write a textbook for use in our public budgeting and financial management course at the Naval Postgraduate School because we could not find another book that covered all that we wanted to teach to our students. However, as we wrote pieces of the book over a period of years, we realized that it would be possible and desirable to produce a book with much broader coverage and relevance.

Budgeting and financial management in the U.S. federal government is highly complex and highly differentiated, e.g., in the processes employed by the Executive branch versus those used by Congress. In this book we attempt to cover the processes of both the Executive and Congress and the relationships between the two. The book provides views from several perspectives, e.g., managerial and political. We attempt to provide readers with an understanding of how federal budget and financial management processes are supposed to operate. However, we then go a step further to show how these processes actually operate often in contrast to the intended template. Additionally, this book is intended to capture and combine the views of the academic and the practitioner, including those of the participants in the process. For the above reasons, we believe this work is unique relative to other books written in this topic area.

The book begins with a lengthy introduction to the basics of federal budgeting and financial management. Alas, even the basics are perhaps too complex for an introduction. This chapter also delves into budget theory to some extent, drawing on the work of Aaron Wildavsky and his theory (or hypothesis) of incrementalism. Chapter II provides a detailed description and analysis of the history and development of federal budgeting, with some emphasis on financial management as well. However, our main focus here is on the evolution of the budget processes of the Executive and Congress. In addition, our intent is to provide analytical and scholarly insight into what happened and why, going beyond the mere facts of history.

Chapter III concentrates primarily on budget formulation, as opposed to budget execution, the topic area covered in Chapter IV. Chapter III delves deeply into the more visible phase of budgeting—budget formulation. However, while the budget debate and critical policy issues are most visible once the budget is under review by Congress, we reach into the intricacies of budget formulation at the agency and department levels because it is here that the framework of many of the most important issues to be decided by the President and Congress are developed and analyzed, a process that culminates in presentation of the President's budget proposal to Congress. We investigate estimation and calculation, negotiation and the tactics and strategies designed to garner the most resources possible for pending agencies. Our purpose is to describe what is done from both academic and practitioner viewpoints. We begin by describing how the process is supposed to operate, and then we concentrate even more on how the process actually works, in some cases in considerable contrast to the formal process template. Similarly, in Chapter IV we dig deeply into the less visible but perhaps most critical phase of budgeting—budget execution. We show that regardless of the myriad of controls and constraints imposed by Congress and Executive control agencies, there is a great deal of effort exerted by managers responsible for executing budgets to obtain as much flexibility and discretion as possible in implementation. A primary reason for this effort is not to disobey the wishes of Congress or Executive control agents, but to obtain the best value for the dollar in meeting the contingent requirements that emerge as spending occurs.

The budget as appropriated by Congress and apportioned and allocated within the Executive branch provides a great deal of instruction on what can and cannot be done with appropriated funds. Moreover, the Anti-deficiency Act and the rest of federal Appropriation Law constrains much of what managers can do to match budget plans developed years before enactment into executable spending methods, using all the cash flow management skills required to meet the needs of program managers and service providers and, ultimately, the public. The intricacies of budget execution are fascinating, at least to us. We hope they will be perceived as such by readers.

Chapter V deals with the extensive portion of federal spending that flows through entitlement programs, also termed direct spending. Our perspective is on control of the growth of entitlements that have expanded to more than 54% of federal spending annually. Rather than describing entitlements programs, material that is covered well in other texts we cite, our focus is on alternatives that may be considered to control the growth of entitlement spending in the twenty-first century when the greatest demand for such expenditures will result due to population demographics and other factors.

Chapter VI focuses on budget analysis and budget analysts. Our intent is to demonstrate how budgets are analyzed and the characteristics of budget controllers and analysts. We analyze the incentives that cause budget control agents to do their jobs as they do. Budget controllers are "gatekeepers" and play the role of protector of the public fisc. Their motives are at once simple (to constrain spending) and complex (to influence program delivery and performance). We demonstrate with examples the strategies and tactics employed in budget review, in justification and defense.

Chapter VII investigates aspects of budget strategy including strategic representation and misrepresentation. Various ploys are used regularly in the budget process by both controllers and spending advocates. These ploys typically are an accepted and legitimate part of budget competition that is inevitable between programs and spenders and cutters. The chapter also addresses patterns of strategy, contingency as a major factor influencing strategy, and how strategies are advanced and negotiated. The chapter ends with prescriptive comments about budget analysis. Managers choose their budget strategies and preferred levels of risk; some will be more aggressive, some less. There are distinct differences between proactive and reactive strategies in budget advocacy and defense.

Chapter VIII delves into approaches to budgeting under conditions of fiscal restraint and stress. Phases of recognition and response to fiscal stress are defined along with the means used to cope with varying degrees of fiscal stress and crisis. These methods range from across the board budget cuts to intricate strategic planning and proactive management responses. The chapter differentiates more versus less successful approaches to the management of fiscal restraint. The most prominent restraint management strategy employed in the past several decades, restructuring, is described and analyzed in detail.

Chapter IX provides a review of budget process reforms, past and present. It attempts to show why and to what extent various reforms succeeded or failed. An investigation of budget process reforms recommended by Caiden and others is rendered. Analysis of the Chief Financial Officers Act (CFOA) and some aspects of the Government Performance and Results Act (GPRA) is provided, thus broadening the scope of our reform review to include financial management initiatives beyond but influencing budgeting.

Chapter X investigates new and emerging approaches to budgeting for results and performance. Responsibility budgeting and accounting is treated in detail as a means for implementing results-oriented budgeting. The chapter that follows reviews and analyzes approaches to performance budgeting, illustrating various approaches with examples from federal agencies, particularly from the largest, the Department of Defense. Chapter XII provides perspectives on budgeting, contracting and management control to demonstrate that there are critical choices to be made by government with respect to the use of different budgetary control structures and means for funding activities, including contracting out.

Chapter XIII provides an overview of financial management reform in the federal government, concentrating on the major changes enacted and implemented roughly over the past decade. Extensive description and analysis of the Chief Financial Officers Act (CFOA) is undertaken, investigating the various aspects of this legislation and implications it has for federal accounting and budgeting. Chapter XIV follows this analysis with an evaluation of the implementation of both the CFOA and GPRA to date. We find reasons to be pleased with the results of implementation of some parts of these Acts while providing criticism of some of the expectations promised to result from adoption that have not and may not be realized. Criteria are applied to evaluate the relative success of these initiatives, finding both positive and less than positive results. We end with cautious optimism about the long-range impact of these measures, reinforced by examples, while offering a warning that unless Congress adopts and uses the analysis provided by the Executive, the results achieved will be less than desired and promised.

The book concludes with three appendices consisting of an example of a public financial management curriculum and two full-length case studies. The first appendix articulates one approach to the design of a Master's degree level public financial management curriculum based upon a management control model. The second appendix provides a detailed case analysis of budget execution and cash flow management, demonstrating the difficulties of budget execution in the "real world" in a single Navy command within the Department of Defense. The third appendix provides the background and the detail to understand the complexity and difficulties encountered in implementing the CFO Act in a defense command.

As noted, this book was written over a considerable period of time. Over this period we have benefitted greatly from counsel and advice from a number of colleagues including Fred Thompson, John Mutty, Richard Doyle, Irene Rubin, Justine Farr Rodriguez, Virginia Robinson, Michael Curro, Edmundo Gonzales, Steven App, John Mercer, Edward DeSeve, Alvin Tucker, John Raines, Michael Bourgeois, Sean O'Keefe, Philip Joyce, Greta Marlatt, anonymous reviewers from the Office of Management and Budget and the Senate Appropriations Committee and other anonymous referees. In addition, we wish to acknowledge the co-authorship of portions of two chapters and authorship of two appendices. John Mutty, former Conrad Chair Professor, Graduate School of Business and Public Policy, Naval Postgraduate School, contributed to Chapter IV on budget execution and Fred Thompson, Goudy Professor of Public Management and Policy at the Atkinson Graduate School of Management, Willamette University contributed to Chapter X on budgeting for results and Chapter XII on budgeting, management control and contracting. In addition, Appendix B was written by Lt. William E. Philips, USN and Appendix C was authored by Lt. Martin Sable, USN, both under the guidance of the L. R. Jones and Jerry L. McCaffery as part of Master's degree thesis work in the Graduate School of Business and Public Policy at the Naval Postgraduate School. To all of these colleagues we owe considerable appreciation.

Jerry L. McCaffery
L.R. Jones
Monterey, California

CHAPTER I

AN INTRODUCTION TO PUBLIC BUDGETING AND FINANCIAL MANAGEMENT

AN OVERVIEW OF THE BUDGET PROCESS

Government budgeting is a process that matches resources and needs in an organized and repetitive way so that collective choices are properly resourced. The product of this process is the budget—an itemized and programmatic estimate of expected income and operating expenses for a given unit of government over a set time period. Budgeting is the process of arriving at such a plan and executing it. Once a fiscal year has begun, the budget becomes a plan for tracking and managing the collection of taxes, fees, and other revenues, and for distributing and disbursing these revenues to attain the goals specified in the budget. A variety of financial management functions is performed throughout the fiscal year in conjunction with taxing and spending in an attempt to coordinate the financial activities of government, and to insure accountability, safety, legality, and propriety in the raising and expending of public monies. At the end of the year, the budget process produces reports that allow for comparison of the achievements of government relative to the commitments made when the budget was enacted. In democratic systems, these commitments represent the will of the people as expressed during the politics of the budget process.

Budgeting and financial management are not performed in a vacuum. They are part of a public policy cycle in which (a) public service demands and preferences are articulated, (b) public policy is developed to respond to these demands and preferences by elected officials, (c) resources are

1

generated and allocated to various public and private purposes, (d) programs and implementation strategies and tactics are developed and executed, (e) spending is incurred in the delivery of services and benefits, (f) the outcomes of policies and programs are reported and analyzed. Citizens consume this information and respond to the manner in which services are delivered and the amounts of services supplied, and again articulate their service demands and preferences to their representatives in government. In democratic political systems, it is assumed that the role of government in large part is to meet the demands and preferences of citizens with the resources afforded relative to the condition of the national economy, and to do so in a manner that promotes social equity, economic efficiency, and social and economic stability.

Public policy in this context consists of a set of goals or objectives, strategies and tactics to obtain these goals, a commitment of resources to achieve goals and objectives, an implementation plan based on strategy and limited by resource availability, and a means for measuring, reporting and evaluating the extent to which goals have been met and other outcomes achieved. If these basic components are not present, then policy may be viewed as not properly formulated. Unfortunately, policy analysis often determines that important components are omitted in government policy development and application. Analysis of policy outcomes may reveal that the costs of service development and delivery by government are lower than the benefits achieved. However, in some cases, benefits are exceeded by costs, i.e., net negative benefits have resulted from government action. Where this occurs, policy and service delivery may be questioned relative to their effectiveness. In democratic systems of governance, it is intended that such questions be addressed regularly in the public budget process.

The budget process may be understood to operate in two main phases, formulation and execution. The model of the budget process shown in Exhibit 1 is useful for delineating the sub-phases of the budgetary process.

While the exhibit is linear, readers must clearly understand that at least three budget years are in play at any one time. First is the budget under execution; it has various reporting dates and deadlines, quarterly plans, and reports to both the Office of Management and Budget (OMB) and Congress. It could also include responses to the Appropriations Committees and to the General Accounting Office (GAO) audits made on the prior year. Second is the budget under review in Congress. This includes hearings at several committee venues. To some extent what these committees say about the budget proposal under discussion must be considered by the agency as it begins preparation of its budget for the coming year. Hearings usually begin late in February and feature the Department Secretary and bureau chiefs. In most cases, key bureaus are heard on separate days. These hearings last until early May and may be understood to be part of the nego-

EXHIBIT 1
The Phases of the Budget Process Cycle

I. Budget Formulation
   A. Preparation of Estimates (Executive branch)
   B. Negotiation
      (1) Executive
      (2) Legislative
   C. Enactment
      (1) Legislative
      (2) Executive
II. Budget Execution
   A. Apportionment to agencies, allotment within agencies and Spending
   B. Monitoring and Control
   C. End-Year Accounting and Reconciliation to Appropriations, Financial Audit, Management Audit, Program Evaluation and Policy Analysis

tiation process noted above. In May, the Departments review their Congressional testimony and prepare written answers for questions asked at the hearings. As the appropriation bills progress through Congress, the Department begins to prepare its initial obligation plan for OMB in mid-August with the final plan due October 1 or within 10 days of passage of the bill. Agencies within the department also have to prepare a departmental financial and staffing plan for the coming fiscal year for the Department Budget Office; the final plans are due two weeks after enactment of the bill.

Thirdly, the budget preparation process for the following fiscal year is running concurrently with the execution of the current budget and testimony on the next budget. Budget preparation begins with a Guidance letter and topline allowances from OMB in winter, is followed up with a Spring Preview session where the Department and OMB may work certain issues at dispute and concludes with the routines of budget preparation as dictated in OMB circular A-11, the budget preparation circular. In 1999, A-11 was issued on July 12 and contained more than 580 pages of explanation, definitions, and instructions. In 1999 and 2000, efforts were made to rewrite A-11 in plain language to make it more accessible to the departments and agencies who must use it. This has been largely successful, but the budget process remains a stunningly complex process, where confusion abounds and the necessity for negotiation is obvious. Various amendments and clarifications are added to A-11 during the year as is necessary.

Each new Presidential regime requires a transition year employing ad hoc budget procedures. In 2000, departments prepared their budgets as current services budget (very little or no policy change) and thus an early amendment to A-11 was issued by Mitch Daniels, President Bush's OMB Director on February 14, 2001 to Departments to carry on with the GPRA initiative and to surface the Bush Administration priorities. This transmittal letter said, in part:

> Most agencies submitted an initial version of their FY2002 performance plan to OMB last Fall. The performance goals in this initial plan were set using a current services funding level, and did not anticipate policy and initiative decisions by the new Administration. You should immediately begin making all necessary changes to your FY2002 performance goals to reflect both the agency's top-line allowance and any applicable policy and initiative decisions. The top-line allowance will need to be translated into goal target levels for individual programs and operations. Your FY2002 performance plans and budget materials should reflect the focus on bringing about a better alignment of performance information and budget resources ... These plans should be sent to OMB at least two weeks prior to being sent to Congress to ensure that the President's decisions, policies, and initiatives are appropriately reflected.[1]

Notice that this letter sent in February 2001 was intended to have an impact on the appropriation bills that would be passed in the summer of 2001 to fund the departments beginning in October 2001. This shows the desire of the new administration to get its priorities imprinted on the budget as soon as possible.

Normally, for the U.S. federal government, each year the programs and spending that departments initially propose to begin the budget cycle are prepared and reviewed in close detail first by agency and then department budget staff. These budgets are based upon instructions from the executive so departments will have some notion of how much they may ask for in total, thus the Spring preview by OMB and the Mid-session reviews. The instructions include policy guidance and directions about the form and format of the budget. The federal budget process did not always operate in this top-down manner, but it has done so since the early 1980s. After this review, budgets are sent to the President's Office of Management and Budget (OMB) where hearings are held, decisions made and passed back to the departments and appeals are heard. December is spent preparing the multiple products that comprise the President's budget, updating and locking-up electronic databases, and preparing Congressional justifications. Even in normal years, this process lasts until the end of January.

By the first Monday in February, the President is required by law to submit to Congress his proposed budget for the next fiscal year. As part of his submittal, he delivers a myriad of exhibits, tables, graphics, and thousands of pages of text that show where revenues come from and on which programs he proposes they be spent. For fiscal year 2002, the federal budget was composed of four volumes, the *Budget of the U.S. Government: FY2002; Analytical Perspectives; Historical Tables;* and *A Citizen's Guide to the Budget.* These are presented to Congress and widely disseminated in the media because they are supposed to make the gargantuan sums of money collected and distributed by the federal budget comprehensible to the average citizen. Unfortunately, given the complexity of the data and the general absence of knowledge and interest of the citizenry in budgeting and what the government does with money, it is doubtful that this objective is achieved to any extent.

It is important to understand that Congress never appropriates the President's budget proposal exactly as proposed. This is because the Constitution provides the power to enact taxes and budgets to the Congress, and not the President. An old and true budget aphorism is, "The President proposes and the Congress disposes." Congress spends eight or more months of effort each year scrutinizing the President's proposal in great detail in numerous committees and subcommittees, debating alternatives and amendments of its own origination, asking questions of witnesses called, and listening to testimony from the President's administration and a variety of other advocates and interest group lobbyists in hearings on the budget. Congress then writes separate authorization and appropriation bills that include substantial changes to what the President proposed, votes to approve these huge bills (typically there are thirteen separate appropriation bills alone) and sends them to the President for his signature or veto. In addition to appropriation bills, Congress may also have to pass other legislation to complete the budget plan, for example, bills that change existing tax laws, enact new ones, or modify benefit structures for entitlement programs (e.g., social security). Because Congress rarely passes budgets before the beginning of the fiscal year, departments and agencies often begin each fiscal year under a Continuing Resolution Appropriation (CRA), spending according to instructions passed to them from OMB (and technically from the Treasury) before appropriations are actually enacted. These instructions provide spending flexibility to keep the government operating and are made possible by passage of temporary spending authority by Congress in the continuing resolution appropriation when appropriations have not been approved prior to the beginning of the fiscal year (October 1 to September 30).

BUDGET EXECUTION

After the formal appropriation has been passed and signed by the President, the process for providing spending authority to departments and agencies begins. OMB apportions money to the Departments who in turn allot money to their subunits. Each Agency head then uses allotments to delegate to subordinates the authority to incur a specific amount of obligations. These allotments may be further subdivided into allocations for lower administrative levels. Following these allotments and allocations, obligations can be incurred (e.g., a contract let) and outlays paid when the work or service is completed or the equipment delivered. The apportionment, allotment, and allocation processes are the actual planning for when funds will be spent, by quarter or month and by administrative level.[2] This process also requires departments to resubmit their budgets to OMB for approval, indicating how actual appropriations, rather than the proposals included in the President's Budget, will be spent. The department requests must be approved jointly by OMB and the Treasury before money is approved for expenditure and made available for obligation in department and agency accounts maintained by the Treasury. In effect, the apportionment/allotment process represents a separate mini-budget cycle within the executive, although its major focus is on when dollars will be spent within the fiscal year and to a lesser extent what the mix of consumables will be within the categories approved in the appropriation bill.

Once the appropriations have been allotted, departments allocate their budgets outward to their subunit agency budget staff, who then prepare and issue spending authority and guidance to the various program components where spending obligations are incurred, services delivered and resources consumed. It is important to recognize that some agencies are very large and have huge budgets. In the Department of Defense (DOD), the Office of the Secretary of Defense and the DOD Comptroller receive and allocate the budget for national defense appropriated by Congress. Among the agencies to which funding authority is provided are the Departments of the Army, Navy, and Air Force, each of which may spend more than $70 billion annually.

In allocating the budget, the central budget staffs of departments and large agencies do not completely free the programmatic side of their enterprises to spend as they wish, despite the desire for such flexibility on the part of those who spend. Rather, spending is accompanied by constant monitoring and control by central budget office staff as well as by budget, accounting, and audit staff internal to the program units. Spending is monitored in terms of actual rates versus those projected, and by other variables including of utmost importance, legality and purpose of expenditure (it has to conform to the appropriation and other attendant control language), schedule and timing, location, measures of production and volume, and other variables. In essence, monitoring looks for variances between planned and actual spending that then have to be accommodated through management and control. Where funding is not available in places most needed, reprogramming or transfers (defined subsequently) are requested. Where funding is exhausted due to exceptional circumstances (e.g., natural disasters), supplemental funding requests are sent to and approved by Congress. Moving money to the highest priority and executing the full amounts appropriated are the key tasks of budget execution, perhaps the most important phase of the budget cycle because it is where services are either provided or not, are provided efficiently or not, and where needs are met or neglected.

While the act of budgeting is a planning process, budget execution is a management process. This process is treated in detail in following chapters. In budget execution agencies obligate or commit funds in pursuit of accomplishing their program goals. Following plans made in the budget preparation cycle, employees or contractors are engaged, materials and supplies purchased, contracts let and capital equipment purchased. The basic assumption is that the budget will be executed as it was built once it is approved. In many jurisdictions this concept has legal backing; the summary numbers that appear in the budget documents stand for all the little numbers behind them. Executing the budget simply means going back to the detailed spreadsheets. Many also assume that this execution phase is a relatively simple task compared to preparing and passing the budget, since all it involves is returning to the budget building documents and executing the plans described in them, as modified by the final version of the appropriation bill. The reality of administrative life is somewhat different. A substantial portion of budget execution is driven by the necessity of rescuing careful plans from unforeseen events and emergencies and unknowable contingencies. At the close of the fiscal year, in the aggregate and on average, budget execution may appear to have been a matter of uninteresting routine dominated by financial control procedures, but it is unlikely to have appeared so uneventful to the department budget officer and his staff or the manager charged with carrying out the program. The usual occurrence is for most of the budget year to unroll as planned, but for execution of a small percentage of the budget to consume a major investment of managerial and leadership effort. All jurisdictions have set rules and procedures to help guide agencies through the budget execution process. The tensions in this process involve issues of control, flexibility, and the proper use of public funds.

The final phase of the budget process involves audit and evaluation. In this phase the disbursement of public money is scrutinized to assure officials and the public, first, that funds were used in accord with legislative intent and that no monies were spent illegally or for personal gain and, secondly, that public agencies are carrying out programs and activities in the most efficient and effective manner pursuant to legal and institutional constraints. The first type of audit is called a financial audit. It concentrates on reviews of financial documents to ensure that products and services are delivered as agreed on, that payment is accurate and prompt, that no money is siphoned off for personal use and that all transactions follow the legal codes and restrictions of the jurisdiction. Such audits are generally carried out or supervised by agents external to the entity undergoing audit. These agents include the General Accounting Office and agency Inspectors General at the federal level as well as internal auditing agencies (e.g., the Navy Audit Service), elected or appointed state auditors at the state level and by private sector accounting firms at all levels of government. There is also some accounting between levels of government as the federal government audits use of federal monies in state and local programs and as state governments audit certain local fiscal practices.

Financial audits evaluate honesty and correctness in handling money. As the role of government expanded after World War II, more effort was spent to measure the efficiency and effectiveness of government. This led to experiments with performance budgeting at different levels of government and ultimately to performance auditing. Here the auditor attempts to ensure that the agency is conducting programs in a manner consistent with the laws and regulations that authorize the program and to see if the agency has taken judicious action in resource deployment to attain programmatic ends. Basically, the auditor is attempting to judge efficiency in resource use and effectiveness in program delivery. Findings from such audits help policy makers enhance program outcomes while minimizing the resources required to operate the programs. Often the same agencies responsible for financial audits also do program audits, but since the audit focus is different, different personnel usually do the audit. The reports often become part of the budget process, especially during the legislative stage, and may lead to changes in the laws and rules that guide the program and to the managerial practices of the agency that administers it.

Audit findings may also be reviewed in special hearings by oversight committees, outside the budget process, who want to ensure that agencies behave responsibly. Generally, these audits are published and available to the public. Both financial audits and performance audits help ensure that a jurisdiction is getting the most for its tax dollars. In so doing, they help maintain the vital element of trust in government and in those who disburse its monies and create and administer its programs. In general, the same entities who audit for propriety may also be called upon to audit for performance, including GAO at the federal level and legislative audit agencies at the state level. OMB also has a management review staff and at state and local levels the budget agencies often require that budget analysts combine managerial analysis work with budget analysis.

After all of this activity concludes at the end of the fiscal year and accounts are closed-out to prevent further obligation, budget accounts are audited internally and externally by agency auditors, Inspectors General, the General Accounting Office and other audit agents. In some cases, private firms conduct parts of or all of these audits. After, or in conjunction with auditing, programs are evaluated to see to what extent they have met the objectives and commitments promised to Congress and the executive, and policies are analyzed for their value. All of the information thus developed becomes grist for the mill for preparation of future budgets, as the cycle operates continuously.

A final note is required regarding the revenue side of budgets. In general, it is only at the top level of the budget staff of Congress, the Budget and Tax Committees and Congressional Budget Office (CBO), and the executive Office of Management and Budget (OMB) for the President, where revenue and expenditure estimates for the upcoming year are totaled based upon what Congress passes in appropriations. Simultaneously, as the President and Congress propose and enact the spending plan for the upcoming year, expenditure budgeting management and control of the current year budget is the pervasive activity that occurs throughout the executive branch departments and agencies as organizational subunits compete for their share of funds. Ordinarily, departments and agencies do not concern themselves with revenues other than fees and charges they are allowed to retain in current or future year budgets, and others they collect incidental to their own operation (e.g., National Park admission fees or federal license fees).

For the most part, departments and agencies compete for their share of general revenues accumulated from the tax mechanism. For example, the Department of Defense and the Department of Health and Human Services do not concern themselves much with general government tax policy and revenue generation; they rely on Congress and the President to tell them if their needs can be accommodated within revenues approved for the current and next budget year.

THE BUDGET IN FORM AND DETAIL

The budget of the federal government, indeed of all governments, has many forms. It can be rendered simply as a single line with a few descriptors (e.g., agency name) and funding proposed or available for spending, or as complexly as is imaginable, containing all kinds of programmatic and even performance—related information and associated funding. Essentially, the only constant in budgets is that funding (dollars in the United States) is shown in nominal values, that is, not discounted over time. Exhibits 2A and 2B display President George W. Bush's overall budget plan for fiscal year 2002.

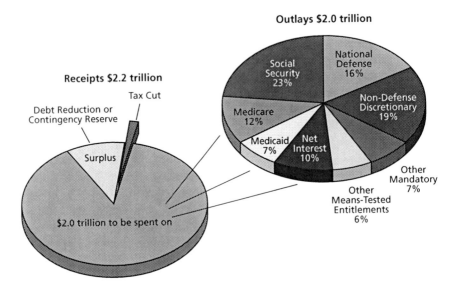

* Means-tested entitlements are those for which eligibility is based on income.
  The Medicaid program is also a means-tested entitlement.

Example 2A

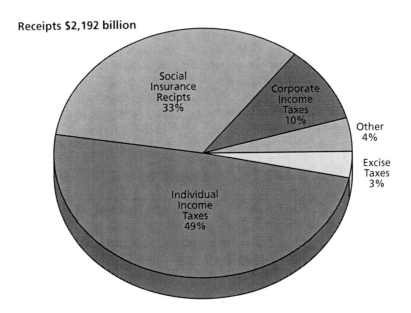

Example 2B
Source: The President's Budget for 2002, Office of Management and Budget

Exhibit 3 shows a relatively uncomplicated object of expenditure budget. The first column represents each object of expenditure upon which funds are available to be spent. This type of budget display is referred to as a line-item budget because each line consists of an item, or more properly speaking, a class of items. For example, the personnel line includes all the personnel positions available to an administrative unit (e.g., clerks, administrative assistants, managers). Usually it includes all benefit costs associated with their employment. In this example, the line displays the total personnel cost authorized for the unit for the current year (CY) and the amount the unit has requested for the next or budget year (BY). As indicated, the spending of this unit is heavily skewed toward personnel.

The second display in Exhibit 3 presents this unit in terms of its programs. This hypothetical unit assesses and collects taxes, and enforces tax law. In the current year, the unit's efforts are evenly divided, judging by dollars spent. In the budget year, the unit intends to emphasize tax enforcement since all of its requested budget increase lies in this category. This display approximates a typical program budget. It reveals far more about what the unit does than the line-item budget, but less about what the unit consumes in performing its function.

EXHIBIT 3
Line-item and Program Budgets

Object of Expenditure	Current Year (CY)	Budget Request (BY)
Personnel	$3,000,000	$3,060,000
Travel	$10,000	$11,000
Office supplies	$15,000	$16,000
Telephone	$12,000	$12,500
Equipment repair	$6,000	$6,000
Capital outlay	$9,000	$5,000
Total	$3,052,000	$3,110,500
Program/activity	CY	BY
Tax assessment	$1,017,334.00	$1,017,334.00
Tax collection	$1,017,333.00	$1,017,333.00
Tax enforcement	$1,017,333.00	$1,075,833.00
Total	$3,052,000.00	$3,110,500.00

The most basic format for display of the operating budget is the object of expenditure budget of the type shown in Exhibit 3. This form of budget display identifies, sometimes in excruciating detail, the items that will be purchased with budget funds. Building, analyzing and making decisions on budgets with this level of detail for large and complex jurisdictions quickly approaches information overload, as reviewers have to struggle to avoid being trapped into questioning inconsequential details about office supplies, while major policy concerns are not fully addressed. To overcome this problem, budgets may be presented in different formats. Table 1 shows spending by department. Table 2 shows spending by appropriation bill and is a snapshot of the House Appropriations target given to its subcommittees (302b allocations) in 2001 for the 2002 budget. Each shows something valuable, but in a little different way.

Table 1.   Discretionary Budget Authority by Agency (In billions of dollars)

Agency	Actual				Estimate				
	1998	1999	2000	2001	2002	2003	2004	2005	2006
Legislative Branch	2	3	3	3	3	3	3	3	3
Judicial Branch	3	3	4	4	5	5	5	5	5
Agriculture	16	16	17	19	18	19	19	19	20
Commerce	4	5	9	5	5	5	5	5	6
Defense-Military	260	275	287	296	310	319	328	337	347
Education	30	29	29	40	45	46	47	48	49
Energy	17	18	18	20	19	20	20	21	21
Health and Human Services	37	42	45	54	57	62	63	65	67
Housing and Urban Development	20	22	21	28	30	32	33	35	36
Interior	8	8	8	10	10	10	10	10	11
Justice	18	18	19	21	20	22	22	22	23
Labor	11	11	9	12	11	12	12	12	13
State	6	8	8	8	9	9	9	10	10
Transportation	13	14	14	18	16	17	18	18	18
Treasury	11	13	13	14	15	15	15	16	16
Veterans Affairs	19	19	21	22	23	24	24	25	26
Corps of Engineers	4	4	4	5	4	4	4	4	4
Other Defense Civil Programs	*	*	*	*	*	*	*	*	*
Environmental Protection Agency	7	8	8	8	7	7	8	7	7
Executive Office of the President	*	*	*	*	*	*	*	*	*
Federal Emergency Management Agency	3	3	4	2	2	2	2	2	2
General Services Administration	*	1	*	*	1	1	1	1	1

Table 1.   Discretionary Budget Authority by Agency (In billions of dollars) (Cont.)

Agency	Actual				Estimate				
	1998	1999	2000	2001	2002	2003	2004	2005	2006
International Assistance Programs	11	31	14	13	13	13	13	14	14
National Aeronautics and Space Administration	14	14	14	14	15	15	15	16	16
National Science Foundation	3	4	4	4	4	5	5	5	5
Office of Personnel Management	*	*	*	*	*	*	*	*	*
Small Business Administration	1	1	1	*	1	1	1	1	1
Social Security Administration	5	5	6	6	6	7	7	7	7
Other Independent Agencies	6	6	6	6	6	6	6	6	6
Allowances	....	....	....	....	5	5	6	6	6
Total	530	582	584	635	661	685	703	720	738

Table 2.   House Appropriations Committee Allocations by Appropriation Bill

Current Status (June 27, 2001)	302(b) Allocation	
	BA	Outlays
Agriculture	$15,519	$15,831
Commerce, Justice, State	$38,541	$39,000
Defense	$300,292	$294,026
District of Columbia	$382	$401
Energy and Water	$23,704	$23,959
Foreign Operations	$15,168	$15,099
Interior	$18,941	$17,768
Labor, HHS, Education	$119,758	$106,238
Legislative Branch	$2,908	$2,855
Military Construction	$10,155	$9,448
Transportation	$14,893	$53,840
Treasury, Postal Service	$16,880	$16,134
Veterans, HUD, Independent Agencies	$84,159	$88,177
Full Committee	$0	$184
Total	$661,300	$682,960

All of the budget formats shown above have their particular uses, as is the case for the myriad of ways in which expenditure plans and programs are displayed. The functional display for Defense (below) includes expenditure in other departments that is defense-related, for example, defense related expenditures in the Department of Energy, civil defense programs in FEMA, Selective Service programs related to the draft, and defense-related activities of some other agencies including the Coast Guard and the FBI.[3] The display by Appropriation for Defense for FY2002 is what the Appropriations Committee has given to its Defense Subcommittee, pursuant to targets given it by the Budget Committee. The total for 2002 in the Departmental display is the amount the President's budget recommended for defense for FY2002. Each of these numbers differs because they measure something different (function versus agency) or the same thing at a different point in the budget process (President's Budget recommendation versus Congressional Budget Resolution totals for the Defense Appropriation bill).

Table 3.   Defense by Function, by Agency and by Appropriation Bill

	2002 Estimates
National Defense function	$319 billion
Defense as an Agency	$310 billion
Defense Appropriation Bill (House 302b)	$300 billion

That the format of the budget depends on its intended use comes as no surprise; what is surprising is that there are so many different venues and contexts in which the budget is used. To understand why this is so requires considerable familiarity with the decision process cycle employed to determine and manage resource allocation. Part of the purpose of this book is to explain the series of decision events that comprise the budget cycle. Additional budget format examples for zero base, line item, performance and program budgets are included at the end of this chapter as attachments A through E. Please note these are for municipalities and not the federal government. They are included because they are good examples of how federal formats might be improved.

BUDGETS AND INFORMATION OVERLOAD

This section explains why so many formats—probably too many—are used in federal budgeting. Technically, the fundamental task in budgeting is twofold; it lies in predicting the future and evaluating the past. Visions about the future are complicated by differing visions of what the future should be, as well as arguments about what it will be given current under-standings of causal relationships. Thus, there is great uncertainty going for-ward; since government is a coercive arrangement and can extract money and time from its citizens and deliver goods and services unequally, say, for example, more to those who are more successful in lobbying and legislat-ing, budgeting tends to be a conservative process where players examine, in excruciating detail, the evidence on decisions that have been made and information about decisions that are about to be made. Consequently, the great problem in budgeting is information overload. Reformers have attempted to address this problem in a variety of ways, with the executive budget movement, the creation of central budget bureaus and legislative staff agencies, public hearings, and published documents describing the budget. Much of this effort involves a rationalistic sense that a better bud-get process results from better information.

Reformers have also attempted to solve the information overload prob-lem by creating better budget systems. Historically, the basic budgeting sys-tem has been an object of expenditure system which features objects of expenditures arrayed in lines of items in spreadsheet format with their names and proposed expenditures, hence the name "line item" budget. The items are usually personnel and supporting expenses, like travel, tele-phone, and offices supplies. In its early form, this type of budget format was closely identified with the accounting system, thus making it relatively sim-ple to execute and audit. In small jurisdictions, with few functions and a lim-ited and homogeneous role for government, this type of budget is still simple to construct, review, execute, and audit. The format of a line item budget presentation includes the line items, what each category cost the previous year, its authorized level in the current year, and the amount requested for funding in the budget year. If this is a biennial presentation, two budget years are shown. Usually, these documents will also show the percentage of change from the current year to the budget year, thus enabling reviewers to scan the presentation and select objects for review, for example, that which increased the most. This type of budget emphasizes control and fiscal accountability, rather than management or planning.[4]

Usually the budget document will have introductory narrative explain-ing the purposes of the unit; this usually changes minimally from year to year and is almost universally referred to as "boilerplate." Budget officers feel that once they have it right, all they need to do is fine tune it with this year's emphasis (buzz words). Most, but not all, line item systems also will have some explanation of changes, usually very brief, and very carefully written. Writers know that readers will not read long justifications, but they also know that the justification will focus how the budget request is per-ceived. In many budget shops, the less experienced budget analysts write the boilerplate and the experts write justification paragraphs. At the local level, the line item display usually carries with it a list of all personnel employed in the unit and their salary cost. This total is transferred to the personal services line on the budget display. There will also be a list of minor capital outlay items (desks, chairs); this may or may not accompany the budget, but the agency budget analyst will use the exhibit to monitor the agency purchases during the budget year. It is easy to see how this type of budget lends itself to control purposes, both for accounting and for managerial control.

THE OBJECTIVES OF BUDGETS AS INSTRUMENTS OF FISCAL POLICY

Political scientists and public administrationists tend to examine budgeting in terms of who gets what, why, and under what conditions. Public administrationists typically are concerned with how the budget is proposed, decided upon, how services are produced, and how budget information is presented and analyzed. They take great interest in the internal workings of government and governance, a propensity shared by political science from which public administration was born. Matters of policy and program effectiveness are of primary concern from this perspective. Public administration attempts to improve the welfare of citizens through attempts to make governance more responsive and government more effective. Often, their prescription for improving effectiveness includes employing more staff and spending more money to achieve unequivocally reasonable and desirable objectives. Criticism of the public administration perspective on budgeting is that it is too much focused on process, overly concerned with function versus output and outcomes, and obsessed with the details of congressional, presidential and agency decision making and service production, to little consequence. However, it may be pointed out that many of the reforms that have made governance more responsive and governments more effective in the past one hundred years or so are wholly or in part attributable to reformist efforts led by public administrationists.

On the other hand, economists tend to examine budgeting from the perspectives of equity (who pays and who benefits, i.e., the distributive consequences of tax and allocation decisions), allocative efficiency, and stability. Our interpretation of this perspective, generally speaking, is that it assumes the role of government is to assess and determine the validity of arguments made by various claimants for shares of the distribution of public money, i.e., to define equity in practice. Equity in the context of budgeting means what is "fair" given that how we define "fairness" is always a debatable question in a democracy and that some degree of competition for resources is inevitable in any socioeconomic system because demand always exceeds supply. How we define what is fair varies over time and is always a primary consideration in the numerous forums of government decision making.

To some, distributional equity refers to policies that transfer income from one set of citizens to another through tax policy, spending and other government actions. Others vehemently disagree with this perspective and generally do not acquiesce to the redistributive role of government. Clearly, how we define what is fair in a democracy is virtually always up for grabs—a work in progress—ever changing relative to the political will of the people and their elected representatives. We are quite aware that fair is sometimes, but certainly not always, defined as equal. But, given variances in need, income, wealth and other variables, distribution of spending based on an "equal share for all" rule would, in many instances, not be judged as fair.

To economists, efficiency means how the decisions of the government affect the productivity of the private sector and the economy as a whole. Efficiency in this context is not concerned with whether the internal operations of government operate in a managerially efficient manner. Rather, efficiency is determined in essence by economic decisions about what should be produced, how, and by whom. The means of production and what is produced is determined through the interaction of the public and private sectors of the economy, and in choices over which goods and services should be provided by government and which are better provided by the private sector. To some, the government is regarded as a net drag on the private economy, causing the sacrifice of efficiency in pursuit of equity objectives. From this view, the best government is that which governs least. To others, the essence of the role of government is to supply equity that can and will never be supplied purely as a function of the pursuit of efficiency in the private sector. The mixed capitalist-socialist form of economy that prevails in the United States represents a compromise between these polar perspectives. As such, the tradeoffs that are forced constantly between equity and efficiency are the very stuff that makes the government budget process intensely competitive.

From an economic perspective, stability refers to policies pursued through the budget to stabilize the economy, in conjunction with the fiscal and monetary policies of the government and the actions and productivity of the private sector. Stability is measured in terms of prices, employment, growth of the gross domestic product and other indices. Just as there are tradeoffs between equity and efficiency, inevitably there will be potential tradeoffs between each of these and stability under some circumstances. Balancing these exchanges is in part a result of decisions made in the ongoing cycle of government budgeting and financial management.

We subscribe to the perspectives of both political science—public administration and economics. Our hybrid view attempts to draw in an interdisciplinary manner on both perspectives, which is to say that neither view is wrong—but that each emphasizes different aspects and ways of understanding budgeting and spending outcomes.

DEFINING BUDGETING AND THE BUDGET

In sending his proposal to create an executive budget system to Congress in 1912, President Taft said: "The Constitutional purpose of a budget is to make government responsive to public opinion and responsible for its acts." (Burkhead, 1959, p. 19). In the proposal, it was noted that a budget served a number of purposes, from a document for Congressional action, to an instrument of control and management by the President, to a basis for the administration of departments and agencies. The multiple purposes of the budget have been noted, but no one has been more eloquent than Aaron Wildavsky in describing budgetary complexity. In his classic 1964 book, *The Politics of the Budgetary Process*, Wildavsky explained that a budget is:

1. Concerned with the **translation** of financial resources into human purposes.
2. A mechanism for making choices among alternative expenditures … **a plan**; and if detailed information is provided in the plan, it becomes a **work plan** for those who administer it.
3. An instrument to attempt to achieve **efficiency** if emphasis is placed on obtaining desired objective at least cost.
4. A **contract** over what funds shall be supplied and for what purposes:
    *   between Congress and the President;
    *   between Congress and the Departments and Agencies;
    *   between Departments and Agencies and their subunits.

    These "contracts" have both legal and social aspects. Those who give money expect results; those who are due to receive money expect to have the funds delivered on time to execute their programs effectively. Both superiors and subordinates have rights and expectations under such contracts, and mutual obligations are present.
5. A set of both **expectations** and **aspirations are contained in proposed budgets** from submitting agencies. Agencies expect to get money, but they may aspire to much more than they are given. The budget process regularly allows them to ask for what they aspire. What they are given in dollars reveals the preferences of others

about the agency's budget. This is important information for the next budget cycle.

6.   A **precedent:** something that has been funded before is highly likely to be funded again (this is defined as budgetary incrementalism).

7.   A tool to **coordinate and control**: to coordinate diverse activities so they complement each other, to control and discipline subordinate units, e.g., by limiting spending to what was budgeted or by providing money to or taking it from pet political projects.

8.   A **call to clientele** to mobilize support for the agency, when programs appear to be underfunded or losing ground to other programs.

9.   "A **representation** in monetary terms of governmental activity..." (Wildavsky, 1964, pp. 1–4).

As explained in the introduction, in the American context under the Constitutional separation of powers between the executive, congressional and judicial branches of government, the budget process begins in the executive branch of government, where the budget plan is developed, and proceeds into the legislative branch where the budget plan is reviewed, reformulated, (sometimes even rejected in total), amended and enacted. The process usually concludes in the executive branch where the President, as Chief Executive of the executive branch (and Commander-in-Chief of the armed forces), signs the budget bill or bills into law. At the federal level, the chief executive may veto appropriation bills he does not like, but eventually he must sign some sort of compromise bill. In contrast, a majority of state governors have an "item veto" authority that allows them to change bills in different ways depending upon the precise nature of the veto power, e.g., in California the Governor can use the line-item veto to cut money from an appropriation for a program approved by the legislature, but cannot add money through the veto.

Budgetary power is shared power, employed under a system of checks and balances made possible by the separation of powers, although the Constitution is clear that taxing power rests with the Congress and, by inference, spending power as well. This is quite different from Parliamentary systems of government, e.g., under the Westministerian form of government. In such systems, the legislative and executive branches of government are, in effect, combined. The political party with the most elected members controls the legislative body or bodies (e.g., the House of Commons and House of Lords in the United Kingdom) and thus obtains the right to form the government and appoint a cabinet of ministers headed by the Prime Minister (PM) as the elected leader of the dominant party. In some instances, coalitions of parties control Parliament where no single party has been able to elect a majority of its members. The various appointed ministers who head the departments of the government (their portfolios) are also elected officials who serve in the legislature. A key committee of Cabinet, chaired by the PM recommends or makes decisions on the budget. The budget represents the government's work plan; if the legislature does not approve it as submitted, a vote of no confidence may ensue, and perhaps lead to the fall of the government and the calling of a general election. In general, the threat of a vote of no confidence holds the majority party together when the budget is in the legislature and prevents any changes except those that the majority party has decided to make itself.

In contrast, in the United States, Congress is free to put its own imprint on the President's budget. Congress may modify only marginally the President's budget in total dollar terms. However, Congress typically takes a position that is very different from the President with respect to agencies and programs. This is particularly true when control of the Congress and the Presidency is divided between the two parties. When one party holds the executive branch and the other party holds one or both houses in the legislative branch, the budget process can be both heated and extended. In the 1980s, several Presidential budgets were termed "dead on arrival" when submitted to Congress, because Congress did not even consider them as a base for spending negotiation. This might have led to a vote of no confidence and a general election in a parliamentary system. Instead, it led to late appropriations of spending bills by Congress, summit meetings between leaders of the executive and legislative branches, and to some extent policy gridlock, sometimes followed by budget process reform efforts. In a parliamentary system, the budget process also begins with the executive branch, but, when the budget is passed to the parliament, the same group of politicians (party) that approved the budget in the PM's cabinet has the power to approve it in Parliament so long as they hold their party or coalition together. Generally, then the budget is passed with little or no change, once it has been announced by the PM. This is the dramatic difference between budgeting in Westministerian versus separation of powers systems.

Once the President has signed the appropriation bills, it is the function of the executive branch agencies to execute the budget as enacted, and not as submitted. This is not as simple as it seems. Changing conditions may lead the executive branch to try to defer spending or rescind (cut) programs; sometimes emergency supplemental appropriations are sought to meet emergencies, e.g., natural disasters or military action. There is a continuous traffic in reprogramming (moving money within appropriations) and transfers (moving money between appropriations), some of which agencies can do on their own and some which Congress must approve. In short, budgeting seems to be a never-ending activity. While the current budget is executed, the budget for the next year is under review in the legislature, and the budget for the year following is under preparation by agencies in the executive branch. Some reformers have suggested that the federal government pursue a biennial budget process where budgeting is done every two years to put more planning and analysis in the budget process. Biennial budgeting is a form of budgeting found in 19 American states in the 1990s. This topic is investigated in depth in a later chapter.

At its heart, the budget process is a planning process. It is about the future and what should happen in the future. For agencies, this planning process may involve agency estimation of the amount of services to be provided in the next year, and to whom services will be supplied; for income security and welfare programs, it may involve estimation of what it will take to provide a decent standard of living for the poor; for defense agencies it may involve estimation of the consequences of U.S. foreign policy commitments and defense resource planning in terms of threat response capacity involving people, major weapons platforms such as aircraft carriers, airplanes, missiles or tanks, and the personnel and support resources necessary for threat management and deterrence. While numbers and quantification give the budget document the aura of precision, it is still a plan; this is most clearly evident in budget execution where agencies struggle to spend the budget they have received in an environment inevitably changed from the one for which the budget was developed. Budget systems provide some capacity to modify the enacted budget during budget execution, e.g., fund transfers and reprogramming, emergency bills and supplemental additions of new funding.

Finally, it is important to recognize that budgeting is not done within government in a vacuum. Both in formulation and execution various stakeholders outside of government attempt to influence budget decisions and outcomes. This environment is depicted in the following "stakeholder space" graphic in which the Boeing Corporation (non-governmental organizations or public interest lobby groups, etc. could be substituted in this diagram to reflect their input) is shown as an example of how private firms play a role in the budget process. What this diagram shows is that before policy can be made, demands and support must be articulated. A "good idea" that gathers little or no support has no chance of making it through the policymaking apparatus whereas an "average" idea that has great support may well become policy. Voters, citizens, lobbyists, political action committees(PACs) all help articulate demands and gather support. The various outlets of the news media are very important in seizing on issues and helping the public understand what is at stake, even if they sometimes prefer the relatively unimportant but titillating, to the important but obscure and complex.

Most observers of the American system assume that nothing is written in stone, thus feedback about current policy outcomes may be immediately fed back into the policymaking mechanism to help correct flaws in current policy. This is not as easy to do as it is to say. Moreover, some things do seem written in stone; subsidy programs and entitlements are very difficult to change. Tax laws, especially when they increase taxes usually only get the necessary support if they are written to occur at a point far enough in the future that a majority of the potential taxpayers feel that they can arrange their affairs so the tax will not affect them. Thus, flawed policies do endure and are hard to change, feedback loop or not, particularly when a small, but intensely vocal group favors the current arrangement. The triangle in the diagram is meant to indicate that there are some focused arrangements that have developed historically where the interests of a particular company or clientele, an executive branch agency and a Congressional Committee or Committees combine to make and sustain policy favorable to those specific parties, perhaps at the expense of the general public. This is true to some extent in all policy areas. These triangular relationships are sometimes referred to as "iron triangles" to denote their power. (The one in our diagram shows the Boeing Corporation, the Department of Defense, and the Senate Armed Services Committee, but it could as well show almost any large company or group of commercial interests or pensioners, their relevant executive agency and their relevant committee.) To a limited extent, the struggle over the deficit in the 1990s, caps on discretionary expenditures and pay-go provisions have changed the dimensions of this struggle so that players within each triangle are forced to limit their aspirations to taking money away from other players within the triangle, rather than preying upon the treasury at large, or another policy area. This is only, however, to a limited extent. Moreover, a policy area that is blessed by

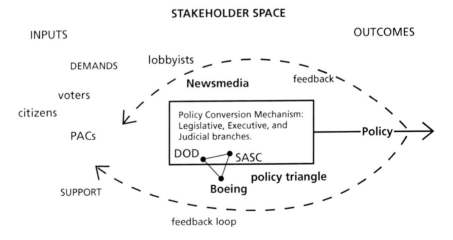

Figure 1.   Stakeholder space.

the President or powerful interests in Congress can be assured of an increasing budget. This is all part of the politics of the budgetary process and serves to remind that real benefits are distributed through the budget process. Citizens who are not aware of this will end up paying for benefits enjoyed by other people as they wonder where their taxes went or how long it will take their children to pay down the national debt.

TYPES OF BUDGETS

Budgets come in different types. There are three basic types of budgets: operating, capital and cash. The operating budget contains funds to be spent on short-term consumables including the personnel payroll and the goods and services that keep government agencies in business on a day-to-day basis, e.g., salaries and benefits for employees, funding for utilities, money to contract for trash management, maintenance and supplies, space rental and lease payments, pens, pencils, copy machine paper and so on. Typically, employee salaries and benefits are the highest cost item in the operating budget, representing anywhere from 60% to 90% of spending. Personnel are usually listed by position by type and grade and perhaps seniority, with a certain percentage added on to cover the cost of fringe benefits including vacation, sick leave, health, life and disability insurance and retirement plan costs.

The operating budget funds the annual operational needs of the jurisdiction, ranging from road maintenance, to park and recreation supervision, tax collection, education, welfare, public safety, and defense. The term for spending the funds in the operating budget is almost always one year. This is so for the U.S. federal government; however, there are options to this arrangement detailed later in this book.

The operating budget usually include minor capital outlay amounts for desks and office machines and the like, below a specified item cost threshold, e.g., $10,000. Consumable items range from computer parts, to telephone installations, to pencils. A budget of this type is called a line item budget, because each item is presented on a separate line in the budget document. The line includes the name of the item, the budgeted amount for the current year and a requested amount for the next year. Many jurisdictions also include what was spent on that item the previous year. Most line item budgets have some brief explanations of the reason for the change from the amount in the budgeted year to the amount requested. Revenue sources may be broken into equally excruciating detail, not only general taxes, e.g., sales, property and income, but also revenue from fees, charges and miscellaneous sources, including parking fines, dog and bicycle licenses, and garage sale permits.

The capital budget contains funding for purchase of long-lived physical assets such as buildings, bridges, land for parks, and high cost equipment such as aircraft, ships, etc. Many, but not all, state government and other jurisdictions in the United States have separate capital and operating budgets. The federal government does not have a separate capital budget, but it has distinct capital accounts, mostly used to pay for acquisition of military hardware in the Defense Department. The capital budget is usually used for long-term investment type functions, including buying parklands, constructing buildings and roads, where consumption spans over a period of years or decades. Thus, the capital budget is appropriated and consumed on a multi-year basis. In state and local governments, capital projects are usually paid for through issuance of bonds whose principal provides the money for the capital budget projects. These bonds normally are paid back over a time period that approximates the consumption of the asset (e.g., thirty years). In contrast, the U.S. federal government appropriates money for capital consumption out of the annual operating budget and outlays it over multiple year terms as the project is executed. Capital and operating budgets must be linked to provide services. Where the capital budget pays for construction of an office building, it is the operating budget that pays for the furniture and equipment to make the building ready for use, and for daily activities of maintenance in and around the building.

Cash budgets are used to manage the cash flow demands of operation on a daily, weekly, monthly and annual basis. The objective of cash budgeting is to ensure the liquidity and solvency of government and its agencies. Liquidity may be defined as having the cash and readily convertible assets that are used to pay the government's bills (i.e., its short-term liabilities). In contrast, solvency refers to the ability of government to sustain operations over the long-term (i.e., greater than one year). Typically, the cash budget is managed in close coordination with the investment functions of the treasury department or other cash controlling entity (e.g., the comptroller or department of finance). The task for proper cash management is to have enough cash available to cover current liabilities, but not too much so that the opportunity to invest and earn interest from surplus cash is wasted. In the private sector, what is termed the "quick ratio" is used as a measure of cash flow management. A ratio of 1.1 or 1.2 cash on hand to 1.00 liabilities is appropriate. Ratios lower than this imperil the ability to meet payment obligations; a higher ratio wastes investment opportunity.

THE PURPOSES OF BUDGETS

In the American system, generalizations may be made about the extent to which different levels of government support different functions. The federal government concentrates on providing national defense, transfer payment aid to education and health, national parks and interstate transportation plus what are termed entitlement programs such as Social Security, Medicare, Medicaid and a variety of social welfare support programs, and national economic and social regulation, e.g., of interstate commerce and transportation, aspects of business competition and competitive behavior, many of the activities of subordinate levels of government, environmental protection, fair labor practices and equality in education. State governments tend to focus budget effort on aid to education (public schools, universities and colleges), state legal and criminal justice systems, prisons, mental health institutions, intrastate highway construction and maintenance, and transfer payments to local governments. State budgets also pay for regulation of electric utilities and other entities including business and local governments. Local (municipal) governments tend to budget for public schools (in cooperation with state government), to provide police and fire protection, libraries, parks and recreation, and to either provide or supervise public utilities including those for water, sewer, and trash collection. Special tax districts provide funding in budgets whose income is derived from either self-generation of taxes, user fees and charges, etc. or transfers from other governments. Special districts have been created in augmentation of county and city governments to provide for water facilities and management (e.g., flood control), fire control, port facilities and management, conservation, capital infrastructure renewal (enterprise zones), and other public purposes. Many states also set up independent school districts with their own budget process and tax powers.

Public welfare assistance for low-income individuals and families, for health and education and numerous other functions including environmental protection, land preservation, municipal sewer construction, flood prevention and other public services is funded across all levels of government in a system of shared tax rights and payments, and guiding regulations. As noted, all governments have regulatory functions; these tend not to cost much in direct funding, although their impact on citizens and the private and nonprofit sectors is great and the cost considerable. Most of the dissension and much of the drama in budgeting revolve around who gets what benefits directly and indirectly from the budgets appropriated at the various levels of government. The inevitable competition over priorities expressed and evaluated in review of the annual budgets of this multitude of governments is fierce, as claims are raised, debated and decided concerning funding for the diverse bundles of goods and services these governments provide.

Table 4 shows the change in support of government functions over time, measured by percent of Gross Domestic Product (GDP). In this table the changes from 1952 to 1993 may be seen. The major change is the decrease in defense spending and the increase in social security spending (41%), Medicare (24%), and state and local medical care (21%). These increases clearly indicate the change in the economy from a defense-oriented economy to a social service-health orientation.

Table 4.   Changes in Functional Categories of Public Expenditure

	Percentage of GDP		
	1952	1993	Difference
Total public expenditures	26.3	33.1	+6.8
National defense	13.2	4.8	−8.4
Veterans' compensation[a]	1.1	0.3	−0.8
Social Security	0.6	4.7	+4.1
Medicare	0.0	2.4	+2.4
State and local medical care[b]	0.0	2.1	+2.1
Welfare and social services	0.4	1.4	+1.0
Primary and secondary education	2.0	3.9	+1.9
Higher education	0.3	1.0	+0.7
Police and corrections	0.4	1.2	+0.8
Net government employee retirement	−0.1	0.6	+0.7
Net interest payments	1.3	1.9	+.06
Unallocable (state and local)	0.2	0.8	+0.6
General government activities	0.9	1.2	+0.3
Residual[c]	6.0	6.8	+0.8

[a] excludes education and health benefits.
[b] includes federal Medicaid grants.
[c] each category in the residual changed by less than 0.3 percentage point of GDP in absolute value.
Source: Rand Corporation (1995).

BUDGET THEORY, INCREMENTALISM AND THE POLITICS OF THE BUDGETARY PROCESS

Budget theory is a somewhat controversial subject. Some scholars continue to search for such theory. However, despite considerable research effort there still is no comprehensive budget theory that will forecast results with reliable predictive accuracy. As noted by V.O. Key more than sixty years ago (1940, 1978, pp. 19–23), the answer to the fundamental question, "On what basis shall it be decided to allocate x dollars to activity

A instead of activity B?"—is no clearer today than ever. The closest approximation to predictive theory we have is incrementalism, a perspective most closely attributed to the work of Aaron Wildavsky. We have noted that budgets tend to be incremental, i.e., that they change by increments, usually small on a percentage basis, thus, what you have this year is likely to be close to what you will receive next year. This is to say that, generally, the best variable to predict the share of an increase or decrease an agency will receive in the budget for the next year is the relative size of the budget for the existing year and past years. This hypothesis has endured despite considerable challenge. Wildavsky's (1964) classic portrayal of the budgetary process suggested that the overwhelming complexity of the budget and man's limited cognitive abilities drove an incremental approach, where programs were reviewed a piece at a time, with different parts being reviewed in different places, with reviewers relying on participant feedback to tell them if they had cut too much from one program or another. The complexity of the budget process dictated that some people had to trust others in this process, because they could only check up on them a small part of the time and because no one can be an expert in everything. In Congress, this usually meant that the many had to trust the few on the appropriations committees to provide cues for voting on appropriation bills.

Wildavsky warned one of the authors as his student many years ago that the search for a general theory of budgeting was a waste of time. He understood the inherent intellectual limits of control as the cause for an incrementalist approach. This view assumes constant making and remaking of the budget, with a heavy concentration of review on what is changed in the current year from the previous year. It also assumes a constant competition between budget spenders and budget controllers. Wildavsky's portrayal of budgeting as an incremental process with specific roles for budget participants was so powerful that it has dominated how people have viewed the budget process in the United States and elsewhere since the mid-1960s. Tracing the development of Wildavsky's understanding in subsequent editions of his classic book and in journal articles approximates a following of the evolution of scholarly thought on the budget process from 1964 to the early 1990s.

The Politics of the Budgetary Process was published in 1964, and revised in 1974, 1979, and 1984. *The New Politics of the Budgetary Process* was published in 1988 and revised in 1992 under his sole authorship. Subsequently, budget scholar Naomi Caiden revised the second book in 1996 and 2001. The genius of the original work was that it spoke to a broad spectrum of interests taking part in budgeting, from the aggressive bureaucrat who wanted to know what was important in getting a budget accepted, to the organizational scholar interested in the possibility of rational and comprehensive budget decision making. For the academic, the original *Politics* appeared contemporaneously with theoretical explorations of complex organization decision making that both supported and critiqued rational and incremental decision making. These works included Herbert Simon's *Models of Man*, (1957), Dwight Waldo's *The Administrative State* (1949), Cyert and March's *A Behavioral Theory of the Firm* (1955), Anthony Downs' *An Economic Theory of Decision Making in a Democracy* (1963), and Charles Lindblom's article, "The Science of Muddling Through" (1959). In characterizing this perspective, Lindblom stated that although comprehensive decision making could be described, "...it cannot by practiced because it puts too great a strain by far on man's limited ability to calculate" (1984, p. 148). Wildavsky subscribed to this perspective.

Wildavsky concluded his own review of this perspective in noting that "...we must deal with real men in the real world for whom the best they can get is to be preferred to the perfection they cannot achieve. Unwilling or unable to alter the basic features of the political system, they seek to make it work for them in budgeting..." (1964, p. 178). Wildavsky suggested that, "...the existing budgetary process works much better than is commonly supposed." However he also noted there is no, "...special magic in the status quo. Inertia and ignorance as well as experience and wisdom may be responsible for the present state of affairs" (1964, p. 178). Thus, he proclaimed that incrementalism should not be viewed as a prescription for what is right; rather it was a description of actual practice. He observed that the major improvements in analysis and decision making suggested by rationalist-comprehensive critics would turn out to be undesirable, infeasible, or both. Instead, to be effective, he felt reform initiatives ought to concentrate on a more thorough comprehension of the complexities of the incremental approach, rather than an attempt to move toward more comprehensive solutions (1964, p. 179). It is this tension between the rational and incremental, between budgetary actors as they are, and as they might be, that provided *The Politics of the Budgetary Process* the theoretical strength to be something more than a catalog of what budget makers said to one another in various meetings in the Executive branch and Congress during the late 1950s and early 1960s.

Conversely, irrespective of its theoretical value, what budget makers said to one another made a real difference for agencies and budget practitioners. Wildavsky captured the essence of the budgetary struggle in two short paragraphs: "Long service in Washington has convinced high agency officials that some things count a great deal and others only a little ... budget officials commonly derogate the importance of the formal aspects of their work as a means of securing appropriations ... 'It's not what's in your estimates but how good a politician you are that matters.'"

However, being a good politician had a special meaning for Wildavsky: it, "...requires three things: cultivation of an active clientele, the develop-

ment of confidence among other governmental officials, and skill in following strategies that exploit one's opportunities to the maximum." Doing
good work was seen as part of being a good politician (1964, pp. 64–65).
Wildavsky viewed confidence and clientele strategies as ubiquitous. Those
strategies that were dependent on time, place, and circumstance, he called
contingent. He argued that the purposes of budgets were as varied as the
purposes of people (1964, pp. 1–3). The words and figures in the budget
represent a prediction about the future; consequently budgets become
links between financial resources, human behavior, and policy accomplishment. Once passed, a budget was also a contract about what government
will do and who will benefit and who will pay. In this sense, a budget represents a series of goals with price tags attached. This formulation has shaped
understanding and analysis of budgeting into the twenty-first century.

In the preface to the original 1964 edition, Wildavsky acknowledged that
his book was not a comprehensive work on the subject of budgeting.
Among other things, it did not deal at all with how funds were raised, or
budgeting for defense. Wildavsky concluded that he would be pleased, "…if
this study came to be regarded as the point of departure" (1964, p. vii) for
more specialized studies.[5] Wildavsky succeeded in liberating the study of
budgeting from the claustrophobic rhythms of formal procedures to focus
attention of observers on the political behavior in the budget process.

The second edition of *The Politics of the Budgetary Process* did not come
out until 1974, but this intervening decade saw a great deal of academic
work done on budgeting. With so much research already published and
more in progress, the tone of the preface of the second edition was under-
standably much more authoritative. It added a chapter on program budgeting, arguing that the rational comprehensive approach would not work
and directing a restoration of the norms of guardianship and reciprocity
against actions of the executive for Congress. His views in this book and in
testimony before Congress influenced the content of the milestone Budget
Impoundment and Control Act passed in 1974, particularly in the establishment of the Current Services Budget to show what it would cost the government if only current policies were funded, with no new programs added
to the budget.

In the 1974 edition Wildavsky also indicated that there was a change in
emphasis from the original *Politics* in the relationship between budgetary
incrementalism and organizational learning: "I would no longer assume …
that organizations, as distinct from individuals, actually make use of the
method of successive limited approximation to move away from the worse
and toward the better" (1974, pp. xii–xiii). Here, he modified and
extended his perspective on incrementalism, indicating in particular how
it impeded evolutionary progress in defining and enacting new and better
policy and the ability of the budget process to be self-correcting.

In the 1984 revision of the *Politics*, for the first time, Wildavsky addressed the question, "Is there a pro-spending bias in the budgetary process." His answer was yes and, consequently, a final chapter was added on spending limits. This chapter noted that the "classic sign of political dissensus is the inability to agree on the budget," and observed, "How we Americans used to deride the 'banana republics' of the world for their 'repetitive budgeting' under which the budget was reallocated many times during the year, until it became hardly recognizable, truly a thing of shreds and patches. Yet resolutions that continue last year's funding for agencies, for want of ability to agree on this year's, are becoming a way of life in the United States. An annual budget is a great accomplishment. Sending out signals on spending that remain predictable so that others can take them into account for a full twelve months is no mean achievement."

Examining the decay of the budget process and the inability of reforms to deal with total spending, Wildavsky predicted that future reforms would deal with the quantity of spending. "Limits on total spending do not guarantee budgetary control, but without limits on total spending there can be no control," Wildavsky intoned (1984, p. 279). In 1985, Congress passed Gramm-Rudman-Hollings the first deficit control measure that capped spending to revenues plus a specified and declining amount of deficit over a five-year period. This was amended in 1987 and replaced by outright spending caps in 1990, 1993, and 1997, each stretching over a five-year time horizon. Once again Wildavsky proved an astute predictor of budgetary events.

The 1984 edition was clearly a transitional work. Wildavsky asserted that the landscape of budgeting in the United States had changed dramatically. Norms of annularity, balance, and comprehensiveness had been shattered beyond repair and the norm of a balanced budget had disappeared in the mid-1960s, replaced with an injunction simply to spend: "Better budgets became those which spent more" (1984, p. xv). With the demise of the balanced budget norm, it becomes more difficult for control agencies to turn back spending requests ... "why take the heat for turning people down?" (1988, p. xxviii). In reflecting on the *Politics*, Wildavsky believed that the sections on calculation were still as relevant as ever, if not more so but, by contrast, the sections on agency strategies for getting funds, "...depends on conditions—trust among participants, ability to anticipate behavior, collective concern for totals, comparability of accounts—that no longer exist" (1974, p. xi) Without limits, there could be no sense of shared sacrifice; without accurate comparisons of budget categories there could be no sense of fair share. To get back to the golden age of incrementalism, where changes were small, alternatives resembled those of the past, and patterns or relationships among participants remained stable, reformers needed to reestablish norms that encouraged such behavior, norms including annularity, balance and comprehensiveness. The last edition of the *Politics of the Budgetary Process* (1988) was prescient. It predicted the direction of reform that Congress and Presidents assented to in efforts to control budget deficits in the 1980s and 1990s.

The Wildavskyian incrementalist perspective on budgeting has not reigned without criticism. Drafts of the original book had "…received an unusually negative response (nine publishers rejected it" (1988, p. xxvii). Readers found it too critical of government (especially if they were in it) or too tolerant of bad practices (if they suffered from them). And stern admonitions were made to abjure frivolity from those who felt that treating budgeting as a game made little of their earnest efforts to develop a comprehensive theory of budgeting. Numerous critics have argued that too much of what is budgeted in contemporary practice is not incremental (see, e.g., Kelly & Wanna, 2001). Therefore, they have rejected incrementalism as a valid thesis of how budgeting works in the contemporary world. Our view comprehends these criticisms. We argue that incrementalism remains accurate and suitable as a general theory, but that there are numerous exceptions where budget amount and content is contingent on other variables more powerful than the base of what was appropriated and spent in the previous year. Thus, our perspective might be viewed as an incrementalist and contingent theory of budgeting.

BUDGET REFORM: A BRIEF SYNOPSIS

Much of the history of U.S. federal government budget reform over the past fifty years has involved attempts at finding ways to present budget information to decision makers in a more meaningful way, so that better decisions can be made about how to allocate scarce resources. These reforms have included performance budgeting, program budgeting, zero-based budgeting, Planning-Programming-Budgeting Systems (PPBS) and various other approaches including those focusing on target-levels, fixed ceilings and mission based budgeting. Allen Schick's (1964) article suggested that all these budget systems embrace control, management, and planning tools and concepts, but that different budget reforms emphasize different concepts. For example, line item budgeting emphasizes control, while performance budgeting emphasizes management. As reform efforts change, so does the central focus of the budget systems.[6] Reform initiatives have been both procedural and substantive. Some reforms have focused on the budget process, in the belief that better staff or a more timely process would produce better decisions. Paramount among these sorts of reforms are the Budget and Accounting Act of 1921 and the Congressional Budget Impoundment and Control Act of 1974.

Dissatisfaction with budget outcomes, primarily with respect to large and growing annual deficits and total debt, has resulted in attempts to mandate a balanced budget, i.e., one where spending does not exceed revenues. Examples of this type of budget reform include the Gramm-Rudman-Hollings Acts of 1985 and 1987, the Budget Enforcement Acts of 1990 and 1993, several attempts at a Constitutional Balanced Budget Amendment, and the 1997 Balanced Budget Act. These reforms have not been undertaken without some adverse consequences. Attempts to meet the GRH targets often involved overly optimistic estimates of spending and revenues and gimmicks such as shifting employees between fiscal years to meet specified ceilings and moving federal paydays to conform to spending ceilings, which probably did more to damage the budget process than improve it, especially since none of the GRH targets were ever met on time.

Only nine times from 1930 to 1998 was the U.S. federal budget in a position where revenues exceeded spending, but by 1998 the budget was in a surplus position, and estimates were offered by CBO in 2000 that this condition could last until 2015. As a result of these surpluses, tax cuts became an issue in the 2000 presidential election and the new President's first policy triumph was the tax cut of 2001. This appeared to substantially shorten the number of years of politicians would have to deal with surpluses.

Dealing with deficits has been a budgetary obsession since the early 1980s. Managing surpluses is uncharted territory for American politicians. The great depression of the 1930s and the intense spending effort of World War II appear to mark a turning point in American society. From this period onward, policy makers appear to have become committed to an increasingly larger role for the federal government in society and the economy. In practice, this has meant that claims on the budget have exceeded available resources and the federal government has been willing to go deeply in debt to meet these claims. In 1995, the national debt stood at $4.8 trillion, after quintupling from 1980, and annual payments for interest on the national debt were the fourth largest category in the federal budget. Whether and how federal policy and budget decision makers will be able to control the total debt of the U.S. government while sustaining the solvency of entitlement programs including Social Security, Medicare and Medicaid is the challenge posed for the twenty-first century.

DEFINING FINANCIAL MANAGEMENT

This book focuses on fiscal policy, i.e., taxing and spending. However, our emphasis is primarily on the expenditure side of fiscal policy. We concentrate on three areas: budget formulation, budget execution, and financial management more generally, of which budgeting is a part. The final two chapters of this book are concerned with financial management and reform exclusively. (See also Appendix A on the design of financial management curricula.)

The scope of public financial management is broad. It includes the finance function (taxation and tax policy, tax administration, generation of non-tax revenues), the treasury or banking functions of government, cash flow management, debt and surplus management, borrowing and investment. Budget formulation and execution are a major part of financial management, for through budgets money is distributed in attempt to meet social demand for goods and services. Public financial management also includes accounting (both financial and management) and auditing, as indispensable tools for achieving accountability and transparency so that the public may understand how the government collects and what the government does with its money.

Under our definition, public financial management includes all of the functions of government that deal with money except monetary policy. Consequently, it includes aspects of personnel management (e.g., salaries and benefits, appropriations and controls pertaining to the amount of employees and workload of agencies), capital asset acquisition and management, fixed asset inventory management and control, risk management and insurance, information systems management and other related financial functions imbedded in the administrative activities of government (see Appendix A for an example of topic areas covered in a model public financial management curriculum).

While public financial management does not include all of the activities performed in each of these areas, it is concerned with the financing aspects of each, particularly from a management control perspective. And as we know, to do anything in government or in any organization, takes money. Money is not the only factor input to government service provision, but it is one of the most important ingredients. Thus, budgeting is a participative enterprise for decision making on the allocation of scarce resources critical to the functioning of democratic political systems. In addition, it is a management control process to insure that funds are spent for the purposes intended without fraud, waste or abuse. Budgeting is not the only financial management function of government as indicated in the definition provided above, but it is perhaps the most important function in determining how the government pursues the objectives of equity, efficiency and stability. For this reason, the primary focus of this book is on budgeting with secondary attention to the other financial management functions of government. Our interest in financial management in this book is constrained to reform initiatives and not in detailing how functions other than budgeting are performed. The chapters that conclude this book provide an account of efforts to improve accounting, reporting, financial management and performance measurement in the U.S. federal government in the post-World War II period.

CONCLUSIONS: HOW MUCH TO SPEND AND WHAT IS WISE FISCAL POLICY?

Ultimately, budgeting always involves a rationing process. Schick (1990a, pp. 1–14) has argued that claiming and rationing are at the center of the budget process. Individuals and groups articulate demands on government for services. If the government can satisfy all demands, no budgeting process is necessary. Conversely, if government is so poor it can satisfy no demands, then no budget process is possible, necessary, or feasible. History offers few examples of societies so rich that all demands could be accommodated, and perhaps even fewer where the power holders of that society wished to accommodate all such demands. The oil-rich states in the middle-east in the late 1970s perhaps came as close in recent history to being able to satisfy all demands, but even here their status was helped enormously by the mix of an abundant natural resource base and a relatively low population. At the other end of the spectrum, are so-called "third world" or developing nations that have such restricted resource bases that they are able to meet few demands and the resources they do raise seem to evaporate under the impact of inflation and corruption almost as soon as they are raised. In neither case does a true budget process exist, as we have defined it.

For budgeting to operate effectively, or at all, not only must demands be articulated as claims for government to meet, but also government must have the capacity to satisfy some, if not most of those claims. Most governments exist in a middle ground, able to meet many, if not most claims, and able to meet more in good years than in bad years.

From a comparative perspective, countries differ in the amount of their wealth they make available to government to solve problems. For example, the United States has consistently allocated between 30 and 35% of its GDP from 1982 to 1998 for federal revenues, while Japan, the lowest, has been around 30% and France, the highest, 50% (Table 2.5, *Guide* FY2001). How they distribute what they are given also differs. For example, while the United States chose to spend 18% of its budget on defense in 1995, the United Kingdom spent 9%. While the United States spent 22% on Social Security, the United Kingdom spent almost 35% (*Guide*, 1996, p. 2; *Budget in Brief*, 1994). The fiscal conditions surrounding the budget process may change dramatically. For example, the inflation rate in Chile was 12,000% a year from 1984 to 1985, but fell to 15% after draconian fiscal reforms in 1985 (*World Press Review*, 1994, p. 20).

The goals that a nation pursues change over time. In 1962, the United States spent 50% of its federal budget on defense; this fell to 16% in the FY2002 budget. Social Security, which provides benefits to more than 43 million retired and disabled workers, is the largest category in the U.S. budget, comprising approximately 23% of all federal spending (*Guide*, 2002). One of the conditions of modern budgeting is the rise of spending on entitlement accounts, such as Social Security, veterans' pensions and benefits, medical care. The growth of the national debt over the last 20 years has brought with it an increase in payments of interest on the national debt. Social Security, Medicare and Medicaid are termed entitlements and result in mandatory payments since they are legal commitments the government must pay as benefits are prescribed in law, along with the conditions of eligibility to receive payments. Government may find legal ways to freeze spending on personnel, capital asset acquisition and other consumables, but it cannot refuse to pay Social Security benefits. For their part, individuals who qualify for such programs are "entitled" to receive payments and may sue government to get what is lawfully theirs. Most governments consider paying interest to their bondholders an absolute must to sustain their credit ratings and reputation. Otherwise, who will buy their bonds the next time they need to offer them?

In the FY2002 budget, mandatory accounts amounted to about 65% of the U.S. budget. The necessity for paying for these programs, and for servicing the debt, limits the flexibility of decision makers to attend to new national needs through the budget. Even where nations make a similar commitment, the resource planning to meet the commitment can vary dramatically. Spending on "social welfare" in Western European nations ranges from about 20% of GDP in Greece to more than 30% in The Netherlands. Within this range, there appear to be four groups, with Germany, France, Belgium and Luxembourg having social welfare systems designed to maintain the income level of the sick, disabled and unemployed. Britain and Ireland rely on general taxation, not to sustain the previous standard of living, but to provide adequate subsistence. Italy and The Netherlands fall somewhere between these two approaches. Spain, Portugal, and Greece are in a fourth group where a high proportion of people are not eligible for benefits. Thus, the gap in benefits can be wide; a disabled person unable to work can receive benefits equal to 97% of the average industrial wage in Belgium, but only 30% in Portugal. An unemployed Belgian will receive 79% of his pay in the first year out of work while a Briton in the same circumstance gets 23%. In general, Western Europe's spending on health care and social security is nearly twice as much as Japan and more than 60% greater than the United States (*Economist*, 1994, p. 57). This diversity in program is an outcome of the budgeting process and fiscal policy decisions.

These data demonstrate that the decision on how much to spend on government, and what programs should be funded differ considerably across nations and regions of the world. They also indicate that the challenge alluded to earlier with respect to the ability to balance demands for spending on social welfare and debt are faced around the world and not just in the United States. Additionally, with respect to the overall thrust of this chapter on budgeting, while the budgets and the budget processes of the nations of the world vary in many respects, the decision cycle explained here in detail for the U.S. federal government approximates that which most nations, and state and local governments in the United States, use to determine the allocation of resources in pursuit of the fiscal policy objectives of government. Nevertheless, important differences do exist between budgeting under the Constitutional balance of powers framework employed in the United States and the Westministerian parliamentary systems used in the United Kingdom, many British Commonwealth nations, and in other countries around the world, as noted previously in this chapter.

NOTES

1.   A-11 transmittal letter from the Director of OMB, Mitch Daniels to agencies for the first Bush budget, dated February 14, 2001.

2.   For more detail on the federal budget execution process, see OMB circular A-34.

3.   See Tyszkiewicz and Daggett (1998, p. 3). FEMA is the acronym for the Federal Emergency Management Agency.

4.   For more on budget formats and what they emphasize, see Schick (1966, pp. 243–258). Also see Hyde, 1978, pp. 71–77.)

5.   Friend and colleague Nelson Polsby related, "I told him not to publish it, for two reasons. First, it did not explain when specific budgetary strategies were used and not used, and when they worked and didn't work. Second, it didn't cover the revolution in the Defense Department with McNamara's institution of PPBS and systems analysis." Polsby recounted Aaron's blunt response, "To hell with you. It's better than anything else out there now and I am going to publish it." Polsby conceded that Aaron was right that it was the best thing written at that time, but did not give in on his two points. The book was a success, of course, and Aaron tried to fill the gaps and correct the deficiencies pointed out to him by Polsby and other colleagues. As it turned out, this took a long time to do this work; *The New Politics of the Budgetary Process,* coauthored with close colleague Naomi Caiden, did not appear until 1988. The most recent edition revised edition by Caiden was published in 2001. Furthermore, Wildavsky never did completely satisfy Polsby's first criterion … and neither has anyone else to our knowledge, although some have come close (see Meyers, 1994). The definitive study of contingent strategy in budgeting has yet to be written in our opinion.

6.   See Schick (1966, pp. 243–258).

ATTACHMENT A:
AN EXAMPLE OF A ZERO-BASED BUDGET FORMAT

City of Wichita, Kansas

TEAM POLICING

Decision Unit

Decision Packages (reflect contingency budgets—different funding scenarios)

ADAM AND BAKER TEAM POLICING
Budget Unit Goal: To protect life and property, prevent crime, respond to all calls for service from citizens, enforce City ordinances, State and Federal laws, investigate and follow-up assigned cases and improve response time.

Year 1978
Budget (000): 4,335.1 millions of $
Positions: 292

1979 Service level options

No.	Cost (000)		Positions		Dept. rank	City rank
	S/L	Cum.	S/L	Cum.		
1.	3,876.6	3,876.6	262	262	1/60	2
2.	338.9	4,215.5	28	290	3/60	7
3.	77.2	4,742.7	2	292	16/60	145
4.	148.9	4,391.6	18	310	27/60	PSP
5.	163.4	4,555.0	12	322	46/60	343

Service level narrative

1. *Quality Reduction and Increased Citizen Risk.* Provides service to the citizens in emergency situations and the officers would respond to cases of a less serious nature. Response time will average 12 minutes per call. This level calls for 256 commissioned officers, 6 civilians, 66 marked (blue and white) vehicles, and 27 unmarked vehicles. These officers provide 24-hour police service to the citizenry. Investigative follow-up and crime scene processing is curtailed.

2. *Minimum Preventative Patrol.* Provides twenty-seven commissioned officers and one clerk typist, who are needed to provide beat officers to answer citizen request calls with a 2 minute per call reduction in the response time from 12 minutes to 10 minutes.

3. *Interaction with USD #259.* Provides for the reinstatement of two school liason police officers who coordinate programs in the schools in two of the team policing areas. At this level, a school liason officer will be available in each of the six team policing areas.

4. *Adds Eighteen Police Officers to Reduce Response Time.* Adds eighteen police officers to provide coverage in the patrol function for vacations, emergency leave, in-service training, and back-up officers. At this level, response time for calls will be reduced from 10 minutes to 9 minutes per call. Positions are funded effective 1 April 1979 (9 months). Costs include $136,049 for salaries and $12,818 for initial uniforms and equipment.

5. *Improved Supervision and investigation.* Adds six detectives to insure more follow-up investigations, to accelerate the investigation process, and to improve clearance percentage; and six lieutenants to provide quality control through supervision and shortened span of control.

Note: S/L-Service level
    Cum-Cumulative (including service levels below the line)
    Dept. rank -Department head's rank of the service package/total number of service packages in the Police Services
        Department (all decision units combined)
    City rank -Executive's rank of the service package out of all service packages forwarded by all City departments for their
        service units
    PSP-Postponed; not ranked
Source: Adapted from Richard Aronson and Eli Schwartz, *Management Policies in Local Government Finance*, 2nd Ed. Washington, D.C.:
    International City Management Association, Figure 5-10, P 112.

ATTACHMENT B.1:
LINE ITEM BUDGET FORMATS
SUMMARY FORMAT

City of St Petersburg, Florida

ALL OPERATING FUNDS
SUMMARY OF EXPENSE BY OBJECT
($000 omitted)

	Actual 1990	Actual 1991	Budget 1992	Estimate 1992	Budget 1993
Personal Services	72,300	77,220	79,160	79,931	83,805
Employee Benefits	25,174	27,437	29,596	30,204	31,931
Services	63,722	67,869	72,340	69,914	70,940
Commodities	9,401	8,843	11,152	10,627	10,605
Capital Outlay	5,668	5,736	5,291	6,410	5,306
Transfers:					
Between Operating Funds	7,983	8,179	7,965	7,991	8,017
To Capital Project Funds	8,594	13,622	10,130	10,130	9,922
To Debt Service Funds	9,660	8,774	9,536	7,722	7,241
To Reserve Accounts	304	2,404	343	3,193	1,351
To Other Funds	2,490	1,879	2,235	1,969	1,841
Other	(306)	0	380	0	0
TOTAL	204,990	221,963	228,128	228,091	228,960

These definitions allow the reader to quickly identify types of expenditures presented in the table above without having to refer to a glossary.

DEFINITIONS:

PERSONAL SERVICES: Services rendered by full-time and part-time employees to support the functions of City departments. Costs include salaries, overtime, shift differentials, and other direct payments to employees.

EMPLOYEE BENEFITS: Contributions made by the City to designated funds to meet commitments of obligations for employee fringe benefits. Included are the City's share of costs for Social Security and the various pension, medical, and life insurance plans.

SERVICES: The requirements for a department's work program which are provided by other entities-either outside vendors and contractors or other City departments. Examples are the costs of repair and maintenance services (not materials); utilities; rentals; and charges from City Internal Service Funds.

COMMODITIES: Expendable materials and supplies necessary to carry out a department's work program for the fiscal year. Such items as repair and maintenance materials, chemicals, agricultural products, office supplies, small tools, and merchandise for resale are included.

CAPITAL OUTLAY: The purchase, acquisition, or construction of any item having unit cost of $100 or more, or a useful life of one or more years. Typical capital outlay items include vehicles, construction equipment, typewriters, computers, and office furniture.

Note: This summary presents expenditures by major objects as well as interfund transfers.

Source: Dennis Strachota, 1994. *The Best of Governmental Budgeting: A Guide to Preparing Budget Documents*, Chicago, IL: Government Finance Officers Association, Exhibit 3-13.

ATTACHMENT B.2:
LINE ITEM BUDGET FORMATS
DETAILED LINE-ITEM OBJECT OF EXPENDITURE BY
ACCOUNT FORMAT

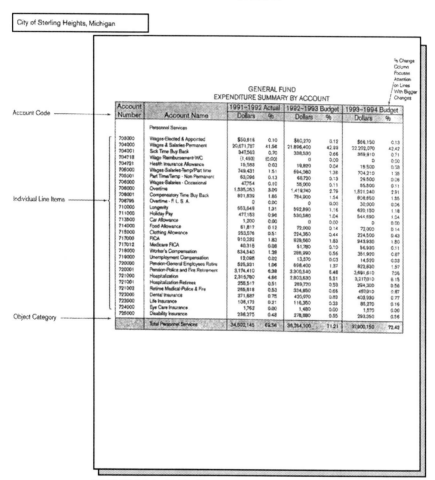

Note: This City's budget contained four object categories: Personnel Services, Other Charges, Capital Outlay, and Transfers Out. Only one category is presented here.

Source: Adapted from Dennis Strachota, 1994. *The Best of Governmental Budgeting: A Guide to Preparing Budget Documents.* Chicago, IL: Government Finance Officers Association, Exhibit 3-14.

ATTACHMENT C:
AN EXAMPLE OF A PERFORMANCE BUDGET FORMAT

City of Fort Collins, Colorado

CITY OF FORT COLLINS

PROGRAM	008301	PATROL SERVICES
FUND	101	GENERAL FUND
DEPARTMENT	800000	POLICE SERVICES

PROGRAM MISSION

To provide a full range of police patrol services, including crime prevention, traffic enforcement, traffic and community problem solving.

The program analysis highlights budget issues and changes in operations from the prior year. It includes information on a staffing reorganization.

PROGRAM ANALYSIS

We will continue using alternative response methods, allowing prompt and effective response to citizen demands for service in the most cost-effective manner. We will continue to emphasize problem-oriented policing whereby issues are addressed through application of problem-solving efforts. Patrol Services' Selective Enforcement Unit (SEU) will continue to concentrate on problem resolution within the community, and the Traffic Unit will continue to address traffic-related issues in 1993. In an effort to expand the application of problem-solving efforts the following changes will take place in 1993: The Records Lieutenant position will move to Patrol to coordinate problem-oriented policing efforts. In addition, the Crime Prevention Coordinator will move from Community Affairs to Patrol, and the Crime Analyst from Records to Patrol – both to be supervised by the Problem-Oriented Policing Lieutenant. For 1993, a DARE officer position has been added to this program.

Line-Item Format
Line-item expenditures and transfers are presented for three budget periods.

EXPENDITURE

	LAST ACTUAL 1991	CURR ADOPTED BUDGET 1992	REVISED BUDGET 1992	APPROVED BUDGET 1993
PERSONAL SERVICES	3,982,715	4,019,890	4,317,320	4,492,928
CONTRACTUAL	857,202	864,040	803,724	830,562
COMMODITIES	186,728	186,639	185,991	181,975
CAPITAL OUTLAY	12,446	0	26,772	0
TRANSFERS/OTHER	0	0	0	0
TOTAL	5,041,091	5,070,369	5,333,807	5,505,465

PERSONNEL

CLASS/UNCLSS	82.00	84.00	84.00	88.00
SEASONAL	.00	.00	.00	.00
HOURLY	.00	.00	.00	.00
CONTRACTUAL	.00	.00	.00	.00
VOLUNTEER	.00	.00	.00	.00
TOTAL	82.00	84.00	84.00	88.00

Personnel Format
Shows the mix of positions allocated to this program (e.g., hourly vs. volunteers).

REVENUE

GENERAL FUND	5,024,206	5,070,369	5,321,015	5,505,465
GRANT	16,885	0	12,792	0
TOTAL	5,041,091	5,070,369	5,333,807	5,505,465

Revenue Format
The source of financing for this program is also displayed.

PROGRAM PERFORMANCE BUDGET

PROGRAM	008301	PATROL SERVICES

OBJECTIVES
1. To meet 100% of citizens' requests for service.
2. Continue to use alternative response methods to most effectively utilize sworn officers.
3. Maintain 1992 response times.

Performance Format
These program objectives for the budget year tie to the performance measures presented.

PROGRAM INDICATORS	1991 ACTUAL	1992 BUDGET	1992 REVISED	1993 BUDGET
DEMAND				
1. Total Incidents	71,188	55,395	76,716	80,550
2. Population Served	89,432	90,709	90,709	92,079
3. Incidents per 1000 Population	796	611	846	875
WORKLOAD				
1. Dispatched Calls Responded to	35,091	39,452	36,845	38,588
2. Dispatched Calls per Non-Supervisory Police Officer and CSO*	516	580	526	546
3. Dispatched Calls Taken by CSO*	6,867	7,200	7,389	7,736
PRODUCTIVE				
1. Per Capita Cost–Patrol	$54.58	$54.14	$57.04	$57.90
EFFECTIVE				
1. Response Times (minutes):				
Priority 1–Routine	17.00	19.86	19.00	19.00
Priority 2–Urgent	7.00	5.41	8.00	8.00
Priority 3–Emergency	4.00	4.00	3.00	3.00
2. % Calls Delayed (tracked) More than 5 Minutes	28.00 %	40.00 %	28.00 %	28.00 %
3. % Dispatched Calls Handled by CSOs*	19.00 %	20.00 %	20.00 %	20.00 %

COMMENTS * CSO is Community Service Officer

Efficiency and effectiveness measures are presented for three budget periods.

Comments Section

Note: In this city, the service format is used for all programs presented within the operating budget.

Source: Adapted from Dennis Strachota, 1994. *The Best of Governmental Budgeting: A Guide to Preparing Budget Documents.* Chicago, IL: Government Finance Officers Association, Exhibit 2-3.

ATTACHMENT D:
PROGRAM BUDGET FORMATS
AGGREGATES FOR ALL PROGRAMS

City of Ft. Collins, Colorado

CITY EXPENDITURES BY SERVICE AREA (PROGRAM)

SERVICE AREA Department	ACTUAL 1991	BUDGET 1992	ADOPTED 1993	% INCREASE OVER 1992
ADMINISTRATIVE				
Administration	$149,138	$149,781	$156,748	4.0%
Employee Development	4,148,114	5,226,301	5,513,717	5.5%
Finance	5,781,888	5,953,984	6,344,255	6.6%
General Services	5,688,288	6,351,566	8,737,459	37.6%
Information & Communication Systems	2,810,260	3,011,117	3,365,212	11.8%
TOTAL ADMINISTRATIVE	16,613,488	20,692,749	24,116,391	16.5%
TRANSFERS TO OTHER FUNDS	(10,109,997)	(11,503,887)	(12,035,104)	4.6%
NET OPERATING ADMINISTRATIVE	$8,503,491	$9,188,862	$12,081,287	31.5%
CULTURAL, LIBRARY & RECREATIONAL				
Administration	$324,364	$324,068	$331,663	2.3%
Cultural Services & Facilities	1,303,519	1,470,435	1,695,228	15.3%
Library	1,556,474	1,475,955	1,652,838	12.0%
Parks & Recreation	7,418,029	7,886,439	8,850,856	12.2%
TOTAL CULTURAL, LIBRARY & RECREATIONAL	10,602,386	11,156,917	12,530,585	12.3%
TRANSFERS TO OTHER FUNDS	(324,751)	(345,298)	(343,949)	-0.4%
NET OPERATING CULTURAL, LIBRARY & RECREATIONAL	$10,277,635	$10,811,619	$12,186,636	12.7%
COMMUNITY PLANNING & ENVIRONMENTAL				
Administration	$164,844	$184,525	$186,808	1.2%
Building Permits & Inspections	614,477	647,587	684,840	5.8%
Economic Affairs	332,053	314,771	344,815	9.5%
Engineering	2,514,753	2,823,280	2,870,447	1.7%
Natural Resources	392,435	494,308	517,591	4.7%
Planning	678,307	721,942	801,939	11.1%
Transportation Services	1,363,529	1,282,466	1,516,715	18.3%
TOTAL COMMUNITY PLANNING & ENVIRONMENTAL	6,160,398	6,468,879	6,923,155	7.0%
TRANSFERS TO OTHER FUNDS	(1,101,501)	(70,969)	(65,904)	2.1%
NET OPERATING COMMUNITY PLANNING & ENVIRONMENTAL	$5,058,897	$6,397,910	$6,857,251	7.2%

Program Area →

Department/ Division Within Program Area →

Note: Existing departments are clustered under broad service area (programs). Departmental lines are maintained.

Source: Adapted from Dennis Strachota,1994. The Best of Governmental Budgeting: A Guide to Preparing Budget Documents. Chicago, IL: Government Finance Officers Association, Exhibit 3-11.

ATTACHMENT E:
PROGRAM BUDGET FORMATS
FOR ONE PROGRAM

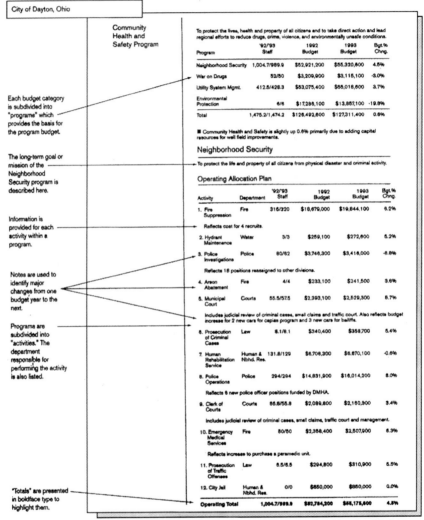

City of Dayton, Ohio

Community
Health and
Safety Program

To protect the lives, health and property of all citizens and to take direct action and lead regional efforts to reduce drugs, crime, violence, and environmentally unsafe conditions.

Program	'92/'93 Staff	1992 Budget	1993 Budget	Bgt.% Chng.
Neighborhood Security	1,004.7/989.9	$52,921,200	$55,320,600	4.5%
War on Drugs	52/50	$3,209,900	$3,115,100	-3.0%
Utility System Mgmt.	412.5/426.3	$53,075,400	$55,018,600	3.7%
Environmental Protection	6/6	$17,286,100	$13,857,100	-19.8%
Total	1,475.2/1,474.2	$126,492,600	$127,311,400	0.6%

■ Community Health and Safety is slightly up 0.6% primarily due to adding capital resources for well field improvements.

Neighborhood Security

To protect the life and property of all citizens from physical disaster and criminal activity.

Operating Allocation Plan

Activity	Department	'92/'93 Staff	1992 Budget	1993 Budget	Bgt.% Chng.
1. Fire Suppression	Fire	316/320	$18,679,000	$19,844,100	6.2%
Reflects cost for 4 recruits.					
2. Hydrant Maintenance	Water	3/3	$259,100	$272,600	5.2%
3. Police Investigations	Police	80/82	$3,746,300	$3,416,000	-8.8%
Reflects 16 positions reassigned to other divisions.					
4. Arson Abatement	Fire	4/4	$233,100	$241,500	3.6%
5. Municipal Court	Courts	55.5/57.5	$2,393,100	$2,529,300	5.7%
Includes judicial review of criminal cases, small claims and traffic court. Also reflects budget increase for 2 new cars for copies program and 3 new cars for bailiffs.					
6. Prosecution of Criminal Cases	Law	8.1/8.1	$340,400	$358,700	5.4%
7. Human Rehabilitation Service	Human & Nbhd. Res.	131.8/129	$6,706,300	$6,670,100	-0.5%
8. Police Operations	Police	294/294	$14,831,900	$16,014,200	8.0%
Reflects 6 new police officer positions funded by DMHA.					
9. Clerk of Courts	Courts	66.8/55.8	$2,089,800	$2,160,300	3.4%
Includes judicial review of criminal cases, small claims, traffic court and management.					
10. Emergency Medical Services	Fire	80/80	$2,358,400	$2,507,900	6.3%
Reflects increase to purchase a paramedic unit.					
11. Prosecution of Traffic Offenses	Law	6.5/6.5	$294,800	$310,900	5.5%
12. City Jail	Human & Nbhd. Res.	0/0	$850,000	$850,000	0.0%
Operating Total		1,004.7/989.9	$52,784,200	$55,175,600	4.5%

Each budget category is subdivided into "programs" which provides the basis for the program budget.

The long-term goal or mission of the Neighborhood Security program is described here.

Information is provided for each activity within a program.

Notes are used to identify major changes from one budget year to the next.

Programs are subdivided into "activities." The department responsible for performing the activity is also listed.

"Totals" are presented in boldface type to highlight them.

Note: Program cuts across departmental lines. The subprogram detail is not presented for the War on Drugs, Utility System Management, or Environmental Protection sub programs.
Source: Adapted from Dennis Strachota,1994. The Best of Governmental Budgeting: A Guide to Preparing Budget Documents. Chicago, IL: Government Finance Officers Association, Exhibit 2-2.

CHAPTER II

THE HISTORY OF BUDGETARY POWER IN THE UNITED STATES

A HISTORICAL OVERVIEW OF BUDGETARY COMPETITION

A review of the history of budgeting in the United States reveals debate over two prominent questions: how should budgetary power be divided between Congress and the President, and how can the budget be employed as a tool to better govern and manage? Although the distribution of budgetary power between the executive and legislative branches of government has changed markedly over the last two centuries, and new methods have emerged to improve governance and management, these two questions remain relevant as they continue to be argued in the context of contemporary budgeting.

The struggle for power between the executive and the legislative branches has been a recurrent theme in the American budget process since the nation was new. Shortly after the Revolutionary War, Congress appeared to have taken the initiative in competition over the proper role of the two branches in debating whether the executive was legally empowered under the Constitution to make budget estimates, and whether the Secretary of Treasury could or should submit a budget framework to Congress (Burkhead, 1959, p. 3). Members of Congress were averse to having the Secretary of Treasury even submit plans to Congress for the next fiscal year (Browne, 1949, p. 12). In contrast, by the late 1960s the steady accretion of power in the executive branch, and within it in the Bureau of the Budget, provided the Chief Executive significant leverage in the budget process. Presidential use of impoundment power and the politicization of the Bureau of the Budget essentially consolidated gains for the Presidency over Congress, and over the executive branch as well.

However, just as nature abhors a vacuum, the American federal system abhors an imbalance of power. The Congressional Budget Impoundment and Control Act of 1974 reestablished Congress's role in the budget process. In 1980, Congress used the provisions of this Act to rewrite the President's budget. While President Ronald Reagan used the Reconciliation Instruction from the 1974 Act to seize a great victory in Congress in 1981, Congress again rewrote the President's budget in 1982. The few years from 1974 to 1980 concluded in a startling reversal in form of most of the twentieth-century practices that had seen Congress increasingly relegated to the role of making marginal and incremental changes in the President's budget.

In 1789, arguments over the balance of power centered on the extent to which the President should prepare a budget, and although this is no longer debatable, the limits to the advantage that preparation gives the executive branch still are arguable. This theme is still as current as it was in 1789. Within this recurrent theme is an idea central to American democracy: power is balanced at the national level between the executive and legislative branches. When a serious imbalance occurs, corrective action ensues to restore and ensure the balance so that when one side is a leader, the other remains a powerful modifier.

The evolutionary nature of American budgeting reveals considerable changes in the uses of budget power and the forms of budget technology. Typically, the developmental context of budgeting is associated with budget reform. However, reform presumes form, and early debates focused on the form of the budget process. During the first century of the nation's existence, simple forms seemed sufficient for simple functions, a premise that held true through the opening decades of the twentieth century. Then, as the functions and responsibilities of government expanded, changes were made in budget technology and technique. This seems to be a linear and expanding process, with more reforms attempted in the last 50 years than in the first 160 of the American experience. Nonetheless, those in charge at the earliest stages of budgeting in this country recognized the need for different budget forms. As early as 1800, civilian agency budgets were presented in carefully detailed object-of-expenditure form, while military expenditures tended to be appropriated as lump sums not unlike specific program categories. Early debate on budget development focused on flexibility and program accomplishments versus strict agency accountability.

Debate about form and content of the federal budget accelerated as a result of local government reforms implemented in New York City and elsewhere during the Progressive era, extending from the mid-1870s through the beginning of the twentieth century, and culminated in congressional enactment of the Budget and Accounting Act of 1921. Passage of the 1921 Act marked the beginning of the federal budget reform movement. The functions of the federal government expanded under the impress of the Great Depression and Presidents Hoover and Roosevelt in the 1930s, World War II and the social service revolution of the 1960s. Parallelisms of state and local to federal reforms became less observable. While local government reform is generally credited with stimulating federal government budget reform during the end of the nineteenth century and early decades of the twentieth century, with the development of the modern post-industrial welfare state and its concomitant assumption of federal government duties and obligations, the need for better federal budget methods and processes became evident. Moreover, reforms enjoying success at sub-national levels of government no longer became automatic candidates for success at the national level. The swift rise and fall of management by objectives as a budget system and zero-based budgeting at the federal level, despite their success in states, are examples. The development of budget form and process is a crucial chapter in the history of federal budgeting and governance, made poignant by the sense that once begun, there was no turning back on budget reform. Decisions on Social Security eligibility made in the 1930s and 1980s, social service programs including Medicare and Medicaid from the 1960s through the 1990s, and the federal budget surplus in the period 1999–2005 will shape tax policy, benefit liability, the budget and the budget process to the mid-twenty-first century and beyond.

EARLY AMERICAN PATTERNS

Early American budgetary patterns were part of and separate from their predominantly English colonial heritage. They were part of that heritage in that the American colonies inherited the full line of English historical experience with a limited monarchy and expanded legislative powers. This historical legacy may be dated to 1215, when a group of dissident nobles forced the King of England to accede to and sign the Magna Carta. Of the sixty-nine articles in this document, the most important is that which stated, "No scutage on revenue shall be imposed in the kingdom unless by the Common Council of the Realm" (Caiden & Wildavsky, 1974, p. 25) The Common Council preceded Parliament, and the statement that revenue could be raised only with the consent of a legislative assembly remained constant. This is often hailed as a beginning of popular government, but it is useful to note that this was basically a sharing of power between the king and the most powerful nobles in the realm, the two top tiers in an elite-dominated society where status was conferred mainly by birth. Nonetheless, by the end of the thirteenth century, the principle was established that the Crown had available only those sources of revenue previously authorized by Parliament.

In England, the Magna Carta was only the beginning of a long process of movement toward popular government, a process completed in the twentieth century when the House of Lords lost the power to reject money bills. By the middle of the fourteenth century, the House of Commons was established and its leaders realized that a further check upon the power of the king would result from legislative control over appropriations. At first, revenue acts were phrased broadly, and once the money authorized was available the king could spend it as he wished. However, Parliament began to insert appropriation language in the Acts of Supply and other similar legislation, stating that the money be used for a particular purpose. Moreover, rules were made for the proper disposal of money, and penalties were imposed for noncompliance (Thomson, 1938, p. 206). Consequently, by the middle of the fourteenth century, fiscal practices included a check on the Crown's right to tax and spend; bills from Parliament carried notice of intent designating what money was to be used for, rules for disbursement of money, and penalties when rules were not followed.

Refinement of this system would take centuries, and its progress was not linear. Some kings were more skillful, personable, or powerful than others, and Parliament's role manifested steady evolution only in the most general terms. Wildavsky suggests that if a benchmark is needed, formal budgeting can be dated from the reforms of William Pitt the Younger (Wildavsky, 1975, p. 272).[1] As Chancellor of the English Exchequer from 1783 to 1801, Pitt faced a heavy debt load as a result of the American Revolution. Pitt consolidated a maze of customs and excise duties into one general fund from which all creditors would be paid, reduced fraud in revenue collection by introducing new auditing measures, and instituted double-entry bookkeeping procedures (Each transaction is entered twice, as a credit to one account and a debit to another.) Moreover, Pitt established a sinking fund schedule for amortization of debt, requiring that all new loans made by government impose an additional 1% levy as a term of repayment (Rose, 1911a, 1911b, 1912). Pitt raised some taxes and lowered others to reduce the allure of smuggling. Because his actions were made in response to the debt load occasioned by the war, however, the model that Americans had to follow was, at best, incomplete. This model encompassed a royal executive with varying degrees of strength and a legislative body attempting to exert financial control over the Crown by requiring parliamentary approval of sources of revenue and expenditure. Approval was provided through appropriations legislation. The model ultimately demanded accountability of administrative officials to Parliament (Browne, 1949, p. 15).

The history of the American colonies has been described as a replication of the struggle between Parliament and the Crown, with the colonies, like Parliament, gradually winning a more independent position (Labaree, 1958, p. 35). The colonies turned the power of the purse against the English Royal Governors. Colonial legislatures voted the salaries of Governors and their agents, appropriating them in annual authorizations rather than for longer periods. Indeed, one colonial governor's salary was set semiannually. In theory, the Royal Governors had extensive fiscal powers, but in fact these powers were often exercised by colonial legislative assemblies. These included raising taxes, appropriating revenues, and granting salaries to the Royal Governors and their officers. Caiden and Wildavsky remark that the colonists were thoroughly in the English tradition of denying supply (budget dollars) to the colonial governors to force compliance with the will of colonial legislatures. Not only were salaries voted annually, but taxes were also often reenacted annually. "Royal Governors were allowed no permanent sources of revenue that might make them 'uppity'" (Caiden & Wildavsky, 1974, p. 25). Appropriations were specified by object and amount, appropriation language was used to specify exactly what funds could and could not be used for, for example, "no other purpose or use whatsoever" (Caiden & Wildavsky, 1974, p. 26) Royal Governors even were prevented from using surplus funds or unexpected balances; these were required to be returned to the treasury. Various mechanisms were used to impose further restrictions on the power of the Royal Governors. In some colonies, independent Treasurers were elected to manage funds. Several colonies required legislative approval prior to disbursement of funds; in emergencies this might necessitate a special appropriation. Some colonial legislatures appointed special commissioners accountable not to the Royal Governor but to the legislature as a further check on the power of the Governor. Caiden and Wildavsky conclude that "…power, not money was the issue" (Caiden & Wildavsky, 1974, p. 32). Thus, from the earliest days of the Americas, budget decisions focused around the issue of the correct balance of power between the colonial legislatures and Royal Governors, setting a pattern that has applied from that time to the present.

Generally, neither expenditures nor taxes were heavy during this period; England did not extract much revenue from the colonies except in periods of war (Browne, 1949, p. 16). What was troublesome to the colonists was that the Crown could and did impose duties and excises intended to regulate trade and navigation without the colonists' approval: hence the revolutionary complaint of "taxation without representation." Before the Revolutionary War, the colonies followed the British pattern of a gradually developing budget power. Decisions about taxation were paramount, and the exercise of budget power was basically sought as a check upon Royal power. Development of the instruments of taxation, appropriations, and accounting were all evidenced in this pattern, but a formal budget system did not yet exist.

The colonies departed from English tradition when they gained independence after the Revolutionary War. Initially, they created fiscal systems from which the executive was virtually excluded. Power was vested in various legislative arrangements in the newly independent colonies. And, as a result of fear of central government inherited from their experience with the British, the powers of the first Congress established under the Articles of Confederation were very weak. In fact, this fear was evident in the manner in which powers were delegated to both the legislative and executive branches. The colonists were also averse to a system of national taxation. Taxation imposed a special hardship on the colonies because hard coinage was scarce and bills or letters of credit were used irregularly. Consequently, the colonies were chronically short of cash and coinage schemes abounded. During the Revolutionary War, borrowing and promising to pay either with bills of credit or by coining paper money became endemic as the colonists pursued the war and made expenditures without tax revenues. Washington's continuing struggle to adequately equip his armies is well known, with the winter at Valley Forge standing for all time as a symbol of heroic efforts to contend with a new nation's ineffectual and rudimentary governmental systems. As Vincent J. Browne observes:

> Until the framing of the Constitution, the future of the States was almost as much imperiled by financial indiscretions as it had been previously jeopardized by the forces of George III. (1949, p. 17)

The costs of war were great. Thomas Jefferson estimated the cost at $140 million from 1775 to 1783. By contrast, the federal government operating budget in 1784 was $457,000. Bills of credit were issued both by the states and by Congress from 1775 to 1779. Bills of credit rapidly depreciated. In 1790 Congress was forced to admit that a dollar of paper money was worth less than two cents and passed a resolution to redeem bills of credit at one fortieth their face value (Dewey, 1968, p. 36). Paper currency did not become legal tender again until after the Civil War.

The Articles of Confederation provided that revenues were to be raised from a direct tax on property in proportion to the value of all land within each state, according to a method stipulated by Congress. These limitations upon congressional taxing power left it dependent upon the states. Congress was not disposed to provide effective fiscal leadership to states, in part because Congress was debating issues related to its own budgetary procedures and its leverage vis-à-vis the states regarding fiscal power. Congress was attempting to act as both the executive and legislative branch in a system where the preponderance of power was held by the individual states.

Table 1.   Revolutionary War Data

	Operating Budgets	Expenditures 1775-1783	Bills of Credit 1775-1779
1784	457,000	$140,000,000	
1785	404,000	(Jefferson est. 1786)	Federal $241,000,000
1786	446,000	$134,645,000	State $209,000,000
1787	417,000	(Hamilton est. 1790)	

Source: Browne (1949, pp. 18–19)

Not only was this a departure from the English tradition but, it was a model of government that would be short-lived in this country.

Constitutional government began, then, with a long history of British practices further shaped by both the inefficiencies of the Confederation and the cost of the Revolutionary War. If American institutions were influenced by an anti-executive trend, they were also affected by the chaotic nature of legislative government under the Articles of Confederation. This period was marked by extraordinary negligence, wastefulness, disorder, and corruption as Congress in its committees prepared all revenue and appropriation estimates, legislated them, and then attempted to exercise exacting control over accounts (Bolles, 1969, p. 358).

Nonetheless, there was an indication of things to come when, in this period of rule by legislative committee, Congress created the post of Superintendent of Finance in early 1781. This was a new approach to the budget, intended to overcome the fear of placing too much power in a single executive. Robert Morris, the first Superintendent of Finance, was charged with oversight of the public debt, expenditures, revenues, and accounts to the end that he would, "...report plans for improving and regulating the finances, and for establishing order and economy in the expenditure of the public money," (Powell, 1939, p. 33) as well as perform oversight of budget execution, purchasing and receiving, and collecting delinquent accounts owed the United States.

The enabling legislation has been referred to as "a bit radical for the times," because of the vast authority it delegated to one man (Browne, 1949, pp. 21–22). Morris's pressure for revenue collection seemed to have angered some members of Congress. Consequently, in 1784, a Treasury Board or committee was established. However, the benefits derived from a single executive, albeit not the President, equipped with broad powers was evident and this pattern would reappear. As a practical matter, the whole period of Confederation was a time of experimentation within the context of anti-monarchical rule. The events of this period seem somewhat confusing, but there existed no model financial system to follow. If William Pitt the Younger's approach was the model, let it be remembered that he was the contemporary of Morris and the Founding Fathers. Pitt did not take office until after Morris, and Pitt's power was exercised in a system where tradition still gave the balance of power to the Crown. Pitt was the King's minister. The Americans were busy negotiating the mechanics of representative government, influenced by the Confederation model of strong legislative assemblies.

CONSTITUTIONAL GOVERNMENT

The Constitution provided the right to tax to Congress and set forth four qualifications on spending power:

1. No money shall be drawn from the Treasury but in consequence of appropriation.
2. A regular statement and account of all receipts and expenditures must be rendered from time to time.
3. No appropriations to support the army shall run for longer than two years.
4. All expenditures shall be made for the general welfare (Article 1, Sec. 8, U.S. Constitution).

The first two points contained in Article 1, Section 8 are the cornerstones of the budget process. On the revenue side, all money bills were directed to originate in the House because of its proportional and direct representation of the people. The role of the Senate was debated, with the compromise that the Senate could concur with the House or propose amendments to revenue bills. Fiscal power would be developed within an environment where the Congress was expected to be supreme at the federal level, and the states were expected to be jealous guardians of their powers. Under the impact of the American Revolution, planning had been nonexistent, management had been a legislative responsibility, and control for propriety was honored more in its absence than in its presence. However, the period 1789 to 1800 marked the beginning of the movement toward executive management and perhaps could be called the first stage of U.S. budget reform. The talents of Alexander Hamilton strongly influenced development in this period (Seiko, 1940, p. 45).[2]

Hamilton was a man of great achievement. He learned applied finance at the age of 11 while a clerk in a countinghouse on the island of St. Croix in the West Indies. He learned quickly and was promoted to bookkeeper and then to manager. Before Hamilton was 21, he had impressed friends with his abilities to the extent that they sponsored him in a course of studies, first at a preparatory school and then at the predecessor to Columbia University in New York. Here he quickly gained a reputation as an adroit protagonist for the cause of the American colonies (Caldwell, 1944/1982, pp. 71–89; Miller, 1959). In 1776, he had won George Washington's eye with his conspicuous bravery as a provincial artillery captain at the Battle of Trenton. Washington used him as a staff officer until 1781 when Hamilton, chafing under the limitations of staff routine, seized upon a trivial quarrel to break with Washington and leave his position. Washington seemed to have understood his impetuous subordinate well. He gave Hamilton command of a battalion that attacked a British stronghold at the siege of Yorktown in October of 1781, a siege that ultimately became the decisive battle of the Revolutionary War.

During the 1780s, Hamilton practiced law in New York City and was active in congressional politics, arguing for a strong central government. Hamilton believed that English government, as then constituted under George III, should be the American model. Hamilton proposed a President elected for life, who would exercise an absolute veto over the legislature. The central government would appoint the state governors, who would have an absolute power over state legislation. The judiciary would be composed of a supreme court whose justices would have life tenure. The legislature would consist of a Senate, elected for life, and a lower house, elected for three years. In this system the states would have virtually no power.

Hamilton's ideas seem to have had little influence upon the Constitutional Convention. However, when opponents attacked the document brought forth by the convention. Hamilton, with James Madison and John Jay, authored *The Federalist Papers*, a collection of eighty-five essays that were widely read and helped mold contemporary opinion; they became one of the classic works in American political literature. This was the man Washington appointed as Secretary of the Treasury in September of 1789.

Hamilton fused his own goals for a strong central government with the new nation's fiscal needs. His first efforts were directed toward establishing the credit of the new government. His first two reports on public credit urged funding the national debt at full value, the assumption by the federal government of all debts incurred by the states during the Revolutionary War, and a system of taxation to pay for the debts assumed.[3] Strong opposition arose to these proposals, but Hamilton's position prevailed after he made a bargain with Thomas Jefferson, who delivered southern votes in return for Hamilton's support for locating the future nation's capital on the banks of the Potomac near Virginia.

Hamilton's third report to Congress proposed a national bank, modeled after the Bank of England. Through this proposal, Hamilton saw a chance to knit the concerns of the wealthy and mercantilist classes to the financial dealings of the central government. Washington signed the bill creating what became the Federal Reserve Bank into law, establishing this national bank and based, in part, on Hamilton's argument that the Constitution was a source of both enumerated and implied powers, an interpretation he used to expand the powers of the Constitution in later years. Hamilton's fourth report to Congress was perhaps the most philosophic and visionary. Influenced by Adam Smith's *The Wealth of Nations* (1776), Hamilton broke new ground by arguing that it was in the interest of the federal government to aid the growth of infant industries through various protective laws and that, to aid the general welfare, the federal government was obliged to encourage manufacturing through tax and tariff policy. Hamilton's contemporaries seem to have rejected the latter view; Congress, at least, would have nothing to do with it. Nonetheless, in little more than two years Hamilton submitted four major reports to Congress, gaining acceptance of three that funded the national debt at full value, established the nation's credit at home and abroad by creating a banking system and a stable currency, and developed a stable tax system based on excise taxes to fund steady recovery from the debt and to provide for future appropriations. Indeed, Hamilton opposed the popular view of war with England in the mid-1790s, at a time when France and England were at war, and England was seizing American ships in the Caribbean. He believed that commerce with England and the import duties it provided were crucial. Hamilton's essays, published in New York newspapers in 1795, helped avoid war with England, thus helping to save his revenue system.

The elements of the new nation's monetary and fiscal policy were bitterly contested issues, and groups began to coalesce around various positions pro and con. Hamilton became the leader of one faction, the Federalists, and because Washington supported most of Hamilton's program, in effect he became a Federalist. The two most prominent individuals in opposition were James Madison in the House of Representatives and Thomas Jefferson in the Cabinet. Madison and Jefferson were the Republican leaders. Hamilton and Jefferson feuded constantly for several years beginning in 1791, as each tried to drive the other from the Cabinet. Finally, tired, stung by criticism of his operation of the Treasury Department, and needing to repair his personal fortunes, Hamilton announced his intentions to resign his post as Secretary of the Treasury at the end of 1794. Hamilton did not, however, retreat to obscurity. He still held presidential ambitions that were narrowly frustrated; he was appointed to high military command, and he remained within the inner circle of the nation's political elite before departing center stage, killed in a pistol duel with Aaron Burr in 1804. Hamilton had made both great accomplishments and bitter enemies.

Hamilton's role in establishing a system for debt management, securing the currency, and providing a stable revenue base make him perhaps the founding father of the American budgeting system. Without faith in the currency, the nation's credit, and the revenue base, it is impossible to make any budget system work. The federal taxing power alone was a dramatic change from the system envisioned under the Articles of Confederation, which approximated a contributory position by the separate states, hectored by the central government. Only a sure and certain revenue base, providing predictable revenue collections, allows the creation and maintenance of the modern nation-state. It was Hamilton's genius to direct the United States to that pathway.

To Congress, Hamilton represented a transitional figure. Before his appointment, the House of Representatives had a tax committee, the Committee on Ways and Means, established in the summer of 1789. But this committee fell into disuse when a Secretary of the Treasury was appointed. At this juncture in history, Congress viewed the Treasury Department as a legislative agency and the Secretary of Treasury as its officer (Browne, 1949, p. 34). The first appropriations bill for an operating budget came about because the House ordered the Secretary of Treasury to "...report to this House an estimate of the sums requisite to be appropriated during the present year; and for satisfying such warrants as have been drawn by the late Board of the Treasury and which may not heretofore have been paid" (1 Annals of Congress, p. 929).

When the articles of the Constitution were being debated, Hamilton wrote:

> The House of Representatives cannot only refuse, but they alone can propose, the supplies requisite for the support of the government. They, in a word, hold the purse ... This power over the purse may, in fact, be regarded as the most complete and effectual weapon with which any constitution can arm the immediate representatives of the people for obtaining a redress for every grievance and for carrying into effect every just and salutary measure. (Hamilton, *The Federalist Papers*, No. 58, as reprinted in Miller, 1959)

Whatever the flaws of the Act creating a Department of the Treasury, it seems clear that its intent was to make the Congress alone responsible for the budget process. That there was little room for executive leadership is demonstrated in the fact that the Act mentions the President only in connection with the appointment and removal of officers. Furthermore, while the act was being debated, opinion was divided over the wording of the duties of the Secretary of the Treasury with respect to whether he was to digest and *report* revenue and spending plans or whether he was to digest and *prepare* plans. Those Congressmen hostile to strong executive power believed that giving the Secretary the power to digest and report plans would take the fiscal policy initiative away from the House. The Secretary would report only what he had already done; this would deprive the House of its ability to exercise a prior restraint on the actions of the Secretary. The word *report* was deleted from the legislation and *prepare* was inserted and carried by the majority (Browne, 1949, p. 31).

Some observers have mistaken Hamilton's approach to appropriation as having established an executive budget system. The traditional model of an executive budget system would encompass a presidential review of departmental documents, revision of estimates, and a unified submission by the President or his agent of those estimates to Congress for approval. As Secretary of the Treasury, Hamilton did not wish the system to function in this manner, and personally he acted as an agent of Congress. The development of an executive budget system occurred in more gradual process, with a steady line of evolution leading to the authorization of a formal presidential budget—but not until 1921.

The first appropriation act of Congress was brief and general:

> That there be appropriated for the service of the present year, *to be* paid out of the monies which arise, either from the requisitions heretofore made upon the several states, or from the duties on impost and tonnage, the following sums. *viz.* A sum not exceeding two hundred and sixteen thousand dollars for defraying the expenses of the *civil* list, under the late and present government: a sum not exceeding one hundred and thirty-seven thousand dollars for defraying the expenses of the department of war; a sum not exceeding one hundred and ninety-six thousand dollars for discharging the warrants issued by the late board of Treasury and remaining unsatisfied; and a sum not exceeding ninety-six thousand dollars for paying pensions to invalids. (I Statutes at Large, U.S. Congress, Ch. XXIII, Sept. 29, 1789, p. 95)

Although salaries are the largest single item in this list (civil list), mandated expenditures—bills and pensions—comprised 45% of the budget, defense 21% and entitlements 14.8%. De facto uncontrollability was high. True to modern practice, this appropriation bill was not the only money bill passed by Congress. Between the summer of 1789 and May of 1792, numerous bills were passed to provide for a variety of expenses, including defense, Indian treaties, debt reduction, and establishment of the federal mint.[4]

The first three bills were written as lump sum general appropriations, for the civil list, the department of war, invalid pensions, the expenses of Congress, and contingent charges upon government. Appropriating by lump sum caused resentment among some congressmen. One wrote of the appropriations bill of 1790 in his diary:

> The appropriations were all in gross, and to the amount upward of half a million. I could not get a copy of it. I wished to have seen the particulars specified, but such a hurry I never saw before . . . Here is a general appropriation of above half a million dollars—the particulars not mentioned—the estimates on which it is founded may be mislaid or changed; in fact it is giving

the Secretary the money for him to account for as he pleases. (Wilmerding, 1943, p. 21)

Notwithstanding their general nature, appropriation bills were linked to estimates of expense as specified in other bills. Expenditures for salaries were generally governed by laws enumerating the salary and number of the officers stipulated; for example, five associate supreme court justices at a salary no more than $3,500 per year. Estimates for the military were assumed to control the appropriations voted for the military. Therefore, even though the appropriations were voted in gross, the calculations adding up to the total were assumed to control the total. By 1792, Congress was appropriating money in gross but stipulating what the money was to be used for, with "that is to say" clauses: for example, $329,653.56 for the civil list, with a "that is to say" clause followed by specific sums attached to an enumeration of the corresponding general items (Fisher, 1975, p. 61; Wilmerding, 1943, p. 23).[5]

Congress was now planning in detail and the executive branch accepted that detail, although knowing full well that the dictates of administering might make it imperative to depart from the detailed plans expressed in the appropriation acts. Budgeting by lump sum was not a characteristic of the routine of American government except in case of emergency appropriations.[6] Congress increasingly specified the itemization of appropriation bills, in part as a strategy to control Secretary of the Treasury Hamilton, who was viewed by some as a member of the executive branch. In 1790, the House had sixty-five members, and most of its business could be carried out as a committee of the whole, but by 1795 it was clear that the Treasury Department could not serve the needs of Congress as well as it could serve the needs of the executive. Therefore, Congress reinstituted the Committee on Ways and Means, initially as a select or special committee, and by 1802 as a standing committee. During this period, Woolcott, Hamilton's successor at Treasury, was embroiled in an increasingly bitter argument with Congress over the transfer of appropriations. Although Congress could appropriate in very specific terms, it could not stop the administration from transferring from one account to another when the situation seemed to warrant such transfers. The War and Navy Departments seemed particularly able to transfer funds, thereby dissolving the discipline of detailed itemization.

In 1801, when the Federalists were defeated and the Republicans took office, Thomas Jefferson spoke to the need for increased itemization of expenditure in appropriations. Nonetheless, the transfer of appropriations was an accepted practice in the administration, albeit an illegal one (Wilmerding, 1943, p. 48). Jefferson himself made the Louisiana Purchase after a liberal interpretation of executive authority to issue stock when government revenues were insufficient to cover necessary expenditures. Congress's insistence on itemization led to deficiencies in accounts. Later, budget practices also became part of developing party politics. The Federalist Party believed in a strong executive, and they preferred lump sum appropriations for activities that would give administrators as much flexibility as possible in managing programs. Meanwhile, the Republican party favored specific line item appropriations that limited department heads to doing specifically what Congress intended. However, Congress found out it could not control everything and, beginning with appropriations for the Army and the Navy, line item controls were relaxed and other controls not invoked (e.g., penalties for unauthorized transfers).

The tension between delegating power to the executive and retaining appropriate congressional control of the power of the purse has remained an issue to current times. Generally, when relationships between the executive and legislative branch deteriorate, because of divided party control or because an executive agency becomes either too aggressive in its budget practices or not aggressive enough, Congress changes the rules to ensure that its intent is preserved, for example, by changing reprogramming within appropriation thresholds (ceilings), requiring advance notification of Congress for reprogramming changes from one category within an appropriation account to another, or by attaching a legislative interest note to an item to ensure that money is spent in a special way, or that a program is executed within the fiscal year.

By 1800, the initial pattern had been set. Appropriation bills were passed and linked to specific estimates for specific purposes, some flexibility was made between military and civil expenditures, and a recognition was established that transfer of funds between categories was technically illegal but necessary to meet contingencies unforeseen at the time of appropriations. The House held major control of the purse. By 1802, it had developed a standing committee to deal with revenues and appropriations, while on the executive side, the Secretary of Treasury had become more and more the President's agent in shaping appropriations bills, collecting revenues, and debt management. Both the legislature and the executive were elected by and responsible to the people. Rudimentary and disconnected as it seems from modern perspectives, no other country had such a budget system.

MAKING THE SYSTEM WORK: 1800–1921

The transfer of power to Thomas Jefferson and the Republicans marked the end of the period of creation of the Republic, the end of the process of separating from England and the setting up of a new government. Much remained to be done, but many of the basic mechanisms of governance, and of monetary and fiscal policy, were now in place. In fiscal affairs the federal government had established its powers to tax and to budget, as well as to issue notes of credit when revenues did not match expenditures. Budgeting was in the main a legislative power. The Department of the Treasury was originally conceived as Congress's assistant. Budgeting power in the Congress was held in the House, which was small enough so that it could operate as a committee of the whole. As the Treasury increasingly served the President, Treasury's power in Congress declined, and Congress chose its own internal review and enactment body, the Committee on Ways and Means, and this committee would gain great power. During the course of the nineteenth century, appropriation bills would be sent to other committees as the Ways and Means Committee work load became heavier, or as political factors dictated. After the Civil War, a committee on appropriations was created. When it used retrenchment powers to reach into substantive legislation under the jurisdiction of other committees, Congress reacted against this expansion of the appropriation committees' powers and diminished the power of the appropriations committee. It seems that whenever a committee role became too important, Congress changed its procedures to move power away from it. Thus, legislative procedure changed, but budgeting maintained eminence as a vital legislative process.

Naturally, the issues of fiscal policy debated by Congress changed with the times. Early debates in the nineteenth century focused on the necessity of budget flexibility in administering the War and Navy Departments. Without these powers it was argued that the new nation could not long survive. Andrew Jackson's presidency changed the focus of debate to internal improvements—public works. Jackson, a conservative, was against extravagance and averred that many of the internal improvement bills were passed to rectify specific situations but did not necessarily secure the general welfare. He tried to veto these bills while Congress sought ways to pass them as riders on other legislation. The Civil War caused great fiscal strain on the Union, and the decades after the war were marked by fierce battles over pensions and veterans' benefits. It is instructive to note that the last Revolutionary War benefit was paid 123 years after the war was over, and that civil war pensions were paid into the latter half of the twentieth century.

Although tariffs, customs, and excises were good sources of revenue, they were not large enough to underwrite the costs of wars, were sometimes changed for political reasons that had nothing to do with balancing expenditure needs and, consequently, did not constitute a stable revenue base. Revenues from other sources were sought. Further, throughout the nineteenth century, federal revenues and expenditures were not coordinated. In addition to the general appropriations bills, there were numerous other bills legislating appropriations passed in each session of Congress. Indeed, it can be argued that an imperative to balance expenditures against revenues did not exist on the legislative level until after the passage of the Congressional Budget and Impoundment Control Act of 1974.

Congress also struggled with other problems during this period, including deficiency appropriations, surpluses that departments carried forward into the next fiscal year, transfers from one military service to another, and expenditures made without the authority of law. Although Congress legislated against these various budgetary sins, it also recognized that it had to leave the Treasury Department some flexibility or it would have to appropriate sums for additional items or expenditures to provide for unforeseen contingencies. Congressional budgeting was reasonably effective in meeting spending needs, special interest influence not withstanding, but not efficient by any measure. This absence of efficiency often led to problems of absence of accountability and insufficient oversight, and illegality in some instances. Fraud, waste and abuse, and naked catering to powerful business and political interests plagued the federal government in this period. Similar problems confronted state and local governments during the nineteenth century. Observance of these problems and others drove forward the movement for reform of systems of taxing and spending at all levels of government, particularly in the last decades of the nineteenth century and the first two decades of the twentieth century.

The Budget and Accounting Act of 1921 is frequently observed to be the watershed in the pursuit of federal budgetary efficiency and accountability, and presidential control. The budgetary practices of the federal government from 1789 to 1921 are sometimes dismissed as unimportant. The functions of government were few, revenues were comparatively small, and debate focused on what should or should not be itemized by Congress. Because taxes were drawn from tariffs intended to protect infant industries, and expenditures spent on pensions or internal improvements, members of Congress could appease all by both increasing tariffs and spending. Furthermore, agencies in the executive branch became expert in the creation of the "coercive deficiency," spending all of the money appropriated to them on "good" projects and then going to Congress for more funding, confident that the particular committee supervising their programs would recommend additional appropriations. The crucial variable in this arrangement was the relationship between the committee chair and the agency head. This interpretation is arguable, in part because it appears to ignore the efforts of both Congress and the executive to budget "rationally" and according to real need through planning, preparation and control of spending. Louis Fisher notes:

We are led to understand that, prior to 1921, Presidents had little to do in framing the financial program of the federal government. Individual spending agencies transmitted their budget requests to Congress in what was called a "book of estimates." The Secretary of the Treasury could have played a coordinating role, but studies conclude that his handling of budget estimates was routine and perfunctory. According to this point of view, Presidents and their Secretaries of the Treasury were passive bystanders during those years, mechanically forwarding budget estimates to Congress without revision or comment. (Fisher, 1975, p. 9)

Fisher suggests that during the nineteenth century a number of Presidents revised departmental estimates before they were sent to Congress, including John Quincy Adams, Martin Van Buren, John Tyler, James K. Polk, James Buchanan, Ulysses S. Grant, and Grover Cleveland, and were assisted in this task by a number of Secretaries of the Treasury. As observed earlier, although the budget process was basically a legislative budget system, the executive branch did play a role in its execution. Some ascribe an even larger role to the executive in this period.[7]

EMERGENCE OF EXECUTIVE POWER IN THE TWENTIETH CENTURY

The first decade of the twentieth century was pivotal in terms of the balance of budgetary power. Government revenues based on customs and excise taxes were insufficient for the task of achieving the nation's "manifest destiny." Although the budget had been in a surplus position from the conclusion of the Civil War to 1893, some policy makers worried that the economy had become penurious and prevented the assumption of new needs. The Spanish American War and the expense incurred in building the Panama Canal created budget deficits. Moreover, customs revenues began to decline. The federal budget was in a deficit position for eleven of the seventeen years from 1894 to 1911, including five of the seven years from 1904 through 1910. The point is that the old revenue system was inadequate to the task of funding America's new and expanding world role. Passage of the sixteenth Amendment by Congress in 1909 and ratified by the states in 1913 permitting a federal income tax, a milestone event in U.S. fiscal policy, was intended in part to remedy this dilemma.

However, it created other problems. With the power of direct taxation of individual citizens, ironically the nation's policymakers feared that taxpayers would become more concerned about where their money was being spent. Thus, passage of the federal income tax must be viewed as contributing to the pressure for budget reform and a stronger executive budget presence. In the years 1919 through 1921, the income tax provided more than 57% of federal government's revenue. The year 1921 is a milestone due to the passage of a watershed budget reform act and the emergence of a major new revenue source.

The debate over strengthening presidential spending power was essentially completed by 1912, with issuance of the report of the Taft Commission on Economy and Efficiency. Taft submitted this report to Congress, along with a plan for a national budget system, but his party did not control the House during that session of Congress and the two branches of government could not agree on a new budget process. The Commission's position was succinctly stated:

> [...the budget is the only] effective means whereby the Executive may be made responsible for getting before the country definite, well-considered, comprehensive programs with respect to which the legislature must also assume responsibility either for action or inaction. (H. Doc. 854,62–2,1912, p. 138; Taft, 1912, pp. 62–63).[8]

Budget reform was further delayed at the national level by the First World War, but reform continued apace at the local and state levels. Indeed, some observers have suggested that budget reform during this period in the American context began at the local level. Reform efforts resulted from indignation over corruption, graft, and mismanagement prevalent in local governments, exposed by journalists and good government movements, and supported by the Progressive party. Budget reform complemented other innovations including establishment of city manager and commission government forms, and the initiative, referendum, recall, and short-ballot electoral procedures. Budget reform in this period may be considered a local affair that eventually carried over to the federal government (Burkhead, 1959, p. 15; see also Schick, 1966, pp. 243–258).[9] The fiscal stress caused by the American commitments to World War I, and President Woodrow Wilson's own interest in budget and administrative reform also precipitated the adoption of the executive budget process.

In his 1917 annual message to Congress, President Wilson stressed his party's platform on budget reform. Although reform seems to have been possible in any of these years, Wilson chose to wait until the end of World War 1. While he waited, the nation incurred a large deficit. In the three years from 1917 through 1919, federal debt grew from $1.2 billion to $25.5 billion. This gave urgency to the case for budget reform. After the peace treaty had been signed, Wilson argued that budget reform would give him a better grasp of the continuing level of defense spending, the effect of the disposal of surplus military property, and the impact of demobilization upon the economy (Fisher, 1975, p. 33).

In 1918 and 1919, a series of bills intended to reform the distribution of budget power were passed, and in 1921 Congress passed the Budget and

Accounting Act (Burkhead, 1959, pp. 26–28).[10] This bill created the Bureau of the Budget (BOB), to be located in the Department of the Treasury with a Director appointed by and responsible to the President. The Bureau was given the authority to, "...assemble, correlate, revise, reduce, or increase" departmental budget estimates (42 STAT. 20, 1921). In view of the Bureau's later move from Treasury to the Executive Office, history judges this first placement harshly. However, the intention of the proponents of the Act was to avoid unnecessary friction between the President and his cabinet officers over budget matters. Providing budget review power within the BOB in Treasury was intended to avoid setting the Bureau against the more powerful cabinet officers. And, placing the Bureau in the Department of the Treasury facilitated the coordination of expenditures and revenues (Fisher, 1975, p. 34). Under any interpretation, establishment of the BOB in 1921 and the crucial tasking of the President to prepare and submit a budget to Congress shifted power to the executive.

Caiden and Wildavsky suggest that the reformers of this era had no conception of informal coordination and communication within and between the branches of government, and that they discounted the possibility that elected officials could make good decisions based on the poor quality of the information which they had been provided prior to passage of the 1921 Budget Act. Reformers were determined to provide a better budget format, believing that provision of better information in plain sight to leaders who were persons of "trained minds" would cause budgets to make better sense, i.e., to be more fair, to respond more genuinely to public service demands, to be more "rational." Thus, reformers were against the existing federal budget system that produced budgets with no standard classification of expenditures by object, no uniform system for recording expenditures against the budget plan, and no budgetary message or summary and no analytic tables. According to Caiden and Wildavsky, reformers also believed that leadership had to come from the executive branch where specialists would put together understandable budgets that balanced. Reformers referred to the "science of budget making" and suggested they would subject budgetary problems to scientific analysis (Caiden & Wildavsky, 1974, p. 35). This view assumed that if goals were agreed to by all, it was just a matter of selecting the best way to attain the goals. Persons of "trained minds" would lead the way. However, critics of reform argued that it was simply a pretext for taking power from the Congress and giving it to the executive (Wildavsky, cited in Chandler, 1984, pp. 379–382). Nonetheless, after the horrendous debt increase resulting from WW1, the executive budget movement was an idea whose time had come, even to Congress.

However, in passing reform legislation that increased the power of the executive, Congress also took something back by creating the General Accounting Office to audit and account for expenditures, led by a Comptroller General of the United States responsible to Congress and appointed for a 15-year term. Any perusal of reports and testimony generated by GAO indicate how important this office has become in providing information for Congress to use in reviewing budgets and making financial management decisions. At the time, creation of the GAO was overshadowed by the attention directed at the Bureau of the Budget.

NEUTRAL COMPETENCE AND EXECUTIVE REFORM: 1920–1970

To a considerable extent, tracing the expansion of executive budgetary power in the period 1920 to 1970 is captured through analysis of the evolution of the Bureau of the Budget. The initial accomplishments of the Bureau of the Budget were not insignificant. Its first Director, General Dawes, instituted significant technical innovations, including the concept of reserves and an allotment system to fund departments and agencies from the Treasury. He also engendered a climate of economy and efficiency. Dawes adopted a technical and nonpartisan profile, describing employees of the BOB as akin to stokers in a ship's engine room, not steering the ship, but simply feeding the fires that drove the engines of government.[11] Dawes' stance defused some potential political problems, but the true usefulness of the Bureau of the Budget would not be seen until the stress of the Depression captured the attention of the nation. In a sense, the turmoil of the first two decades of the twentieth century was followed by a period of relative fiscal calm in the 1920s. The innovations that the deficits of the period of 1903 to 1920 created would not be tested and used until the mid-1930s.

If creation of the BOB appeared to represent a major shift in the balance of budgetary power between the Congress and the executive, what happened then to the Bureau in its early years? For almost a decade after Dawes, the Bureau had no great mission. It spent its time in trivial gestures toward economy in an era when the great impulse toward economy was generated elsewhere, either as a result of the winding down of expenses of World War I or because of the philosophies represented by liberal or conservative Presidents. For example, the Bureau's mandate included authority to conduct government-wide studies to secure greater economy and efficiency, but generally it ignored that aspect of its role. Instead, it proudly announced that it had taken its "own medicine," spending little more than half of its appropriation in 1921 and indulging in such activities as checking employees' desks for excessive use of official stationery, paper clips, and other supplies. It also directed federal employees to use the Army radio network instead of making long-distance telephone calls and to take the upper berth in Pullman train cars when traveling because they were cheaper (Berman, 1979, pp. 7–8).

Faced with the depression in the 1930s, Franklin D. Roosevelt could have strengthened the BOB, but he chose as his first director a conservative with whom he could not work. In 1934, the BOB remained a small, rigid, and inactive agency attached to the Treasury Department. It, however, became the logical candidate for expansion. As a result of the reorganization initiatives contained in the 1937 Report of the Brownlow Committee, the Bureau of the Budget was transferred into the newly created Executive Office of the Presidential (53 STAT 1423, Executive Order 8248: 4 Fed. Reg. 3864; see also Pearson, 1943, p. 126; Smith, 1941, p. 106). This was done under reorganization Plan No. 1 of 1939, which marked the beginning of a truly effective budget bureau in the United States. Under Roosevelt's administration, the BOB employed various fiscal management tools, including practical control over allotments, central legislative clearance, and bill analysis. It was, however, in 1939 a small agency with about forty staff. By the end of World War II, the staff would increase to 600, representing an expansion unmatched before or since.

The halcyon days of the Bureau of the Budget existed from 1939 through the end of the 1940s. During this time, the Bureau built and held a reputation for unsurpassed excellence as a neutral, analytic power operating as a staff instrument for the executive. The reputation for excellence gained during these years of depression and war would mantle the Bureau into the early-1970s. But then, as noted below, its function changed to match the politics of the time. Further, it would become tainted somewhat by the politics of Watergate and the aggressiveness of Richard Nixon in using (or abusing) his Presidential impoundment authority to refuse to spend money appropriated by Congress. It would be accused of exerting too much power, of resistance to change in a world interested in policy analysis instead of budget examination, and failure as an intergovernmental program manager for the multiplicity of programs resulting from Johnson's quest for the Great Society (Fisher, 1975, p. 58; see also Davis & Ripley, 1967, pp. 749–769). However, during this entire period, for better or worse, it functioned increasingly as the instrument of executive budget and policy making power. It was at its height during the 1940s when it still functioned much like it did at it inception, but as noted below, the BOB was to undergo serious modification.

One way to conceptualize budgetary control of the type wielded by the BOB and all central executive budget control agencies in government is to envision it as a tool that operationalizes fiscal values. These fiscal values are basically economizing values. As identified by Appleby, they include fiscal sense and fiscal coordination: "Fiscal sense and fiscal coordination are certainly values. The budgeting organization is designed to give representation in institutional interaction and decision-making to this set of values" (Appleby, 1980, p. 134). Appleby argued that the budget function is inherently and preponderantly negative because it is against program expenditure and expansion. He explained that this is proper because program agencies and pressure groups are so extensive that there is no danger the values they represent will be overlooked or smothered by budgeteers.

Appleby conceded that a budget control agency cannot always be negative, for there are ways to save money by spending money, and the controllers have to be on the lookout for these occasions. In the main, however, budget control agencies will be the aggressors, pushing to cut, trim and squeeze spending. Spending agencies, on the other hand, will temper their requests by their judgment of what is wise and practical, and what policy makers and the budget bureau will accept. The executive budget bureau is at the center of this struggle, and yet it is removed from direct contact with many if not most of the political pressures of the politics of budgeting due to its insulation within the executive and the fact that it works for only one political party (the President's) at a time. Consequently, the budget bureau should act as a counterweight to ensure that economizing fiscal values are entered into the decision making calculus.

Wildavsky (1964) characterized the budget process as a competition between the "spenders" and the "cutters" with BOB and other budget control agencies being the primary cutters in government. However, they are not the only cutters, as the appropriations committees play this role also. When they do, however, it is often to cut one program to add funding to another. With respect to spenders, program agencies are expected to advocate for their programs and constituencies both within and outside of government. Members of Congress and the President, as elected officials, generally are expected to play the role of spending advocate most of the time. Otherwise, how would they get reelected? In a democracy, what do people send their elected officials to Washington, DC to do? The answer in large part is to solve or resolve problems, and to do so requires spending money from the perspective of the clients of governments and many stakeholders in the economy. Consequently, according to Wildavsky, the spenders vastly outnumber the cutters and this creates a pro-spending bias in government. An understanding of the roles, duties and expectations related to the players in the budget process is critical to comprehension of budgetary competition for power. It is also important in attempting to understand the proper functioning of budget control agencies.

Two problems haunted the Bureau of the Budget from its inception. First, if the whole structure is dedicated to economizing, then the role of a budget bureau is preempted. With its role preempted, the usefulness of a budget bureau diminishes. This relationship was true of the period from 1921 until the 1930s, and again during the Eisenhower years, from 1952 to

1960. Secondly, when a budget bureau is very good at what it does, it tends to get drawn into the role of general staff advisor, or even roles that would seem to be more political and belonging to, for example, the White House political staff. This was probably true of the Bureau of the Budget (renamed the Office of Management and Budget or OMB in 1969–1970) during the Johnson and Nixon years from 1964 through 1972, and certainly true during the Presidency of Ronald Reagan in the 1980s.

When a budget bureau serves as political advisor, representation of fiscal values may tend to get suppressed by the necessity of offering political alternatives. In 1967, a BOB self-study described the Bureau's nonpolitical professionalism as an Achilles heel. It acknowledged that although BOB budget examiners were generally knowledgeable about their programs, they did not have a political point of view. This had been seen as the height of professional behavior.[12] The examiners merely presented alternatives, and politicians would make the right decision, a view dating back into public administration history, at least as far as the Prussian general staff model. In fact, some have argued that the entire executive budget process in the United States is based on the Prussian system, with BOB serving the function of the General Staff (Sundelson, 1935, p.1). The concept of neutral competence and apolitical service was typified by the folklore the BOB perpetuated about itself. As Berman noted, "BOB officials often told the story that if a Martian army marched on the Capitol, everyone in Washington would flee to the hills, except the Budget Bureau staff, which would stay behind and prepare for an orderly transition in government" (Berman, 1979, p. x).

Neutral competence was the keystone of the philosophy of the BOB. The Bureau stood ready to serve the master with fidelity and expertise. However, in the late 1960s this was not enough. Fisher concluded that what the BOB lacked in the mid-1960s was political judgment that would allow it to operate in the policy process. Rather, it became a "captive" of "abstract theories of organization, doctrinaire views of management, and impractical claims of constitutional power" (Fisher, 1975, p. 58).

The Bureau was reorganized in 1969–1970 to add political acumen by layering political appointees over the career staff (Reorganization Plan No. 2 of 1970). After 1970, the Bureau's representation of fiscal values would be filtered through nets of political values before they reached the President, a change that may have improved the advice the Bureau could give the President but probably changed the character of neutral competence. Gone was the pure budget technician, lost in part to the era of policy analysis where the ability to detail the consequences of alternative budget decisions was the task at hand. What happened to merely cutting the budget through close examination and intimate knowledge of the program? A reorientation of the role of BOB/OMB probably was a necessary change.

Schick observes that the Bureau as a simple representative of fiscal values could serve every President with, "...fidelity, but it could effectively serve only a caretaker President. It could not be quick or responsive enough for an activist President who wants to keep tight hold over program initiatives" (Schick, 1970, p. 532). As the functions and responsibilities of the Presidency changed, so did the role of the budget bureau.

In the last two decades, the politicization of OMB has accelerated. The President's budget is viewed as an opening bid and the budget estimates in it are often obviously optimistic—sometimes OMB argues that the numbers will come true if Congress adopts the President's program as is, and quickly, at that. Thus, the Budget of the United States has become a marketing tool. In recent years, the Citizen's Guide to the Federal Budget demonstrates this. Much of the FY2002 Guide is devoted to charts and graphs showing how high taxes are. However, chart 2.5: Revenues as a percent of GDP in the FY 2001 Citizen's Guide to the Federal Budget—the last Clinton budget—shows that the United States is second lowest country of a group of Western European nations and Japan in percent of GDP drawn off by taxes for federal government purposes. This chart has disappeared in the FY2002 Guide. The new chart 2.5 shows Constant Dollar Revenue Growth and is preceded by chart 2.4 which is entitled Individual Income Taxes as a Share of GDP at Record High, spiking above the WWII years in 1999. The Clinton chart 2.5 was the wrong message for the Bush administration.

Highly respected budgetary scholar Jesse Burkhead judged the institution of the executive budgetary system in the United States to be a revolutionary change. Burkhead argued: "The installation of a budget system is implicit recognition that a government has positive responsibilities to perform and that it intends to perform them" (Burkhead, 1959, pp. 28–29). To do this would require reorganizing administrative authority in the executive branch, said Burkhead, and an increase in publicly organized economic power relative to privately organized economic power. Thus, the institution of executive budgetary systems in the United States clashed with customary doctrine about public versus private economic responsibility, but more importantly it was fundamentally at odds with the basic organizing precepts of the founding fathers. The budget system after 1921 and particularly in the post-World War II years through 1970 was an integrating system that allowed positive movement toward goals by relatively small groups of participants within the political system. It had to work this way, or it could not be an efficient system. But this kind of organizational efficiency appears to run counter to the Constitutional doctrines of separation of powers and checks and balances. Consequently, Burkhead suggested that not only would the practices of government have to be altered before budget systems could be installed and operated, but their development and installation alone were "revolutionary" in the context of American society.

Burkhead concluded that although budget systems need not be synonymous with an increase in governmental activities (budget systems can be used for retrenchment), their installation is synonymous with a clarification of responsibility in government. It is this framework of goal accomplishment that makes the installation of an executive budget system so important. The role of the Bureau of the Budget was crucial to this system.

SUBSTANTIVE BUDGET REFORM IN THE EXECUTIVE BRANCH

The search for substantive reforms of the budget must also be seen as part of the process shaping a positive executive budget system. Historically, American budgeting systems have represented object-of-expenditure classifications, with each classification given a budget line; hence the name line item. Typical line-item objects include such expenditure items as personnel, travel, rent, office supplies, and the other supporting expenses necessary to support personnel, which was the single largest item in most government budgets until well into the twentieth century. Line-item budgets focus on the inputs bought to perform the functions of government. Line-item budgeting is easy to adapt to different situations, and easily understood. It is appropriate for governments faced with simple, stable tasks. It does not, however, lend itself easily to analysis of what government is doing (i.e., activities) or accomplishing (i.e., results). Neither does it relate the costs of objects purchased with the services performed or the resources consumed.

As government became more complex and its responsibilities for providing a better quality of life increased, the need for budget systems that measured government impact became more apparent. Moreover, as the study of administration, both in the private and public sector, progressed, the budget function fell under increased scrutiny as a managerial tool to help the executive manage government or a large corporation. The trend accelerated in the 1930s and the 1940s with the theories promulgated by the scientific management movement in the private sector and the recognition that public administration was a career field for practitioners as well as an academic discipline with its own theory base for the public sector. During World War II, many of the nation's leading academics moved to Washington to assist the administrative process and took their experiences back to their universities.

During this period, the budget power was expanding and defining its responsibilities. The taxing power was used during World War II to prevent inflation through extremely high marginal rates, a signal that the federal government was committed to maintaining stability in the economy and not just in purchasing inputs. This trend was accelerated with the passage of the Full Employment Act of 1946, which in essence made the President manager of the economy. This legislation entrusted the President with the responsibility to maintain full employment levels. Later, in the 1960s, the President was routinely held responsible for managing supply and demand, using macroeconomic tools to keep the economy on a stable course with neither too much inflation nor too much unemployment. In 1964, on the advice of macroeconomic advisors, the President asked for and received a tax cut that actually resulted in increased revenues (Pierce, 1971). This may have marked the high-water mark of macroeconomic management, inasmuch as the economy has since then become increasingly less tractable and more open to external shocks like oil price increases.

Currently, perhaps the major budgetary responsibility incumbent upon a President is managing the economy, irrespective of the extent of his power to actually affect the economy. On the expenditure side, the passage of the Social Security Act in 1935 and its subsequent expansion has led to commitments for future spending both to its beneficiaries and to other programs developed to transfer income directly to those whose standard of living is below an acceptable minimum level. Health care for seniors and for the poor has become an important and expensive part of this package. These programs commit the government to future expenditures that are not controllable without changing benefits in a separate legislative process. A majority of the annual budget (65% in FY2002) has become uncontrollable (The Budget of the United States Government, 1976, p. 49; see also Blechman, Gramlick, & Hartman, 1975, pp. 193–207; Gist, 1977, p. 342). Periodically the solvency of the social security systems is threatened, studied, and extended, usually by increasing the tax rate or base. Current spending patterns and the aging of the population once again are putting the program in jeopardy as the number of workers to beneficiaries declines. It appears that maintenance of the social security and health care system will test the ingenuity of policymakers over the next two decades.

With the responsibility for macroeconomic management and the growth of social welfare spending, the budget power has been subjected to a revolutionary refocusing of responsibility. This process began with the New Deal programs, was intensified with World War II, and was confirmed by the period of the Great Society. Defense, one of the standard categories of the American budget, gained impetus with the dawning of the atomic age. No longer was defense spending a matter of protecting borders or projecting forces to battlegrounds thousands of miles from the United States. When Russia became an atomic power in the 1950s and then succeeded in beating the United States into space in the same decade, the defense establishment was confronted with defending America from atomic war. Budgeting for this mission required an adjustment so vast as to be revolutionary. Moreover, the problem of defense budgeting was exacerbated by the traditional separations between the armed services, where rivalries sometimes produced duplication and waste. The budgeting apparatus was also used to maintain and improve military services (Gross, 1969, pp.113–137). What budget system could best embrace these enhanced roles for government and cope with these developing strains?

The most current sequence of budget reform starts with performance budgeting and concludes with top-down or fixed ceiling budgeting and the line item veto. Performance budgeting (Burkhead, 1959, Chs. 6–7, and pp. 133–181) connects inputs to outputs.[13] It is typified by indicators of cost per unit of work accomplished and focuses on the activities of government. Its history reaches back to the Taft Commission of 1912, its implementation in the Department of Agriculture in 1934 and the Tennessee Valley Authority in the later 1930s, as well as its being strongly recommended by the Hoover Commission in 1949. In 1949, Congress required that the budget estimates of the Department of Defense be presented in performance categories. Performance budgeting was a manager's budget tool. During the 1950s under the leadership of Bureau of the Budget Director Maurice Stans and others, executive budgeting was transformed somewhat radically through the institution of performance measures into budgets. Many of the measures had already been in use for decades as proxies that facilitated and simplified negotiations between the Executive and Congress. However, in this first wave of performance budgeting (the second wave would hit in the 1990s) great effort was exerted to develop measures of performance and relate these to appropriations and spending. In fact, many of the measures developed in this era did not measure performance. Instead, because it was easier (and perhaps the only approach possible), workload data were used in place of real measures of performance. Still, budgeting in this era moved far from the simple line-item formats of the past. Formulae and ratios between proposed spending and actions were integrated into the Executive budget along with explanations of what the measures demonstrated and how they related to justifications for additional resources.

The emphasis of budget reform shifted in the early 1960s to what was termed "program budgeting." Program budgeting (Mosher, 1954; see Novick, 1969) was and is a variation of or evolution from performance budgeting in which information is collected by program categories, without much of the detail of the performance-budget construction,[14] and then categories of spending are tied to specific objectives to be achieved. Activities are grouped by department, agency, and then by mission objective and sometimes by function and projected out for a five-year period. Program budgeting was experimented with in the Department of Agriculture in the early 1960s as reported by Wildavsky and Hammond (Wildavsky & Hammond,

1962) and later adopted throughout the entire federal government through Executive Order by President Lyndon Johnson in 1966.

The Programming, Planning, Budgeting System (PPBS) (Lee & Johnson, 1983, ch. 5; see also Hinricks &Taylor, 1969; Merewitz & Sosnick, 1972; Schick, 1966, pp. 243–258; 1973, pp.146–156) is a thorough planning system that incorporates many sets of plans and documentation and draws upon various disciplines, including economics, planning, cybernetics, and administration, to set goals and then derive benefit/cost ratios that indicate which goal to choose. Budgeting becomes a simple matter of costing out the goal chosen. In theory, program budgets were supposed to provide the Executive and Congress information on what the federal government was spending for particular categories, e.g., health, education, public safety, etc. across all departments and agencies. Program budgets may best be understood as matrices with program categories on one axis and departments on the other. Thus, in the fully articulated program budget Congress could determine how much was spent on health or education in total to promote deliberation over whether this was enough, too much or too little. Regrettably, although Executives prepared their program budgets and related spending to objectives, like so many Executive reforms, Congress largely ignored what it was presented, preferring to stick with the traditional appropriations framework for analysis and enactment of the budget. Why was this the case? Perhaps program budgets presented too much information to be used and understood by Congress. Or as likely, Congress perceived that program budgeting would reduce the power of members of appropriations committees because the budget in this format was determined too much by formula, thus decreasing the political spending discretion of Congress (Jones & Bixler, 1992). Although this experiment was suspended by President Richard Nixon in 1969 for political reasons, and because it was perceived as paper-heavy and consuming too much staff time for preparation and analysis, the system continues to be used in the Department of Defense (DOD), in part because DOD purchases substantial long-lived capital assets and program budgeting requires long-range planning as its first component, i.e., it suits the needs of the Defense Department. This system reached its zenith under Robert McNamara in the Department of Defense in the early 1960s and, as noted, still is used by DOD today.

Nixon instituted a new Executive reform—Management by Objectives (MBO), and with it came budgeting by objectives. Just as PPBS grew to some extent out of performance budgeting, budgeting by objectives retained two key components of PPBS—the focus on objectives related to spending and the multi-year framework. MBO is a work-planning system, equivalent in some respects to performance budgeting. It was used by the Nixon administration to bring business principles to government. It featured setting program objectives and stressed evaluation of program accomplishments in a contractual process between supervisor and subordinate. Its failure was in large part due to the stigma of the excesses occasioned by Nixon administration (Jun, 1976, pp. 1–45; Rose, 1977, pp. 64–71). It also did not handle large policy questions very well. One administrator complained that the central budget office rejected his budget package and told him the policy question had been settled and they did not want to see any more of those little milestones and numbers. His comment was that the numbers proved the policy probably would not work.

Zero-based budgeting features zero-based analysis, decision packages, and funding at various levels of effort, including levels below the accepted budget base (Pyhrr, 1977, pp. 1–8; Schick, 1978, pp. 177–180).[15] It is a retrenchment-oriented system used in many states and local jurisdictions. Many consider ZBB too small a system to encompass the problems of the modern welfare state, the Social Security system, or even the major elements of economic management. In 1977, President Jimmy Carter mandated its use by all federal departments and agencies. President Reagan ended the brief, paper-heavy experiment with ZBB in 1981.

The reforms noted above were attempted as a result of executive branch initiative. And in the 1980s under Reagan another executive reform crept into the process. It has been termed "top-down" budgeting. This name came as a description of how the Reagan administration initiated the annual budget process through OMB. In essence, departments were told how much they would have to spend, i.e., given their top line. Then it was left to departments to propose what they wanted to spend on under these ceilings. Top-down budgets were stipulated according to the ideological and political priorities of the Reagan administration, e.g., they raised defense spending dramatically while either capping or cutting spending for domestic discretionary budget programs. This approach to budgeting placed OMB in the role of explaining, advocating and even negotiating the President's budget before Congress in a way it had never done before. OMB Director David Stockman would present testimony and then respond to members' questions about spending and deficits using a pocket calculator to estimate the consequences of various alternatives. OMB's forecasts of balanced budgets were heavily criticized by the CBO as too optimistic about the economy and revenue projections. And, in fact, CBO proved to be right as the combination of entitlement program growth, defense spending increases and revenue shortfalls placed the federal budget into unprecedented non-wartime deficit. Stockman himself said that he warned the administration to no avail that its policies would produce, "endless deficits as far as the eye can see" in a memoir written after he left office (Stockman, 1985). As we note, the deficits did not last forever, but it took until the beginning of the twenty-first century to balance the budget and accumulate a surplus.

Finally, a word about the ill-fated Presidential line item veto. It is useful to compare the options for budgetary control in most state governments in the United States to those proposed, enacted and then found to be unconstitutional by the U.S. Supreme Court due to their judgment that the measure violated the Constitutional dictates of separation of powers. It appears to some people, former Presidents Reagan and Bush, Sr. for example, that there could be lower deficits if the U.S. president had an item veto. This measure would permit the president to reduce or cut entirely the budgets of specific programs (line items) within the appropriation legislation sent for signature into law after passage by Congress. We must remember that the U.S. Constitution provides all authority to appropriate spending to the Congress and none to the president—thus the phrase "Congress proposes, the President disposes."

There is reason to doubt the assertion that the line item veto would reduce or control government spending significantly. First, there is a very important distinction between the right to veto a particular item of appropriation and the right to let it stand but to diminish it. On the basis of U.S. state government experience, where many governors have line item veto authority, it might be assumed that, because an item veto increases the power of a governor, it does decrease spending. But, we must remember that governors are elected officials just as are legislators. They have high priority programs they want to spend more on if they can. More refined analysis shows that in actual use in states that have it, the item veto is generally weak in limiting overall government spending. However, the line item veto is very strong when it comes to reducing the spending and activity of specific programs and agencies. Thus, the device is employed as another weapon in the politics of the budgetary process and its application is often likely to be related intimately to political ideology and the tradeoffs of power politics.

At the federal level, it is inevitable that a president would wish to spend more or less on some programs than the amounts appropriated by the Congress. He could use the item veto as leverage with Congress to persuade party leaders to cut and redistribute spending more in line with his priorities before the budget ever reached his desk. He could play "hard ball" with Congress—he could say "you either cut or add money to this or that program or I will whack out the things you love most, the 'pork' for congressional constituents."

There appear to be some other potential problems with the item veto. For example, state legislators appear in some instances to vote higher appropriations and to exercise less spending discipline because they can then pass on the heat and responsibility for cutting budgets to the governor. This allows legislators to take credit for attempting to meet the needs of the people while the governor catches the wrath, amplified by the media, of those who perceive that they have been wrongly penalized by item reductions or eliminations. This is useful for legislators in particular when one political party controls the legislature and the governor is from the opposing party.

In state legislatures, the avoidance of fiscal responsibility is not desirable. Moreover, if one is an advocate of increased spending to meet many worthy and unmet needs that cry out for attention, then it is a shame to do nothing about it. Faced with an item veto, what is a logical response? One possibility to increase the chances of success would be to form a larger instead of a smaller coalition. In the past, a coalition just large enough to get expenditures through was needed. Under a new system with an item veto of the type some propose for the United States, a two-thirds majority would be required. Consequently, elected officials would have to promise even more spending to more potential program beneficiaries. Thus, it is quite possible that an item veto would be met with what is described previously, termed "logrolls" in the budgetary parlance of the United States. Larger bargaining coalitions would produce much higher spending. Both democratic government and spending control would be furthered more by giving the central government power to require budgets to be voted up or down as a whole. This, in our view, is more likely to force spending accountability and control onto elected officials than narrower measures such as the item veto.

SUBSTANTIVE BUDGET REFORM IN CONGRESS

Perhaps the reason why no single and dominant budget system has sprung forth and remained intact on the executive side is that Congress reasserted its power in the period after 1970 beginning with the passage of the Congressional Budget and Impoundment Control Act of 1974.[16] This Act sought to correct certain abuses of presidential impoundment powers, but more important, it also sought to reorganize the Congressional budget power to give Congress a better chance at full partnership in budgeting for the modern welfare state. If the Full Employment Act of 1946 gave the presidency responsibility for managing the economy, the Congressional Budget and Impoundment Act of 1974 extended the same opportunity to Congress. In addition, Congress equipped itself with more analytic power by creating the Congressional Budget Office, comprising a neutral staff imbued with a sense of high calling and professionalism similar to that found in the Bureau of the Budget of the 1940s but in a somewhat more complex fiscal world.

The Congressional Budget Act centralized the budget power in the House and Senate Budget committees. These two committees have the responsibility to develop a target resolution in the spring of each year containing detailed appropriation targets to guide the work of the appropriations committees. The target resolution shows the overall situation, total spending, including the level of spending by function, taxing projections, and the level of surplus or debt forecasted. Then, in September, the budget committees were to shepherd a second resolution through Congress that matched the early planning target to the final appropriation bills. This second resolution process was meant to reconcile bills passed at the end of the process with the budget resolution targets, but it was never quite used that way and was discontinued after 1981. In June of 1981, Congress attached reconciliation instructions to the first resolution and in effect dictated what would be done later that year in appropriations committee work. Through the reconciliation process, the budget committees ask Congress to tell its appropriation, taxing, and authorizing committees (for entitlements) to set spending, taxing, and program levels for entitlements that will bring the appropriations, tax collections and entitlement spending in at the budget resolution number. Points of order are available during the session to enforce this discipline.

The reconciliation instruction of June 1981 marked a turning point in the American budgetary process. For the first time in the history of the United States, the legislature set binding budget targets for taxing, spending, and debt, and thereby had a sense of what the national budget ought to be before it started enacting appropriation bills. At no other time since 1789 had this been done. The budget resolutions of 1976 did provide recommended targets from 1976 to 1980, but it took the passage of the reconciliation bill in 1981 to make these targets binding. After 190 years of titular vesting of the power of the purse in Congress, Congress organized itself to pursue a budget prospectively, rather than adding up the total appropriations and expenditures and calling it a budget.

The 1981 budget was essentially an executive budget, but it was endorsed in Congress only after a bitter struggle. President Reagan won his tax cut victory in the summer, but passage of the other appropriations bills took until late December. By this time, the President in his insistence on reducing domestic expenditures had squandered much of the good will his victory in the summer had provided. In fact, his next budget would be declared dead-on-arrival. In 1982, Congress used its newly developed budget power to develop Congressional budgets basically different from the proposed executive budgets of 1980, the final Carter budget, and again in 1982, the second Reagan budget (Peckman, 1983, p. 19). Congress has exercised its budget power both with and against the executive. Although the power to prepare and submit budgets remains with the executive, and

a formidable power it is, Congress has evolved into a powerful and systematic modifier of budgets. There are some indications that suggest that the
outcome of the Congressional Budget Reform of 1974 has been to give
Congress a tool to systematically increase spending beyond that which the
President has requested over the last 25 years. The difficulty with this measurement is that Presidents Ford, Carter, Reagan, and Bush Sr. either pre-
sided during conservative eras or were more conservative in terms of
spending than was Congress. Then in the last years of the 1990s with a surplus in hand, Congress felt little need to be frugal and consistently and significantly increased appropriation bills over the amounts planned for in
the budget resolution and over the President's budget request. This was
especially true for defense spending.

From 1950 to 1970, Congressional scrutiny of budgets was characterized
by students of budgeting as one of incremental review and marginal adjustments by appropriation committees to whom the other members of Congress deferred. Incremental behavior was rational, according to Aaron
Wildavsky, because in reviewing that in which he or she was most interested, members allowed individual self-interest to protect the public good.
Richard Fenno documented the success of final adoption of appropriations committees' recommendations as 87%. Ira Sharkansky observed that
congressional behaviors could be summarized as the concept of contained
specialization, meaning elite status, specialized expertise, deference to the
acknowledged experts, and conflict management (Fenno, 1966; Sharkansky, 1969; Wildavsky, 1979). These descriptions still hold true: decisions are
still incremental, appropriations committees are still very powerful, and
legislators adopt strategies to contain conflict. But major changes have
occurred; OMB must be seen as a major lobbyist of Congress and Congress
itself has a centralized mechanism to set and drive and enforce budget
goals it may choose with the budget resolution, reconciliation and points
of order based on budget targets. This is a different situation than that
which Wildavsky, Fenno, and Sharkansky described.

Moreover, during the period from 1950 to 1975, enormous changes were
taking place within society, and the composition of the budget reflected it.
Social service expenditures increased dramatically, medical care was added
to social security guarantees and social security itself was given an automatic
cost of living adjustment. Defense expenditures decreased as a share of the
federal budget and along with the rising social service expenditures came
an increased percentage of the budget dedicated to mandatories. With
mandatories and their COLA's came mandatory increases, which in some
years were larger than the discretionary increase.[17] Moreover, the budget
process itself was less satisfactory. Although each appropriation bill was
intensely scrutinized, no one knew what all the appropriations bills would
total until they all had been passed, usually well into the new fiscal year.

Moreover, the bulk of the mandatory expenditures were not reviewed annually and did not fall under the jurisdiction of the appropriation committees. Thus they were often blamed when spending increased, but when it was due to mandatory increases, as it often was, they had little or no control over it. Moreover, as macroeconomic management became more important to the nation, Congress had no apparent forum of its own to make and enforce economic policy through the budget. Thus, the budget process became less and less useful to the realities of managing a modern welfare state. Seizing on the Nixon abuses of the impoundment power to reorganize the budget process and make itself a full partner in the process once more was an outcome not totally anticipated. Some thought that Congress had merely changed the fiscal year in an attempt to give itself more time to process appropriation bills to offset its difficulty in passing them on time. Others saw it as a weighting of the budget power in favor of Congress at the expense of the executive. Although the act does improve congressional potential, it need not be said that it usurps executive prerogatives. There is more than enough budget power for both branches to share. Congress does become a powerful critic, however. It has the power to redevelop the budget when the President's original submission does not match congressional interpretations of the needs of a particular year. The battles over the deficit exemplified this.

THE BATTLE OF THE DEFICIT: 1985–2001

President Reagan's creation of large annual deficits was surprising at first, given that he had campaigned for President in 1980 on a platform that included a call for a balanced federal budget. And once the deficits began to materialize, the administration tried to capitalize on them by proclaiming that they would be cut by more stringent cutting of a bloated federal bureaucracy. Not to be outdone in top-down budgeting, Congress jumped into the fray, attempting to do what Reagan could not, i.e., balance the annual budget. In 1985, after much haranguing and negotiation, a Republican led coalition passed the Gramm-Rudman-Hollings Act (GRH) that set specific future year targets for deficit reduction. GRH II was passed in 1987 to eliminate conflicts over executive-congressional jurisdiction and, notably, to extend the deficit targets that neither Reagan nor Congress could meet. These targets were further extended in the Budget Agreements of 1990 and 1993.

In 1990, President Bush agreed to tax increases despite his "read my lips—no new taxes" campaign promise of 1988. While this may have contributed to his defeat by Bill Clinton in 1992, tax increases had to be part of the overall package to balance the budget, all parties admitted. Entitlement controls also had to be imposed. The 1990 Budget Agreement created the "Pay as you Go" (PAYGO) rules for entitlements that required any increases in entitlement spending to be offset either by new taxes or cuts in other programs. Congress did not always obey these rules, but overall they helped to restrain entitlement growth. The effort to control the deficit culminated in 1997 with passage of the Balanced Budget Act negotiated between a Democratic President and Republican Congress with a goal of balancing the budget by 2002. Fortunately, and due primarily to the robustness of the private economy and the large tax revenues resulting from strong GDP growth and private sector productivity increases in the United States in the 1990s, by 2000 the federal budget was in a surplus position, what some call "balanced." This culminated a fifteen-year effort by both political parties, and by the executive and Congress to increase revenues and curtail federal spending while protecting important entitlement programs including Social Security, Medicare and Medicaid.

Deficits and the National Debt

Thomas Jefferson estimated the costs of the Revolutionary War at $140 million from 1775 to 1783. Bills of credit to help pay for the war were issued both by the states and by Congress from 1775 to 1779. Since they would be honored only if the revolutionaries won, their probable value changed with the fortunes of war and with the economic problems of the new nation. As a practical matter they depreciated rapidly. In 1790 Congress agreed to redeem bills of credit at one fortieth of their face value. Even with this devaluation, it is estimated that the new American government began with a public debt of about $78 million in 1789. Today, this sum seems tiny compared to the current deficit, as does the operating budget of $326,000 in 1788. If all 2001 current revenues could be diverted into paying off the national debt accumulated up to 2001, it would take about 2.5 years; by the same measure, paying off the Revolutionary War debt with the 1778 revenues would have taken 240 years. No wonder the Founding Fathers worried about balanced budgets.

In the matter of debt, nations are not unlike individuals; they go into debt in emergencies, when their usual income sources are inadequate, to make major purchases and to keep promises like sending children to college. For a nation, the comparable events include war, depression, infrastructure building like interstate highways, and social security and medicare programs or other entitlements the nation intends to pay for in good times and bad. Some debt is allowable; a lot of debt is not good. In the United States, most states have statutory or constitutional provisions against a deficit in their operating budget. When their revenues do not meet forecasts in a budget year, they implement routines to decrease the rate of spending, like purchasing and hiring freezes, limits on travel, and the suspension of certain personnel actions that cost money. Some also issue short term debt until the start of the new fiscal year when management efforts prove inadequate. The American federal government is not prohibited from running a deficit, and, in fact, it has done so in emergencies and for most of the twentieth century as a result of wars, both cold and hot, and unfavorable economic conditions.

While the annual deficit or the accumulated debt can be measured in nominal dollars, a better indicator is a measurement against the productive capacity of the country as measured by its gross national product. Figure 1 presents the annual deficit or surplus as a percentage of GNP from 1797 to 1997. When a surplus occurs, the line moves above the zero point, and when a deficit occurs the line moves into minus territory. The sharp spikes below the zero line represent the impacts of World Wars I and II, the War Between the States, the War of 1812, and the increasing costs of the cold war and the Reagan military buildup. While there were periods of surplus, prior to and after the War of 1812, after the War Between the States, and for shorter periods after WWI and WWII, there is no period of surplus with the same amplitude as the deficit spikes after the War Between the States and World Wars I and II.

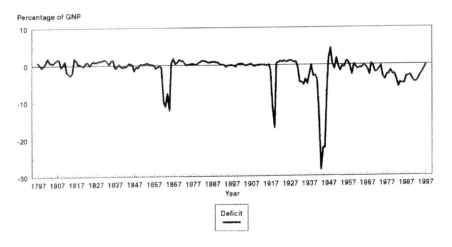

Figure 1.   Annual deficit as a percent of GNP (1797–1997).
Note: Figure 1 and Figure 2 are from the testimony of Paul L. Posner, Director, Budget Issues, GAO, before the House Committee on Ways and Means, June 24, 1998 and may be found in Budget Issues: An Overview of Federal Debt, GAO/T-AIMD-98-221 on pages 15 and 14 respectively.
Source: P. Posner. June 1998. GAO/T-AIMD-98-221.

Throughout its early history, U.S. federal budgets were small and deficits were created by emergencies like wars and depressions. When the emergency had passed, the debt it had caused was generally paid down—but not off. Except for periods of war (when spending for defense increased sharply), depressions or other economic downturns (when receipts fell precipitously), the Federal budget was generally in surplus until the Great Depression of the 1930s and World War II. While still stabilizing the currency and paying down Revolutionary War debt, the United States generated its first deficit in 1792 and there were deficits during the war of 1812, the recession of 1838, the Civil War, the depression of the 1890s and World War I. For the first 60 years as a Nation (through 1849), cumulative budget surpluses and deficits yielded a net surplus of $70 million. The Civil War, along with the Spanish-American War and the depression of the 1890s, resulted in a cumulative deficit totaling just under $1 billion during the 1850–1900 period.

Between 1901 and 1916, the budget hovered very close to balance every year. World War I brought large deficits that totaled $23 billion over the 1917–1919 period. The budget was then in surplus throughout the 1920s. However, the combination of the Great Depression followed by World War II resulted in a long, unbroken string of deficits that were historically unprecedented in magnitude. As a result, Federal debt held by the public mushroomed from less than $3 billion in 1917 to $15.4 billion in 1930 and then to $242 billion by 1946. In relation to the size of the economy, debt held by the public grew from 16% of GDP in 1930 to 114% in 1946.

Figure 2 shows the effect of the accumulation of these deficits. It measures debt held by the public as a share of GNP for the same period. The

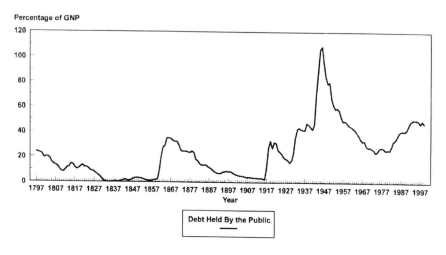

Figure 2.   Debt held by the public as a share of GNP (1797–1997).
Source: Paul Posner, GAO, June, 1998.

good news is old news: around 1830 debt held by the public as a percentage of GNP approaches zero. Obvious paydown periods can be seen after each of the wars cited above, but the trend from 1917 onward was certainly upward. Notice again what a strain WWII was.

Deficits

A deficit results when spending is greater than what is received in revenues for a fiscal year; a surplus results when revenues exceed spending. When spending and revenues are equal, the budget is said to be in balance or balanced. In government, a deficit results when revenues do not equal expenditures at the end of the fiscal year. This is called an operating budget deficit. This deficit must be financed somehow; otherwise suppliers, employees, and others who depend on the commitment of government resources could not be cared for or paid. Usually governments issue debt instruments to pay for the deficit. Some jurisdictions have rainy day funds to provide for emergencies where more revenue is needed than provided by the current year's taxes. States and local governments are often prohibited by law from going into debt for operating budget expenses, but for the American federal government operating budget deficits have been a fact of life. For their part, even though guided by statutes forbidding deficits on operating budgets, state and local governments do not find it easy to come out even at the end of the fiscal year; often they must take draconian actions to cut down expenditures and sometimes they still run short term deficits which are paid for out of the next year's funds; when their resources are not up to the burdens that political choices have imposed on them they may face various conditions of fiscal stress and their ability to finance capital improvements by selling bonds may be impaired as their credit rating falls. Using a separate capital budget for planning and financing capital purchases like parks, highways, and buildings helps state and local governments keep their operating budgets in balance. The federal government does not maintain separate capital and operating budgets.

During much of the nineteenth century, revenues could be raised from customs fees and import duties. This allowed policy makers to raise revenues from external sources while protecting the nation's infant industrial base and pay out benefits internally. This was a relatively easy political choice. This system worked because the federal government's functions were few and favorable geography separated it from foreign entanglements not of its own choosing. As a result, in 1930, federal government outlays totaled 3.3 billion; the budget was in a surplus position (receipts were $4.1 billion) and the total debt held by the public was $15.4 billion. New deal programs led to a doubling of federal expenditures by 1934 ($6.5 billion) and a near triple by 1940 ($9.5 billion). The shock of the second world war almost quadrupled federal outlays by the end of 1942 ($35.1 billion) and that amount more than doubled by the end of 1943 to $78.6 billion. By the end of 1945 federal out-lays were $92.7 billion and the deficit for that year was $47.6 billion. In this year alone, the operating deficit was larger than all the stock of debt prior to the beginning of WWII and the total national debt had reached $235.2 billion. From 1930 through 1996, surpluses occurred in only eight years; in 58 of these 66 years the budget was in a deficit position.

These trends are documented in Table 2. The chart illustrates the growth of deficits and debt. While total debt was small in 1940, its percentage of GDP was high (44.8%) illustrating the cumulative strain of the Great Depression. In 1945 and 1946 the cumulative debt was actually greater than the total GDP for those years; this is some indication of the cost of becoming the arsenal for democracy to the United States during WWII. The year 1943 represents the worst operating deficit year, where the deficit amounted to 31.1% of GDP. This level of effort would never be approached again in this century.

What the years 1980 through 1994 illustrate is the impact of relatively modest annual deficits; at the end of this period debt as a percentage of GDP had grown to just over 50%. When operating deficits are built into the budget year after year, they are referred to as structural deficits. Deficits that occur as a result of emergencies or underperformance in the economy so that revenues are less than predicted and unemployment and/or welfare expenditures more may be called frictional deficits. Despite efforts to contain annual deficits, the last two decades of this century must be seen as a period of structural deficits.

As the responsibility of the federal government grew and the size and complexity of the budget increased and deficits became an annual event attention changed from the dollar amount of the deficit to measurement of the deficit as a percentage of gross domestic product. The theory was that the size of the deficit only mattered in relation to the ability of the country to carry the debt load.

Table 2.   Deficits and the Growth of Debt

Year	Outlay $ in billions	Deficit $ in billions	Deficit as % GDP	Total debt as % of GDP
1930	$3.3	+$.7	.8%	15.9%
1940	9.5	−2.9	−3.1	44.8
The Impact of WW II				
1941	13.7	−4.9	−4.4	42.9
1942	35.1	−20.5	−14.5	47.8
1943	78.6	−54.6	−31.1	72.8
1944	91.3	−47.6	−23.6	91.6

Table 2. Deficits and the Growth of Debt (Cont.)

Year	Outlay $ in billions	Deficit $ in billions	Deficit as % GDP	Total debt as % of GDP
1945	92.7	–47.6	–22.4	110.9
1946	55.2	–15.9	–7.5	113.8
The Deficit Years				
1980	590.9	–73.8	–2.8	26.8
1981	678.2	–79.0	–2.7	26.5
1982	745.8	–128.0	–4.1	29.5
1983	808.4	–207.8	–6.3	34.1
1984	851.8	–185.4	–5.0	35.2
1985	946.4	–212.3	–5.4	37.8
1986	990.3	–221.2	–5.2	41.2
1987	1003.9	–149.8	–3.4	42.4
1988	1064.1	–155.2	–3.2	42.7
1989	1143.2	–152.5	–2.9	42.3
1990	1252.7	–221.4	–4.0	44.0
1991	1323.4	–269.2	–4.7	47.4
1992	1380.9	–290.4	–4.9	50.6
1993	1408.7	–255.1	–4.1	51.9
1994	1461.9	–203.1	–3.0	50.1
1995	1515.8	–163.9	–2.8	50.1
1996	1560.6	–107.5	–1.4	48.5
1997	1601.0	–21.9	–0.3	46.1
The Surplus Era				
		Surplus	Deficit/GNP	Debt/GNP
1998	1653.0	69.2	0.8	42.9
1990	1703.0	124.4	1.4	39.7
2000	1788.0	236.9	2.4	34.7

Source: Extracted from A Citizen's Guide, FY 1996. Historical Summary, pp 12–14; Financial Report to the Citizens, U.S. Dept. Of Treasury, Receipts, Spending, The Annual Budget Deficit, 1996–2000; Revenues Outlays Deficits, Surplus, Debt held by the Public, Fiscal Years 1962–2000.Congressional Budget Office, Table 4, Appendix F. The Budget and Economic Outlook, FY 2001–2011. Congressional Budget Office, Jan. 31, 2001.

Aaron Wildavsky has argued that one of the legacies of the revolutionary war period was the creation of a balanced budget ideology in the United States that has basically been honored except in times of emergency (Wildavsky, 1988, Ch. 2). The history of the deficit seems to support his argument. Steven Mufson has noted that from 1947 through 1980, both Democrats and Republicans tacitly agreed that the deficit should not exceed 1% of GDP in time of prosperity; in fact, the average for the entire period was less than 1% of GDP (.86%) (Mufson, 1991, p. 6). Thus while actual outcomes resulted in a marginal deficit, the ideology of a balanced budget continued. This profile changed in the 1980s with the election of President Reagan and the combination of the defense buildup, an income tax cut and a recession. Deficits in the early 1980s reached sizes basically unknown since the Second World War, reaching a high of 6.3% of GDP in 1983 and averaging 4.1% from 1980 through 1994. This accumulation of annual deficits caused the national debt to quintuple from 1980 to 1994. The size of the annual deficit and the growth of the debt became powerful political issues that were almost always at center stage from 1981 through 1997. Some observers believed that these issues pre-empted other policy issues and that efforts to contain the annual deficits prevented policy makers from considering other national issues. Some analysts believe this was an intended outcome of the Reagan revolution; if government could not be shrunk directly, then diminishing its revenue capacity would ultimately force the national government to do less. Others suggest that the real villains in this picture were entitlements, the growth in entitlement qualified people, the rising costs of medical care and its reflection in medicare and medicaid costs, and the perceived ownership of a full annual cost of living increase for people in entitlement programs and on public pensions (e.g., social security).

National Debt

Congress has imposed a limit on the amount of gross public debt outstanding. The first limits came in 1917 and were set to help plan during WWI a time of unprecedented debt expansion. Prior to 1917, Congress approved each debt issuance. By setting limits substantially higher than the current amount of debt, Congress avoided having to authorize the expansion of debt piecemeal, with each act of legislation that would have exceeded the current limit. Congress this avoided having to make two major decisions on a piece of legislation: first, is it a good bill in its own right and second, is it worth raising the amount of public debt for, and perhaps third, is it worth creating new debt at this point in time given the current state of the economy? Without some headroom in the debt limit, some legislative enactments might have failed simply because of timing; more debt would be inflationary in a time when further expansion might overheat the economy. Setting debt ceilings also gave the executive branch flexibility to meet its obligations without worrying about the debt limit in addition to the problem at hand, very useful in time of war or depression, or when payment of entitlements enacted in past years come due in the present, but threaten to exceed the current amount of allowable debt. Thus a debt ceiling was both a limit on the amount of debt and an empowerment that allowed a certain flexibility until the ceiling was obtained.

Debt ceilings were raised several times between February 1941 and June 1946, when a ceiling was set at $275 billion. This limit remained in place until August of 1954. The first temporary limit was enacted in 1954, an expansion of $6 billion, to $281 billion. From 1954 to 1996, Congress enacted about 60 permanent and temporary increases to the debt ceiling. The idea of a temporary ceiling is that Congress will be forced to vote soon on the proper level of debt. It also carried with it some hint that debt might be paid down. In various years politicians have used the approach of a debt ceiling limit as an action forcing mechanism—a club to make the other party or other chamber of Congress or other branch of government compromise. The threat of defaulting on part or all of the debt by not approving a new debt ceiling favored the status quo and forced a proponent of action to compromise to get something new enacted that would be agreeable to both sides; otherwise the other party would not agree to vote to extend the debt ceiling. In 1985 such a struggle resulted in a debt ceiling crisis and the Treasury was unable to follow its normal trust fund investment and redemption policies. Instead, to avoid breaching the debt ceiling, it suspended investing certain trust fund receipts and redeemed some trust fund securities earlier than normal to pay fund benefits. Congress subsequently provided the Secretary of Treasury with legal authority to use the civil service trust funds to avoid exceeding the debt.

An extended political clash of wills between the Congressional Republicans and a Democratic President in 1995–6 again put the debt ceiling in jeopardy. Neither side was willing to compromise and each bet the other would capitulate under the threat of exceeding the debt limit. However, using the tools provided subsequent to 1985, Treasury Secretary Robert Rubin was able to maneuver adroitly around the debt limit. The Republicans basically lost their bet; President Clinton was not forced to settle for fear of exceeding the debt limit and much of the onus for the extended budget battle fell on the Republicans when it was finally all over in April of 1996, seven months into the new fiscal year. As had the Treasury in 1985, Secretary Rubin took action in 1995–6 to avoid defaulting on the debt. Asked to evaluate these actions, GAO concluded that they were in accordance with statutory authority provided by the Congress and the administrative policies and procedures established by Treasury. Moreover, GAO said: "These actions helped the government to avoid default on its obligations and to stay within the debt ceiling." GAO added that after the crisis had passed the Treasury was able to restore the proper amounts to all the accounts from which it had borrowed.

This era (1985–2001) has been characterized by the battle against the deficit. The surpluses of 1998 to 2001, the biggest surpluses in history in 2000 and 2001, the $5.1 trillion surplus estimated from 2000 to 2010, and the tax cut of 2001 seemed to indicate that this battle had been won. However, with any victory comes new dilemmas. The era of the beginning of the millennium has witnessed strong disagreement over what to do with the surplus. Democrats leaned toward increasing domestic and some defense spending and paying off the cumulative national debt. Republicans favored higher defense spending increases, large tax cuts and debt reduction as well. Both parties claimed a desire to protect Social Security from attack by the opposing party. Neither Congress nor President Clinton was willing to compromise much in deliberation over the 2001 budget, leaving tougher negotiation until after the general election in November 2000. Republicans continued to hold a majority in the House in 2001 and the Senate was evenly split at 50–50 for the first time in history as a result of the election. The Republicans elected a president from their party and counted on the vice-president to break any tie votes in the Senate. Early in the year, one of the Republican Senators defected to the Democrats, thus they became the majority party in the Senate and the policy apparatus was split, with the Republicans holding the House and the Presidency, but not the Senate.

Decisions about the disposition of the deficit would continue to be fought over in the early 2000s. President George W. Bush proposed a sweeping tax cut that Congress pared down and debated at length before passing. CBO reduced its projected surplus estimates through 2010 in early 2001, leaving many to wonder how much tax reduction the nation could afford. The slowing of the economy caused the Federal Reserve Board to cut interest rates and the tax cut was portrayed as a complimentary measure to insure continued economic growth. Even so, the tax cut, a flat economy, rising medical care costs and the impact on the social security trust fund of the coming retirement of the baby boom generation raised the specter of deficit politics in the fall of 2001, as both parties promised not to touch the Social Security fund surpluses, knowing full well that if they had to, they would.

Procedurally, top-down budgeting reigns in both the executive and Congress. With Congress this is the result of the authority given to the Budget Committees in the 1974 Budget Act. Budget Resolutions (BR) carry multi-year targets for revenues, spending, and debt or surplus, and government borrowing authority. The BR thus sets the ceilings that appropriations and other committees use to formulate their revenue and spending actions. Moreover, our impression is that the budget resolution has become a force to be reckoned with after the budget battles of the 1990s, especially after the Balanced Budget Agreement of 1997, where the Republicans in Congress forced the President to agree to a path to a balanced budget over a five-year time horizon. In the 1980s the BR was seen as a nice thing to do, but without any real authority, something that was important in the spring, but something that vanished in the summer. This appears to have changed. On the executive side, Presidents since Reagan have continued to employ a top-down or fixed ceiling approach enforced through OMB. Gone are the days when spending proposals made by departments and agencies and negotiated with the BOB/OMB created the base of the President's budget request to Congress, a base which Congress only slightly modified. Now top-down guidance comes first and Congress can and does act as a powerful modifier to the President's proposals. Moreover, OMB itself is heavily involved in the budget process at all stages in Congress. In the summer of 2001, in a bill covering OMB's own budget, Republicans from the President's own party, on the House Appropriations Committee stuck in a clause that said no money could be used for the salary of a budget office worker who "prepared what Congressional officials considered too-detailed instructions to appropriations committees" (Schlesinger, 2001, p. 1). This was later removed in the Senate.

Currently, the federal budget apparatus uses an amalgamation of many of the techniques analyzed above. Line-item budgeting is an underlying theme, with elements from other budget systems adopted to suit individual agency preferences. However, remnants of program budgeting (the Department of Defense continues to use PPBS), budgeting by objectives and even the ceilings of ZBB remain. And with passage of the Government Performance and Results Act of 1993, in conjunction with the Chief Financial Officer Act of 1990 (CFO Act), federal budgeting embraced a new phase of performance budgeting, using an approach that seems to be an amalgamation of the initiative of the 1950s combined with the ethic of strategic planning. One of the clear trends is toward multi-year budgets directed by both the President and Congress. Some requests for authorization are moving toward annual review in an effort to reduce the number of uncontrollable accounts, while planning appears to be moving toward multi-year consideration. Inevitably, as the Congress and President attempt to grapple with the question of what to do with the budget surplus and how to maintain the solvency of entitlement programs as they face the challenge of an aging populace, multi-year and longer-term budgeting perspectives must be employed.

Federal budgets dominated by the macro problems of inflation and unemployment, and by huge deficits or surpluses, have forced the budgetary system to adopt a crisis posture at the top, while the more mundane agency-level routines of budgeting are carried out by using managerial budgeting systems with no guiding theory. What we learn from this experience is that theories are sometimes replaced by events and that no one system is appropriate for all events, but consideration must be given to the use of some elements of several systems. It is also useful to reflect that the modern welfare state provides a vast array of services and is held responsible for societal welfare. Some budget systems simply do not lend themselves to these responsibilities. From this perspective, zero-based budgeting and management by objectives would seem to be less useful as national budgeting systems, but the top-line spending constraint embedded in both the processes used by the Executive and Congress remain a critical part of the budget process.

CONCLUSIONS

Many dysfunctions still exist within the budgetary process (Caiden, 1982, pp. 516–523; Comptroller General of the United States, 1981). From 1962 to 1981, 85% of the appropriations bills for federal agencies were passed after the beginning of the fiscal year. Passage of the Congressional Budget Act of 1974 reduced this percentage to 65 but has not eliminated the problem. It still disrupts agency workload planning cycles, especially those involving new programs. Critics have suggested that the budget is made on an installment plan, emphasizing continuing resolutions in Congress and deferrals and rescissions from the Oval Office.

The Gramm-Rudman-Hollings Act of 1985 and subsequent deficit control measures further complicated budget choice even as it simplified choices. By linking deficit reduction to across-the-board cuts, it struck at the heart of the budget decision: selective choice. Moreover, Gramm-Rudman-Hollings with its annual allowable deficit targets encouraged gimmicks to meet the annual target, such as optimistic revenue estimates, understated outlay totals, and expense shifting (e.g., DOD paydays) to fit outlay totals within a targeted year. While GRH has long since been replaced, the history and practice of budget gimmickry remains alive and well.

Other dysfunctions include the constant temptation to use off-budget spending, the growth of tax expenditures, and the impact of interest expenditures caused by the growth of the national debt. Although substantial amounts of the debt were paid off from 1998 through 2001, it is unclear how much more will be paid down subsequent to the tax cut of 2001. Interest still will have to be paid on what is left. There is also a constant traffic in supplemental appropriations for various purposes—emergencies, economic stimulus, and defense and foreign policy matters unanticipated in the annual budget process. In 2001, mandatory expenditures consumed about 65% of the budget, thanks largely to entitlement programs, and interest on the national debt. As a practical matter, these, with defense procurement contracts, and civil service salaries, make about

90% of the budget uncontrollable in any particular year. The same factors indicate that for each annual increment, a high percentage of the increase will be uncontrollable. Thus, Congress's choice of alternatives is limited, or guided, by its previous choices.

So long as social welfare spending and defense appropriations comprise so large a portion of the budget, it will remain relatively intractable. In defense, expenditures escalate as systems become more complex and more expensive than originally calculated. In social welfare, expenditures have to be made when people qualify. Definitions of the point at which people may fend for themselves may shift somewhat, but the basic policy is unlikely to be changed. The basic commitment to a Social Security system that provides for a dignified and healthy retirement should remain intact. All of these factors only compound the budget problem. The struggle over defense and social welfare programs may seem grim and repetitious, but the stakes are high and the outcome worth the struggle. The social security program alone provided income that kept about half of the nation's senior citizens above the poverty level in 2001.

What else is there to observe in 200 years of budget history? Budgeting began in this country as a legislative enterprise. The people exercised the power of the purse through elected representatives. Effective representation of demands was emphasized over the needs of executive efficiency. Our experience with a prominent executive budget power is relatively limited. In periods of extreme crisis, the legislature has tended to cede power to the executive and reclaim it after the crisis has passed. Although there is a good deal of conflict in the budget process, there is also a good deal of reconciliation and adaptation.

The United States was a country born poor. There were no crown jewels, no colonies to exploit. As a consequence of the Revolutionary War, the currency was a wreck and the colonists owed a substantial debt. Alexander Hamilton's efforts have long been recognized for paying down the debt and stabilizing the currency, in effect, putting the country on a sound, but not rich, fiscal footing. This uncertain fiscal history may have been the start of the balanced budget ethic which dominates so much of American budgetary discussion and practice. A country born poor, or just out of debt, must live within its means. How this has turned out is interesting. Aaron Wildavsky compared American National budgets to their European counterparts. He found that U.S. budgets have been more consistently balanced and that per capita revenue and expenditure ratios consistently lower than that of our European counterparts. What could explain these differences? Wildavsky suggests it comes about as a social legacy rising out of the revolutionary period.

Wildavsky observes that the winning side Revolutionary America was composed of three groups. The first, the *social hierarchs*, wanted to replace the king with a native variety better suited to colonial conditions. The second were *emerging market men* who wanted to control their own commerce. The third were *egalitarian Republicans*—a legacy of the continental Republicans. They stressed small, egalitarian and voluntary association. What allowed these three groups to coexist, create, and operate a successful government was agreement on a balanced budget at low levels of expenditure, except in wartime. Wildavsky suggests that there was no formal declaration of this agreement, nor was it done on a single day. However, this agreement lasted for 150 years until a new understanding was forged in the 1960s. The social hierarchs would have preferred a stronger and more splendid central government, and the higher taxes and spending that went with it. But the emerging market men would have had to pay, thus they preferred a smaller government, except where taxing and spending provided direct aid. Together this coalition led to spending on internal improvements, like railroads, canals, and harbors. However, it was the egalitarian Republicans who did not believe that government spending was good for the common man, meaning the small property-holder and/or skilled artisan. They suggested that unless the scope of government spending was limited, groups of these common men would withdraw their consent to the union. Limiting, not expanding, government was their aim.

Out of these three strains came the impetus for a balanced budget at low levels of taxing and spending. Egalitarian Republicans were able to place limits on central government. Market men won the opportunity to seek economic growth with government subsidy, but the extent of this was limited by an unwillingness to raise revenues. The social hierarchs obtained a larger role for collective concerns provided they were able to convince the others to raise revenue. Wildavsky suggests that no group got all it wanted, but all got something. The Jacksonian belief that equality of opportunity would lead to equality of outcome helped cement this outcome observed Wildavsky. The result has been an ethic of a balanced budget at comparatively low levels of taxing and spending. Moreover, what is balanced in this equation, according to Wildavsky, is not only the budget, but also the social orders and their supporting viewpoints that helped found the country.

Of the men and eras surveyed, Alexander Hamilton seems to have been uniquely placed. Budget history has tended to give more prominence to Charles Dawes, the first Director of the Bureau of the Budget, thanks to the importance of the Budget and Accounting Act of 1921. We feel Hamilton was a far more important figure on the budget stage. It is clear that at some time during the mid-twentieth century the budget power assumed burdens that made it different in kind from anything that had gone before. The coming together of responsibilities for social welfare, macroeconomic management, and defense strategies precipitated the modification that strengthened executive power in the process. No convenient date appears to mark this change, but it probably occurred somewhere between 1946 and 1964. Still, Congress retains the power of the purse and is increasingly able in matters of budget analysis and action, and its decentralized and disconnected budget review and enactment process is no longer so disorganized.

The most important function the federal budget has at this juncture in history is the pursuit of economic stability, what this chapter has called macroeconomic management. It is a goal that the federal government attempts to achieve by making minuscule shifts in the federal budget to stimulate contraction or expansion of the economy. Such a goal seems outside the ability of any single nation to achieve through fiscal policy. At this juncture in history, monetary policy seems to dominate. Prospectively, honoring the commitments made in social security legislation and the expectations of its current and future beneficiaries seems to be going to take increasingly creative policymaking.

The long sweep of history teaches us that techniques of budgeting are not as important as the purposes for which the money is spent. The process itself is a resilient and flexible procedure able to accommodate changing conditions. Part of the genius of the American character resides in its impulse to find a better way, but not to depart radically from tried and tested methods. Social engineers, rationalists, and autocrats might have done better, but experience with the budget process leaves us with a demonstration that representative government works. Government of the people, by the people, and for the people is a strong and durable form of government.

NOTES

1.   The best recognized biography on Pitt is Rose (1911a). See also Rose (1911b, 1912).

2.   For an excellent biography of Hamilton, see Miller (1959). For a summary of Hamilton's thought on executive leadership, see Caldwell (1944, pp. 71–89).

3.   Hamilton's program was outlined in four reports: *Reports on the Public Credit*, January 14, 1790, and December 13, 1790; *The Report on a National Bank*, December 14, 1790; and *The Report on Manufactures*, submitted to Congress, December 5, 1791.

4.   There were fifteen appropriations bills passed between the founding of the Federal government and May 8, 1792. A listing of these may be found at 3 Annals 1258–1259. From 1789 to 1792, the United States had a surplus of $21,762 on revenues of $11,017,460. (3 Annals: 1,259) During this period, general appropriations grew steadily from $639,000 in 1789 to $1,059,222 in 1792, and ranged from a high of $2,849,194 for payment of interest on the national debt in 1790 for 1792 to a low of $548 for sundry objects in 1790. Protection of the frontier was a growing expense: $643,500 in 1792, not included in the general appropriation. In 1791, Congress appropriated $10,000 for a lighthouse; in 1792, $2,553 was appropriated for a grammar school. Of the $11 million raised to the end of 1792, more than $6.3

million was applied to the debt, either interest or principal. It is clear that these were still transitional years for the federal budget.

5.   Fisher notes that lump sum appropriations are especially noticeable during periods of war and national depression, when the crisis is great and requirements uncertain. At these times, the Congress tends to delegate power (Fisher, 1975, p. 61).

6.   The description in this section is summarized from Browne (1949) and Wilmerding (1943).

7.   This position was supported by both academics and public administrators. Notable among the former were Smithies, *The Budgetary Process in the United States* (1955, p. 53); and White in his four-volume history of the federal government, notably, *The Jeffersonians* (1951, pp. 68–69); *The Jacksonians* (1954, pp. 77–78); and *The Republican Era* (1958, p.) 97. The bureaucrats who argued this included two budget bureau directors, Maurice Stans and Percival Brundage; see Fisher (1975, pp. 269–270). Fisher describes the growth of executive budget power as a steady accretion manifest in numerous statutes, financial panics, wars, "...a splintering of congressional controls," and demands from the private sector for economy and efficiency.

8.   This commission report was submitted to Congress on June 27, 1912. See also Taft's message, *Economy and Efficiency in the Government Service* (January 27, 1912).

9.   Burkhead (1959, p. 15) suggests that the interest of the business community in reform was the crucial element in this mixture. Business expected lower taxes. To understand other variables at work, see also Schick (1966, pp. 242–258).

10.   Burkhead suggests the primary motive of Congress in passing the budget act was to reduce taxes, not to improve executive leadership.

11.   53 STAT 1423, Executive Order 8248: 4 Fed. Reg. 3864. For an expansion on this theme and perspective on the expansion of the role of the BOB, see Pearson (1943, p. 126) and Smith (1941, p. 106). Pearson and Smith provide in depth descriptions of the Budget Bureau. Smith was Director of the Bureau in this period. Both authors make a strong case for the "neutral competence" of BOB staff. For a later assessment of this neutral competence, see, for example, Heclo (1975, pp. 45–72).

12.   For a description of OMB at work in the 1960s, see Davis and Ripley (1967, pp. 749–769). Perhaps it was the BOB leaders who failed to make political shifts; or it may have been that the problems they faced were intractable relative to their power and domain.

13.   The literature on these budget reforms is voluminous. The citations listed here are intended as an introduction to the subject. For performance budgeting, see Burkhead (1959, Ch. 67, also pp. 133–181).

14.   On program budgeting, see Mosher (1954). See also Novick (1969).

15.   See also U.S. Senate, Subcommittee on Intergovernmental Relations, Compendium of Materials on Zero-Base Budgeting in the States (1977).

16.   Perhaps the most comprehensive coverage of the Congressional Budget and Impoundment Control Act is Schick (1980b). For a description of reconciliation, see Schick (1982a).

17.   COLA is the acronym for cost of living adjustment.

CHAPTER III

THE STRUCTURE AND PROCESS OF BUDGETING

INTRODUCTION

This chapter extends the analysis of budget preparation and enactment process presented in chapter one to better explain what is an overly complex process so that it may be more easily understood. The chapter describes in detail the basic stages of budgeting with emphasis on the politics and strategy imbedded in the process.[1] The primary focus of this chapter is on the federal government, but state and local practices are noted when they differ greatly from federal patterns.

Generally, the executive branch agency in charge of coordinating the budget issues a memo to start the budget process. Detailed instructions are sent to all agencies about how to prepare a budget. Then agencies prepare budgets. For discretionary accounts, budgets focus on price increases, workload changes and desired new efforts. Each agency has an internal budget process to build the budget it will present to the executive and the legislature. After all its decisions have been made, the final agency budget is sent to the central budget office where it is reviewed. This usually results in decreases for many program requests. Hearings or meetings may be held with the agency to discuss budget issues, review problems and perhaps to hear appeals over items that have been reduced. The final budget then is combined with other agency budgets. Revenue structures are reviewed and the need for new taxes is assessed. The final budget sent to the legislature will normally include summarized data about all agency budgets and any new taxes or tax increases.

The budget package is then sent to the legislature. Here it is referred to committees where it is reviewed. Hearings are held with executive agencies, budget bureau representatives, experts on the economy and with other interested parties affected by the agency budget. Committees review and revise budgets. At the U.S. federal level a Budget Committee is charged with overseeing the passage of a general budget plan to set targets for total spending and for the detailed appropriation bills that will come later in the session. The Appropriations Committees in the House and the Senate and their staffs are responsible for creating these appropriation bills. Once these have been written and the dollars set for each account ("marked up"), they are reported out of committee and sent to the floor of each chamber for debate and passage. When each chamber has passed a bill, a conference committee is created to resolve the differences in the bills. Their report is then taken back to each chamber and voted on. Once this conference committee is approved, it is sent to the executive for signature or veto. In some jurisdictions, an item veto is available. The budget is then executed as it was enacted.

THE FISCAL YEAR BUDGET CYCLE

While it is easy to erect a linear model of the budget cycle from preparation through execution, in reality these budget cycles overlap in annual budget systems. For example, at the federal level, in the Spring, a budget officer will be executing the current year budget and preparing to testify on the budget just submitted to Congress, beginning to construct the budget for following year and may be responding to audits and reviews of past budgets from Congressional and executive branch sources.

The budget cycle provides a set framework allowing for regular review of policy and program. Budget cycles are based on a fiscal year calendar. The federal budget fiscal year runs from October first of each year through September 30 of the following year. The fiscal year is referred to by the date of the year in which it ends. Thus, a fiscal year beginning in October 2002 and ending in September 2003 is called FY 2003. Until the Congressional Budget Act of 1974, the federal government operated on a July 1 to June 30 fiscal year, as do all states except Alabama, Michigan, New York, and Texas.

To understand the complexity of the overlapping budget cycles, each of which lasts for a period of from 2-1/2 to 3-1/2 years (depending on whether one counts the audit year as part of the cycle), we will review the process from the variety of perspectives that must be managed simultaneously in federal government budgeting. For example, any time from April to August of 1998 agencies planned and prepared their FY 2000 budget that was submitted to OMB in the fall of 1998 and delivered to Congress by the President in February 1999. In August and September 1998 managers completed execution of the FY 1998 budget. They also provided information to Congress in support of their FY 1999 budget, which was in the final stages of Congressional review. At the same time they may have been defending their decisions on their FY 1997 budget in the audit process. With the development of future budget year requirements, a budget administrator may have five or more fiscal years to keep straight.

While some or most of this is done in different offices, decisions made about almost any of these budgets can influence all budgets. If a spending proposal is accepted by Congress—or Congress adds a special interest item that is not fully funded—in the current appropriation bill, (for FY2001), there may be associated overhead or supporting expenses that need to be inserted in the FY 2002 budget before it goes to OMB for review. In addition, a program under executed (not fully spending its appropriation) in FY 1998 may lose funding for FY 1999 or FY 2000 and perhaps even face cancellation. Consequently, in order to discharge their legal responsibilities and to be effective players in the budget process, participants have to know where they are in the budget process and what is expected of them and what others are doing in the budget process. While state and local budgets are less complicated, the same principles apply, but generally fewer offices have to do the work, so the burden of calculation is almost the same.

While most jurisdictions in the United States use an annual fiscal year, nineteen states use a biennial budget process (Kearns, 1994). Annual budget processes are designed to lead to a review and passage of a budget each year. Biennial processes lead to a new budget every two years and have a definite on and off cycle: executive branch preparation and legislative review occur every other year as opposed to an annual cycle where the executive is always building a budget and the legislature is always reviewing a budget.

Biennial budgeting is basically a state form of budgeting, although some local governments use it, but states are not entirely consistent in the way they implement biennial processes. Some states adopt two one-year budgets while others adopt a single budget for the two-year period. In the former case, any surplus would go back to the general fund at the end of the first fiscal year; in the latter case any surplus could be used in the next fiscal year. As a practical matter, the routines of budget execution (apportionments, allotments, quarterly and annual reconciliation of accounts) make execution of biennial budgets similar to execution of annual budgets. There is a substantial difference in the preparation cycle, however, since the second year of the biennium is a full year farther into the future than it would be in an annual budget system. This means that it is more difficult for administrators to predict changes that will occur in their programs in the second year. It also means the system must have procedures to cope with emergency situations. These range from calling special sessions of the legislature, to empowering a legislative committee to meet in the off-session to react to changing financial conditions and perhaps provide agencies with some extra funds to meet unanticipated events, to granting power to the Governor to manage state spending to cope with economic changes.

Since annual budget systems are seen as more flexible, the major trend in the twentieth century has been for states to adopt annual budget systems. In 1940, forty-four of the 48 states had biennial budget systems; only four had annual legislative sessions and consequently annual budgets (New Jersey, New York, Rhode Island, South Carolina). Kearns (1994) found that annual and biennial formats each had proponents among state budget officials. Some preferred the biennial pattern because they believed that budget preparation costs and budget expenditures were lower and that more opportunity existed for long range planning and legislative deliberation and program evaluation and oversight. Others favored the annual pattern, citing increased time for legislative consideration of the budget, increased accuracy of revenue estimates, the reduced power of the executive branch (since the legislature remains in session and can continue its routine oversight responsibilities or react to emergencies), and the elimination of many special sessions and supplemental appropriations. Kearns submits that some part of the move toward annual budgets results from the desire of state officials to be able to respond more quickly to federal policy adjustments in order to be eligible for more federal funds.

Dialogue over a biennial budget for the federal government has centered on the improvement in Congressional oversight that would result under a biennial pattern when Congress had the off year to review and consider how well the programs it had legislated were working. Proponents also believe that biennial budgeting would decrease the tremendous annual effort now devoted to developing and implementing the annual budget in both the executive and legislative branches of government. For example, in 1996, Senator Pete Domenici (1996) commented that each year the Army Corps of Engineers prepares and submits to the Appropriations Committee an eight-volume budget justification amounting to more than 2005 pages for a budget that is equal to two tenths of 1% of the federal budget. Domenici noted that the Senate debates and votes on the same issue three or four times a year "...once on the budget resolution, again on the authorization bill and a few amendments on the floor and again on the appropriations bill." Domenici observed that by his calculation the Senate devoted roughly 40% of its time to debating budget resolutions, reconciliation and appropriations bills in 1993. Domenici suggested an annual budget is not really necessary for most budget functions, since he considered that only 4% of discretionary spending required annual funding because of unpredictable funding patterns. Finally Domenici argued that Congress does not spend enough time reviewing federal government operations and, furthermore, oversight within the annual framework is not as good as it should be, nor as good as it could be in a biennial cycle (Domenici, 1996).

While the federal budget runs on an annual cycle, it is complicated by the use of five year "outyear" projections for the annual congressional Budget Resolution under the responsibilities of the House and Senate Budget Committees, involving multiple year spending, revenue, borrowing, debt or surplus projections and other estimates. Both Congress and the executive branch use multiple year budget estimates in internal documents in budget preparation, during testimony before appropriators and as required by statutes governing the budget process. The Budget Resolution established by the Budget Reform Act of 1974 requires a display of revenue and spending levels for a multiple year period; this has usually meant five years, although Congress is free to choose the time period to agree with policy goals. For example the FY 1996 Budget Resolution used a seven-year forecast to illustrate how a balanced budget would be achieved by 2002. The Senate Armed Services Committee has required a biennial budget presentation by the Department of Defense since 1987, while the Defense Department uses a five to six-year financial planning horizon in its internal budget process and a five to ten-year time horizon in its planning processes. Thus budget makers must know not only what step in the process they are dealing with, but also what fiscal year. Years beyond the immediate budget request year are called "outyears," and while they are as good as estimators can do, they are commonly acknowledged not to be as accurate as the numbers in the budget year. Figures in these years are said to be "not of budget quality." This is substantially different from biennial budgets that legislate detailed appropriations for all accounts for the second year of the biennium; the numbers for both years are necessarily of budget quality.

Executive Preparation

At the federal level, the process of formulating the executive budget begins in the spring of each year, at least nine months before the budget is transmitted to Congress and at least 18 months before the fiscal year begins. The executive process begins with the setting of Presidential priorities and the transmission of those priorities to the agencies. While much of this is done verbally, there is an instructional circular to be followed (OMB A-11) and OMB also holds a Spring preview with agencies to identify issues and get agreement on directions. This preview usually occurs in the middle of the agency budget process, after agencies have begun their budget process, but long before that process is finished. Agencies build their budgets from the late winter (March) through the summer. In late July or early

August, OMB does a midsummer budget review whose focus is mainly on the state of the economy and how changes in economic conditions impact the budget under consideration in Congress and could impact budgets being constructed. Agency budgets are submitted to OMB for review in the fall, a dialog ensues, and decisions are made and incorporated into the final draft of the budget document. The process concludes with fine-tuning in December and January and the assembling, printing and transmission of the Presidential budget document to Congress on the first Monday in February. Subsequently the President may also submit budget amendments to Congress. President Carter submitted two comprehensive budget amendments in 1980 due to quickly changing economic conditions; President Clinton submitted a substantial amendment to his budget in 1995 to match Congressional pursuit of a balanced budget by 2002. The first year of a new Presidency is also likely to see substantial budget amendments sent to Congress. Once an appropriation bill has been passed, the President may still seek to amend it through a supplemental appropriation bill, basically adjusting the appropriation during the execution phase. Supplemental bills are commonly used for emergencies like disaster relief.

Prior to the start of the budget process, the President establishes general budget and fiscal policy guidelines. These may result from conversations with close advisors such as the Director of the Office and Management and Budget (OMB), the Secretary of Treasury, the Chairman of the Council of Economic Advisors and key cabinet officials from important agencies in which the President has taken a strong substantive interest, like defense or health. Recent elections also influence priorities; a newly elected President may have made promises he wishes to implement or an off-year election result may lead him to modify his program. These guidelines are transmitted to departments and agencies by the Office of Management and Budget. During the budget preparation process, OMB works with agencies to convert the President's general policies into specific policy directions and planning levels, both for the budget year and for the following four years. Specific instructions and forms are circulated to the agencies as part of the general budget circular controlling budget preparation (A-11). In general, Presidents seem to be most active in budget making in the first years of their terms; in later years they pay less attention to solving problems through the budget process, to some extent because so much of the budget is "fixed" or mandated by law and made up of entitlements supported by powerful clientele groups.

Once general guidelines have been set, agencies begin their internal budgeting process. Taking cues from the President's priorities, agency heads set priorities for their own agencies. Agencies concern themselves with personnel staffing levels and supporting expenses. They may ask about the number and type of personnel required, labor-saving efficiencies, program intensity levels and clientele demands. Budget change requests are then built in terms of additions or reductions to the ongoing staffing levels and supporting expenses. Agencies whose responsibility is to distribute money directly to citizens through pension funds, health care payments, subsidies, contracts, insurance programs, grants, loans, and credit programs will often ask the same kinds of questions, but the focus will be on efficient processing of checks and vouchers and auditing to ensure that those who are eligible receive what is due them and that those who attempt to defraud the system are thwarted. In these cases the administrative budget to disburse funds may be only a small percentage of the total funds disbursed or collected. For example the basic administrative expenses (salaries and supporting expenses) for the Farmer's Home Administration were only 3% outlays in 1985 (Meyers, 1994, p. 23).[2] In this process, budget makers are heavily dependent upon calculations and numerical relationships that have worked in the past. For example, tax collection agencies carefully monitor their cost to collect a dollar of taxes; welfare agencies tend to focus on number of clients served and fraudulent claims; libraries focus on circulation figures and police and fire protection agencies may keep response times as key budget indicators. Reviewers tend to monitor the same vital statistics, both within the agencies and in the legislature. Recent trends in performance measurement at all levels of government have enhanced this trend as decision makers try to assess what indicators will enable them to understand how to get the most for what is spent (Gore, 1995, p. 5).[3]

Agency budget processes usually combine *centralized* and *decentralized* elements. The budget process proceeds on a top down basis for some decisions and a bottom up basis for others. For some decisions, a high degree of centralization may be necessary, particularly in large procurement programs that are unique or experimental; top down processes usually dominate jurisdictions under fiscal stress, where the chief executive and the budget bureau will issue guidance about how much agencies can ask for or how much budgets might have to be reduced or what kinds of programs might have a higher priority. For other decisions, input from field level commands and district and regional offices are more appropriate; these might include decisions on local maintenance items or local service or clientele needs. Philosophically, the argument is sometimes made that decentralizing the budget process spreads the organization's goals and objectives throughout the organization and helps train future managers by making them sensitive to cost tradeoffs and forcing a more general view of organizational goals. Most agencies use a mix of centralized and decentralized patterns. The basic questions that need to be answered remain focused on what needs to be done, by whom and for how much. These questions should be focused on the level of organization that can best answer them.

Agencies have their own budget process calendar, generally beginning with the guidelines of the chief executive and proceeding through a series of steps culminating in the agency budget. In the federal government this process takes place from spring through early fall, when the budget is presented to OMB. Agencies typically build their budgets using numbers from the current budget as their base and modify it by what they see needs to be done as revealed by problems in current administration or, perhaps, by direction from clients or clientele groups important to the agency. Once the budget has been pulled together, it goes through various review phases to perfect it and to integrate and co-ordinate one program with another. In major agencies, the internal budget process typically involves a series of hearings, budget presentations, reviews and appeals at several levels before the final agency budget is ready to be transmitted to OMB.

In Exhibit 1 there is a neatly packaged summary of the agency budget process from the Department of Education. Exhibit 2 illustrates the complexity of the Department of Navy's internal review process.

EXHIBIT 1
Budget Formulation within the
U. S. Department of Education

Preparation of the budget begins in the Department of Education during May, when the Secretary sends a letter to the Senior Officers kicking off the process. This is roughly 1–1/2 years before the beginning of the fiscal year in question. The agencies begin to make their plans, set their priorities, and develop their budget requests, which are submitted to OMB, usually in early September.

After the Secretary's transmittal of the budget, OMB examiners will schedule hearings or informal discussions to obtain a better understanding of our request and to allow the Department to defend it. By late November or December, OMB examiners have made their recommendations to the Director of OMB, and decisions on budget levels are made.

Once final decisions are reached, the Department begins preparation of materials to be included in the printed President's budget and special analyses that explain and justify the budget. These documents include appropriations language; technical financing schedules; narrative explanations of the President's requests and policies; and special exhibits for such items as research and development activities, Federal credit programs, civil rights activities, and tax expenditures that aid education.

Current law states that the President must transmit the budget to the Congress after the first Monday in January but not later than the first Monday in February.

Source: U.S. Department of Education, Budget Home Page, Stage One: Formulation.

EXHIBIT 2
Tentative Department of Navy Budget Review Calendar

Control Numbers Issued to Budget Submitting Offices	May 15
Budgets Submitted to Navy Budget Office	June 30–July 10
Analyst Review	July 1–July 29
Mark Distribution	July 31–August 8
Appeals on marks	August 6–August 13
Major Issue Meetings	August 12–August 20
Briefings to Senior Navy Leadership	August 24–August 31

(The budget is briefed up through increasingly higher levels of command, both civilian and military, beginning with the Deputy Secretaries of Navy and concluding with the Chief of Naval Operations, the Commandant of the Marine Corps and finally the Secretary of the Navy. The budget is 'perfected' at each step.)

Final control numbers issued	September 1
Budget Submission to the Office of Secretary of Defense/OMB	September 15

Source: Adapted from Department of Navy Budget Guidance 98-1, April 16, 1998. Local offices may start the budget process before May 15 in order to have their submissions to those offices charged with formal submission of a portion of the budget. For example, the budget office for the Pacific Fleet consolidates and submits budgets for a number of smaller units. A "mark" is usually a cut in the requested number, although a few may be increased. After the budget is submitted to the Office of Secretary of Defense, there is another process of analyst review, hearings, marks, and appeals that takes place.

While budgeting is taking place deep within the agency on matters so mundane as the need for one additional worker or the correct cost ratio of office supplies to workers, there is also a continuous exchange of information, evaluation and policy decisions at the highest level of government, among the President, the Director of OMB, White House staff, agency heads and secretaries of departments. These decisions result from how the previous budget was treated by Congress, debate over the budget currently in Congress, and projections about the economic outlook that are prepared jointly by the Council of Economic Advisors, OMB and the Treasury Department (see *Analytical Perspectives*, 1996, p. 311).

In the fall, agencies submit their budget requests to OMB where they are reviewed by budget analysts. OMB's review is first done at the staff level where issue papers are prepared in consultation with the agency and recommendations made. A Director's review is held to discuss major issues with the agencies, where the analysts defend their recommendations. The OMB director then makes his decisions and the numbers are passed back to the agencies; if agencies disagree with the passback numbers, they can appeal to the Director and, if not satisfied, to the President. Large agencies may have teams of budget analysts assigned to them responsible for different functional areas. In smaller governments, one analyst may handle several agencies. Usually budget analysts are in close touch with their agency and its programs throughout the year on matters of budget execution as well as budget preparation. A large part of their job entails understanding the agency program and its budget needs. The analyst tries to help shape the agency budget before it gets to OMB to enhance programs the President desires or the analyst thinks are in line with Presidential priorities. Both in execution and preparation, the budget analyst is a communicator of policy during the year. This ongoing dialogue is beneficial to both parties since it allows the agency to inform the OMB analyst early in the process of problem areas and both sides can work to shape the areas of disagreement and agreement.

Many issues are solved at the analyst level in concert with the budget office in the agency. Other issues are not so easily solved and may go to higher levels between OMB and the agency. Unresolved issues of major significance may require the involvement of the President and White House officials as well as the Director of OMB and the relevant department Secretary. At these later stages, the large agencies are expected to solve their own problems; they usually have a short list of items they can appeal and when they appeal they usually are required to have a solution within their own agency budget; usually they cannot look to anyone to suddenly find extra money in another agency to solve a problem for them. When an agency gets less than it wants at this stage in the process, it does not mean that the issue is closed. Most agencies have strong linkages to Congress, to their authorizing and appropriating committees and may be willing to allow the President's people to make changes they estimate may be restored by Congress. Moreover, the perspective of the Department Secretary is not necessarily the same as that of the lower level program administrator who may have firm believers in his program on the appropriation committees.

As the process begins to move into its final stages in December and January, it is not unusual to have budget proposals leaked to the press as trial balloons. Most of these trial balloons are quickly exploded, as opponents in Congress speak out directly against them and lobbyists orchestrate letter writing and faxing campaigns to illustrate the disruption that would occur in a program if the hypothetical solution proposed in the leaked communiqué were adopted as policy. While it is wise not to put too much credence in these early December budget solutions, a large part of budgeting does involve consensus solutions, and such agreement is only gained by justifying early and often what is about to happen. Later in January leaks should be taken more seriously as "anonymous sources" representing administration officials, congressional aides and lobbyists speak to the media "on the condition of anonymity" and with the understanding that "some details are still being fine tuned." Congressional leaders may also speak directly to Presidential suggestions, giving signals about what might or might not be acceptable. For example, in January 1997, a story quoted anonymous sources as saying that President Clinton wanted to restore about $16 billion to welfare programs that had been changed in the summer of 1996. Senate Majority Leader Trent Lott (AP, 1997, p. 5) was quoted in the same story as saying it "...was too soon to start fiddling with welfare." This may or may not dissuade the President from including a modified proposal in the budget. It does, however, indicate the outlines of the coming budget struggle.

Once the policy decisions have been made, the numbers have to be calculated and totaled and the actual budget story written for the budget documents. While much of this is automated and only needs updating, it is still a time-consuming process accomplished in a short time period. Cynics observe that the real end of this process occurs only when the government printing office must have copy to print the final version of the budget that will be presented to Congress. This usually happens late in January and marks the close of the executive budget process for the agencies and OMB. Meyers notes that budget participants want to be seen to be meeting the budget process deadlines, thus they may accept some accounting gimmicks in the budget process in order to do so. Meyers (1994, p. 54) cites an OMB political appointee who remarked that the Spring Preview was a time for serious analytic work with "no gimmicks there," but the December stage was pure gimmicks: "...We'd always do net outlay gimmicks, and we'd boost the income tax receipts and slow down the military's miscellaneous procurement accounts."

The late December time frame gives decision makers one last chance to examine the state of the economy and consider the effects of such economic and technical factors as interest rates, economic growth rates, the rate of inflation, unemployment levels, and the size of beneficiary populations. As the federal budget has become dominated by mandatory payments to people who are entitled to claim benefits, as benefits have been linked to cost of living adjustments, and as deficits increased the national debt and the amount of interest paid on it, seemingly small changes in the numbers that measure the performance of the economy (inflation rate, unemployment rate, GDP growth) can mean large dollar changes in revenue and spending.

Schick (1990b, pp. 164–169) has argued, for example, that the change from a predominance of discretionary spending to mandatory spending in the federal budget has made a substantial difference to OMB and to what budget analysts do. Schick notes the old routines of budgeting that focus on justifying new personnel or a new capital equipment item are not as important as the factors that drive the economy and changes in budget categories related to the economy. Furthermore, while OMB could deny a personnel increase request and tell the agency to absorb the workload or find a labor-saving device, it is far more difficult for OMB to make an unfavorable trend in the economy vanish. Traditionally budget analysis was dominated by calculations about what was actually spent and the relationships between personnel and supporting expenses where historically derived ratios would be applied to the new budget request. With the growth in entitlement programs including Social Security and Medicare and other inflation adjusted programs, the art of budget analysis becomes the craft of forecasting what will happen in the economy over the next three to five years. Past costs are not as relevant as future estimates. Unfortunately, forecasting is imprecise and different forecasters can come to slightly different results which, while differing only slightly in absolute terms, can lead to billions of dollars of difference when applied to the budget and to multiple year baselines.

In general, OMB has been accused of being more optimistic in its economic projections than the Congressional Budget Office. In a study of deficit estimates, CBO was found to be more correct than OMB in 16 out of 20 deficit estimates from 1993–1996, although OMB tended to be more correct in estimating income shares (Budget Newsletter, 3/17/97). OMB has suggested that the reason its estimates are more optimistic than CBO is that they assume a fiscal dividend from the timely adoption of the President's recommendations for the economy as provided by his budget message. Unfortunately, Congress rarely adopts these precisely as submitted and the very makeup of the bicameral legislative system that emphasizes committee work and deliberation and discussion precludes maximizing timeliness. In any case, the point is that small changes in these assumptions can affect budget estimates by billions of dollars. Recognizing the importance of these economic factors, each year the Budget document explains in great detail its economic assumptions (*Analytical Perspectives*, 1996, Ch. 1).

If forecasting for one year is difficult, multi-year estimates are even more complex. These multi-year forecasts are called baselines.[4] Baselines are projections of future spending if existing policies remain unchanged. The Congressional Budget Act of 1974 required OMB to prepare five-year forecasts of a continuation of the existing level of government services. They estimate the receipts, outlays, and deficits that would result from continuing current law through the period covered by the budget. For receipts and mandatory spending, which generally are authorized on a permanent basis, the baseline assumes they continue in the future as required by current law. For discretionary programs, which generally are funded annually, the baseline assumes future funding will be equal to the most recently enacted appropriation, adjusted for inflation. Because most receipts and mandatory programs adjust automatically for inflation, the baseline represents the amount of real resources that would be used by the Government over the period covered by the budget on the basis of laws currently enacted.[5]

OMB provided its first projection in 1974 and CBO in 1976. The two agencies differed on how to treat inflation. From the start CBO's projections assumed all appropriations would keep pace with inflation; OMB however did not adjust discretionary appropriations for inflation. In 1985, this practice became law in the Balanced Budget and Emergency Deficit Control Act (Gramm-Rudman-Hollings), only to be quickly reversed with the amendment to GRH in 1987 to allow baseline calculations for discretionary appropriations to be adjusted to keep pace with inflation. Subsequently adjustments were made to refine the inflation adjustment index. After 1990, personal services were adjusted by the employment cost index and non-personnel spending by the GNP fixed-weight price index.

Baseline forecasts are useful for several reasons. They warn of future problems for individual tax and spending programs or for Government fiscal policy as a whole. They provide a starting point for formulating and evaluating the President's budget. A baseline may be used as a "policy-neutral" benchmark against which the President's budget and alternative proposals can be compared and the magnitude of proposed changes assessed. Additionally, the Budget Enforcement Act of 1990 requires the use of a slightly different sequestration baseline to determine how much to cut and how much to leave in each account if spending limits have been exceeded.[6]

OMB and CBO develop official baselines. In dealing with programs that are related to an index like the cost of living, as are many benefit programs, different estimators may make different predictions about the rate of change. Notwithstanding the official baselines, different players in the budget process may make their own baseline estimates in order to argue for more or less money for a program. The Budget Committees have tinkered with baselines from time to time, adding and subtracting items in the baseline in an effort to conceal increases or decreases in spending or the magnitude of deficit reduction sought (Van De Water IEPPA, p. 242). These are tactical positionings for the annual budget struggle. For example using a baseline that will lead to a higher total in the outyears may make a program seem generously funded, thus supporting a cut in the outyears and perhaps in the present year. Then, too, a reduction in the current year which results in a cut from an inflation indexed baseline may give a program more than it had the previous year, but less than a full inflation adjusted increase.[7]

Schick has termed this phenomenon baseline alchemy and suggested that in the 1980s both parties used baseline alchemy to argue over program incrementalism; some calling real increases cuts (up from the actual amount in the current year but down from the baseline amount) while others used the same numbers to exaggerate the amount of savings made in the budget process by focusing on the amount cut from the baseline, rather than the amount of increase over the current year appropriation. Thus increases could be called cuts and cuts increase, as negotiators positioned themselves to gain support for a particular policy and level of spending. Competing baselines from the executive branch and Congress and the argument over inflation adjustments and what indices to use for what accounts have added further complexity to the budget process. In 1994 the House passed a bill that would have eliminated inflation adjustments for baselines, but the Senate took no action. In 1996 the House inserted in the Budget Resolution Report a sense of the House provision that baseline budgeting was biased against policies that would reduce the projected growth in spending because "such policies are portrayed as spending reductions from an increasing baseline ... [causing] ... Congress to abdicate its constitutional obligation to control the public purse for those programs which are automatically funded" (Report 1997, p. 33). The public has taken ownership of these baselines as they apply to cost of living adjustments in benefit programs and legislators rightly fear adverse electoral consequences when they cut below the cost of living baseline. Thus current policy—and the current policy baseline—is to give a full inflation adjustment in entitlement programs. Irrespective of the confusion different baselines may cause, baselines do indicate where a program is headed and how much it will cost without any policy change; this is particularly valuable information for policy makers in a system like the U.S. federal government where about 65% of the outlays (2001 and 2002) were mandated, with most indexed to inflation as well as impacted by demographically driven increases in caseload and medical costs.

The transmittal of the President's budget to Congress is scheduled in law for the first Monday in February. For FY97, President Clinton's budget comprised six volumes and more than 2100 pages, "...a complex and daunting array of tables and charts which provided both summary overviews and detailed breakouts of federal revenues and spending for the budget year" (Currow et al., 1996). Amendments to it may also be sent Congress at any time until almost the end of the summer, while OMB carefully tracks the progress of the appropriation legislation in order to make the President's preferences known on key issues. While some states resemble the federal government in budget preparation, this pattern is not universal. Clynch and Lauth (1991) suggest that some states may be classified as executive dominant systems like those in California, Illinois and Ohio. In these states the process resembles the federal process: Governors prepare a unified budget to serve as the legislative budget agenda, deny the legislature access to original agency requests and possess strong vetoes. However, in other states, legislative leaders or key committees develop a unified budget that serves as the legislature's budget agenda; these include Florida, Mississippi, Texas and Utah. In these states, the executive budget proposal plays a marginal role. A third group of states mixes the two patterns with the Governor preparing the budget and holding a strong budget power, but allowing the legislature access to agency budget requests.

There is almost no sensible way to encompass the budget practices of the tens of thousands of local governments and special districts (fire, flood, irrigation, recreation),[8] other than to say that they all have a budget process. In the main, local governments have an annual budget process embedded within the laws of the state within which they exist, for local governments are creatures of the state, and how they operate is fixed in the constitution and organic laws of their state. Historically, many local governments relied upon property taxes and balanced operating budgets; as they grew, the demands for service growth were funded by the appreciation of property. This led to a neat equation where additional spending had to be balanced by additional resources or spending was constrained by resources. Without the ability to go into debt on the operating budget, spending discipline was tight, balanced budgets were presented and steps taken during execution (hiring, travel, and procurement freezes) to attempt to avoid overspending if revenues did not come in as predicted. Many jurisdictions maintained "rainy day funds."

The quasi-neatness of this system has declined under the demand for more and different services (for example toward more welfare and social services and away from property protection and development functions) and the increase in intergovernmental revenue flows. Now local governments receive a substantial portion of their revenues from federal and state governments. This has complicated both the budget process and execution for recipient governments. First, they must anticipate what the granting government is going to give and when the funds will arrive. Secondly, some grants are given in the expectation that the subordinate government will gradually assume more of the costs of the program. Ultimately this may impose a burden on the recipient government greater than it anticipated. Moreover, it is not unknown for federal and state governments to simply impose mandates on local units and let them worry about funding the mandates. The intercession of courts to provide certain remedies (e.g., handicapped access guarantees or restrictions on the number of prisoners per cell) has also complicated state and local government budgeting.

In general, the smaller units of government, towns, townships, rural counties, and independent school districts, tend to have a legislatively dominated process where program administrators present budgets to elected boards (see, Sokolow & Honadle, 1984). The budget may be voted on in an annual meeting. Metropolitan counties and cities may have an executive budget process that resembles that of the federal government: budget instructions, budget guidance, strategic planning, agency procedures and hearings, executive review and a budget office charged with assembling the budget document and presenting it to the governing board for approval. Then there is a wide range of situations in the middle, where even very small localities can hire managers to give professional guidance to the budget process and where even relatively large localities under professional management may make imprudent or inappropriately aggressive decisions.

LEGISLATIVE REVIEW

Congress is an important player in the budget process. It considers the President's budget proposals and can approve, modify or reject them. It can change funding levels, add programs not requested by the President and eliminate Presidential favorites. It can make changes in taxes and other receipts that fund government. In the U.S. system of shared powers and checks and balances, Congress should be seen as a powerful player in the budget process with rights and responsibilities of its own, focused on protecting the power of the purse. Fundamentally the power of the purse is given to Congress by Article I of the Constitution. Section 8 provides that Congress shall have the power to provide for common defense and general welfare and Section 9 adds that no money shall be drawn from the Treasury but in consequence of appropriations. Until the passage of the Budget and Accounting Act of 1921 that created the Bureau of the Budget and an organized executive budget process (and the General Accounting Office), Congress tended to deal directly with the agencies. It could be argued that Congress was more important in the budget process than the President. From 1921 to 1974 the executive budget power was clearly ascendant, but the Congressional Budget Act of 1974 increased the strength of Congress by organizing its efforts and improving its information resources. The outcome is that the two branches clearly share the budget power. This division of power makes for a complicated budget process and in times when party control is divided in Congress and between Congress and the White House, the orderliness of the budget process appears to suffer as neither party nor branch of government can force a conclusion entirely favorable to its side and on a timely basis. Another way of looking at this problem is that the rich diversity of the country sometimes manifests itself in an inability to produce budgets on time and to find clear lines of public policy to which all can agree. Reformers who focus simply on the construction of a linear and clean budget process must be cautioned that the process must serve the country it reflects; where there is no clear consensus on policy, it is not useful to expect a clean and simple budget process.

The legislative budget process has a definite beginning, middle, and end. The beginning starts with the receipt of the President's budget and concludes with the passage of a concurrent resolution on the budget. The middle is that period of time usually from April through mid-September when committees review and markup appropriations bills and the House and Senate debate and amend the appropriation bills and pass them. The end occurs when the same bill is passed in each chamber, usually in the form of a vote on a joint conference committee report, and sent to the President and signed. The rules of the Congressional Budget Act of 1974 indicate this should occur before October first of each year, but in most years most appropriations bills are passed late. Thus the end game usually lasts from mid-September until mid-November while participants seek to resolve issues in controversial bills. During this end game, those agencies for which the President has not signed an appropriation bill receive their funding through a temporary, stopgap measure which enables the work of government to continue, called a Continuing Resolution Appropriation (CRA). These will include all appropriations not yet signed and are usually set at the current year's funding level, although Congress has discretion about what level to choose. CRA's may last a day, a week, or a month; there may be only one CRA or as negotiations over budget issues are prolonged, several CRA's might need to be passed. Since most legislators recognize the futility of government shutdowns as an action forcing mechanism, CRA's are usually not controversial, although the President has vetoed CRA's and some non-emergency functions of the federal government have been shut down for short periods of time when the President and Congress were unable to agree on appropriation bills and CRA's.

Upon receiving the President's budget, the first task of Congress is to write a Budget Resolution as required by the Congressional Budget Act of 1974. This Budget Resolution is a Congressional rule and does not go to the President for approval. Each standing committee of the House and the

Senate is required to recommend spending levels and report legislative plans within their jurisdiction to their budget committee. These are called "views and estimates" letters. The House and Senate Budget Committees hold hearings, usually beginning with the Director of OMB and the Secretary of Treasury and the Chairman of the Council of Economic Advisors and continuing with other experts both in and out of government. They draft separate versions of the Budget Resolution and bring them to their chambers for debate, discussion and passage. Differences between the versions passed by each chamber are ironed out in a conference committee and then the consolidated final version is passed by both chambers. The Concurrent Resolution is supposed to be passed by April 15, but it is often late. From 1976 through 1996, Congress has been on time with the Budget Resolution three times (Domenici, 1996, p. 22). In 1985 the budget resolution was 139 days late (Schick, 1990b, p. 174) and in 1990 Congress could not agree on a Budget Resolution and each chamber passed a "deeming" Resolution which was deemed the Budget Resolution and allowed the budget process to go forward. The actual Concurrent Resolution passed the House on October 8 and the Senate on October 9, (179 days late), expanding from $1.23 trillion to $1.5 trillion in the process. Schick (1994, p. 13) notes that the Budget Committees have a hard time attracting support and Budget Resolutions typically squeak through on party-line votes in contrast to appropriations bills that are normally supported by majorities of both parties and are often approved by lopsided majorities.

The Budget Resolution becomes Congress' spending plan. Actual appropriations must still be provided in separate appropriation bills. Tax law and entitlement changes assumed by the Budget Resolution also must be passed in separate vehicles. This is most often done by one or more reconciliation bills, constructed pursuant to reconciliation instructions developed by the Budget Committees and included within the conference report on the Budget Resolution. The FY98 budget resolution set total targets for the years 1998 through 2002 for federal revenues, new budget authority (some budget authority is provided by permanent authority), budget outlays, deficits, public debt, direct loan obligations, and primary loan guarantee commitments. The Budget Resolution also set targets for social security revenues and outlays. The levels on new budget authority, budget outlays, new direct loan obligations and loan guarantee commitments are then subdivided into 20 major functional areas, ranging from national defense, agriculture, energy, natural resources, health, and income security to net interest, allowances and undistributed offsetting receipts. The 1998 Budget Resolution Conference Agreement also displayed these areas in terms of discretionary and mandatory totals; for FY98 about 33% of total spending was classified as discretionary.

As required by sections 302 (1974) and 602 (1990 amendment) of the Congressional Budget Act of 1974, the Joint Statement of the Managers of the Budget Resolution includes a statement of the levels of total budget authority, total budget outlays and for the House only, total entitlement authority, allocated to each Committee. These allocations are divided between mandatory and discretionary totals. For the House, the allocations are broken down by budget function. Most committees have budget authority and outlays in several functional areas; for example, the House Agriculture Committee draws from nine functional areas. The House Appropriations Committee draws from 18 of the functional areas (but not allowances and offsetting receipts) and has almost all of the discretionary new budget authority (98.5%). Section 602 requires the House and Senate Appropriations Committees to allocate their totals among their 13 subcommittees, thus creating a control mechanism which links budget totals to specific spending measures (Schick, 1994, p. 88).

The tasks of the Appropriations subcommittees vary in their jurisdictional reach. In 1995, Curro and Yocom reported that seven major federal organizations fell under the jurisdiction of only one subcommittee. They were the Departments of Commerce, Housing and Urban Development (HUD), Justice, Labor, Treasury, the Veterans Administration and the Environmental Protection Agency. Six others had to deal with two subcommittees. These included Agriculture, Education, Energy, State, Interior, and Transportation. The Department of Defense and the Department of Health and Human Services had to report to five Appropriation subcommittees! This structure poses information coordination problems for both the departments and the subcommittee members. Conversely, while five subcommittees deal with two or fewer agencies, eight have multiple agencies reporting to them, with four of them making decisions on budgetary resources for "a half-dozen or more major federal organizations and literally dozens of subordinate bureaus and independent agencies" (see, Curro & Yocom, 1996, p. 45). Managing information in this setting becomes very complex. Curro and Yokom suggest that this may be a particularly difficult problem for crosscutting initiatives where programs affect different subcommittees or levels of government and could, perhaps, result in more unintended than intended consequences. Later we discuss how GPRA also has to cope with the fact that many federal programs are provided across agency and jurisdictional lines and how this makes it very difficult to measure performance metrics such as efficiency, effectiveness and more global outcome measures. Curro and Yokom note that for the Appropriations Committees, the political tradeoffs that are inevitably made across subcommittee boundaries may lead to a suboptimized mission or function results due to the fragmented nature of the subcommittee missions as lawmakers find it difficult to schedule hearings, pick out the crucial bits of information from a plethora of witnesses and mark up and report out their appropriations bills on time.

The Budget Resolution does give a top down number and discipline to this process. The appropriations bills built by the subcommittees may not exceed the subtotals allocated to them (602b allocations); the amounts distributed to the subcommittees may not exceed the total given to the full committees (602a allocations) and the amounts allocated to the full committees cannot exceed the budget authority and outlay totals in the Budget Resolution. House and Senate procedures differ slightly and the Senate is generally recognized as having a tougher set of enforcement rules (Schick, 1994, p. 88). Schick compares the 602b allocations for subcommittees to a bank account; the allocation endows the account. Whenever a subcommittee produces spending legislation, it is charged against that account. The subcommittee is not permitted to overspend its account; when its account reaches zero, it is out of business for that year (Schick, 1994, p. 91).

The Appropriation Committees' subcommittees write the appropriations bills and they do it in accordance with the dollar allocations they have been given. These 602b allocation numbers (subcommittee allocations) are used by participants in the budget process for scorekeeping. At any point in the floor discussion of an appropriation bill, a point of order may be brought by a member that a committee has exceeded the target number given it. If the point of order is held to be well founded, the bill will have to be modified. In this way the Budget Resolution passes responsibility to the committees who are its experts in substantive areas to build appropriation bills and then holds them accountable by dollar totals for what they have developed. The House and Senate Budget Committees are the principal scorekeepers; they issue reports as the passage of legislation dictates, assisted by the Congressional Budget Office that provides cost estimates for legislation reported out of committees for floor action. The scorekeeping reports help in sustaining or rejecting points of order against bills that might appear to break the Budget Resolution discipline. Since 1990, additional mechanisms have been created to control the budget process in Congress in addition to scorekeeping and points of order. These include spending caps for discretionary appropriations, where defense and nondefense discretionary expenditures have been given a ceiling number beyond which they are not supposed to be able to go, and the reconciliation process and pay as you go provisions (PAYGO) for mandatory expenditures in the Senate. Pay as you go provisions force Congress to find "billpayers" for tax or entitlement changes so that new provisions are paid for by the elimination of old provisions or the creation of a new revenue source. This is a way to keep the effect on the deficit neutral. Setting specific targets for discretionary expenditures capped their growth rates and helped retard the growth of the deficit in the mid-1990s and beyond.

In the 1980s Congress had to solve the dilemma of integrating appropriations, spending authority carried by permanent law (e.g., permanent authorizations provides for entitlement spending and permanent appropriations provide appropriation from past years for the current year), tax policy and the level of deficit. It did this by using the reconciliation provision of the Congressional Budget Act of 1974. By adding reconciliation instructions to a Budget Resolution, Congress instructs specified committees with jurisdiction over entitlement laws to restructure their programs so that the rate of spending will be reduced; thus the Budget Resolution is aimed at the appropriations committees and the reconciliation instructions are aimed at committees committing federal resources through other means.

Reconciliation bills originate from reconciliation instructions developed in the Budget Resolution and are drafted under the aegis of the Budget Committees acting from the guidance of the committees to whom reconciliation instructions were sent. Section 104 of the FY98 Conference Report sent reconciliation instructions to eight standing committees in the Senate asking for a reduction of specified amounts of spending from the programs within their jurisdiction, one revenue reconciliation instruction to reduce taxes, and one pay as you go instruction providing that the Committee on Finance could be a bill payer for a children's health initiative costing not more than $2.3 billion in 1998 if it could reduce other expenditures by a like amount. The pay-as-you-go provision is a Senate practice enforced by a point of order which was extended through the year 2002 by the FY96 budget resolution (H.C.R. 67, 104th Congress Section 202) and reiterated in the FY98 Budget Report (Report: 1997, p. 109).

In the House, reconciliation instructions were issued for two separate reconciliation bills, one for entitlement reform and the other for tax relief. Instructions for the former were given to eight committees for each bill. In general reconciliation instructions direct a committee to report changes in laws within its jurisdiction such that the total level of spending does not exceed a given amount, thereby reducing future spending in that area. Generally, reconciliation instructions indicate the dollar amount to be saved, leaving specific program changes to the particular committee. These may include changing tax laws and fees and various entitlement program changes, including benefit formulas, eligibility requirements and shared cost percentages. The first Clinton budget-tax battle in the summer of 1993 was a reconciliation bill and the major welfare restructuring of 1996 was entitled a reconciliation bill. Reconciliation bills are major bills, but it may be said that they exist outside the normal appropriations process, since they are an attempt to get at programs and funding not reviewed in the normal appropriation process. Conversely, the reconciliation bill may include all of the budget process; in 1990 an omnibus reconciliation bill was passed that included reconciliation directives affecting taxes and deficit reduction, all the appropriations bills and changes in the budget process. This package implemented a summit agreement made between the President and Congress.[9] In 1987, similar events occurred, but these were not normal budget years.

As can be seen, Congress does not pass a budget per se, rather it passes spending authority for specified purposes in Appropriations Acts each year. There are usually 13 Appropriations Acts. They carry *budget authority*, the legal power to incur obligations that will result in immediate or future *outlays*. Outlays are the amounts of money a program is actually expected to spend in a given year. Congress votes budget authority and its staff estimate when the outlay will happen based on historical data. For example, most budget authority for salaries is spent out in the year for which it is voted; however a contract to repair a facility may be let late in the fiscal year and the actual outlay of dollars may occur in the next fiscal year.

Wildavsky (1988, p. 11) indicates this practice of voting budget authority has historical roots dating from when the country was large, infrastructure primitive, and communications slow, and Congress wanted to provide budget authority so that work could be begun and funds obligated through contracts or hiring of personnel and outlays would be paid as the work was completed. Once an obligation is made, the actual payment can occur in the current or the next fiscal year as appropriate. An additional complication is that appropriation bills can create budget authority for the budget year and for future budget years, thus what an agency has to outlay (total obligational authority or TOA) depends not only on the budget for the new fiscal year, but obligational authority that has been passed in previous years to be spent in the new fiscal year.

The House initiates appropriation bills. The Appropriations Committees in each chamber have jurisdiction over the annual appropriations. Traditionally these committees have been divided into subcommittees that hold hearings and review detailed budget materials developed by the agencies under the subcommittee's jurisdiction. While the agency witnesses are most central to the subcommittee deliberation, other witnesses also submit testimony before the subcommittee to support or amend some part of the agency request. James Payne (Meyers, 1994, p. 180) compiled data showing that pro-spending witnesses at appropriations committee hearings outnumbered anti-spending witnesses by 145 to one. While this data was received with few gasps of astonishment, the size of the disparity is astonishing.

The Department of Defense budget is first presented by the Secretary of Defense and the Chairman of the Joint Chiefs of Staff. Then the Secretary of the Navy, the Chief of Naval Operations, and the Commandant of the Marine Corps will appear on the Department of Navy budget. The sequence is much the same for the other military departments. As questions get farther down into the details of the budget, budget officers and program managers from various levels will be called to testify. In addition to hearings, Congressmen and Senators submit written questions to the agencies, and staff spend many hours on the telephone getting answers to questions. Many hours are also spent by analysts and managers within the agency trying to convince the committee staff and members to see issues the way the agency sees them. Each department has a budget office, but it also has legislative liaison offices dedicated to servicing the information needs of Congress.

Congressional staffers work hard to ensure that the right issues get raised at hearings, that answers are given to the right questions and that all sides of an issue are explored. This is important to staff, for later in the session, when they brief their Congressmen on an issue, before mark up or floor action, they can refer to what witnesses said in committee hearings to refresh their memories.

At the beginning of each Congress, committee membership is organized to reflect the outcome of the last election. Committees are divided between majority and minority party members so that the majority party has control and the minority party is well represented, generally in proportion to the seats each party holds in the chamber. Staff for committees and subcommittees is similarly divided. This makeup is critical to the policy making process. Congressional control does change, so completely excluding the minority would not be a good idea, since in most years some votes from the minority side are important to pushing a bill through when some members of the majority party do not believe they can support it. The appropriations committees in particular like to get as much bipartisan agreement over issues as they can in committee in order to come out with a united front on complex budget issues. Indeed, some issues will even be presented as "nonpartisan," as just a matter of good fiscal management. Nonetheless, it is the majority chairman who controls the committee markup process and if worst comes to worst, he can ignore the minority members on some issues. To do so on all issues would mark him as an ineffective chairperson.

After the hearings, the subcommittee marks up the bill by approving or disapproving or modifying numbers and programs, writing instructions or limitations in the appropriation bill language or for the report that will accompany the bill and sends it to the full committee. The full committee then scrutinizes the bill, mostly from a perspective of how this bill will fit in with the other bills in terms of its allocation and the total allocation given the committee. It then reports out the bill to the full chamber. Here the bill is scheduled for debate, amendments are offered and voted up or down, and then the bill is voted on for final passage as amended. The same process ensues in the other chamber. When a bill has passed each chamber, a conference committee will be appointed to resolve the differences between the two bills. The report of the conference committee resolving the differences is taken back to each chamber and voted on. Once this is accomplished, the bill is sent to the President for approval or veto. When appropriation bills are not passed on time, Congress enacts a continuing resolution appropriation (CRA) to fund the affected agencies so that they may continue to administer their programs. CRA's must be presented to the President for approval or veto. In some years a portion or all of the government has been funded by an omnibus continuing resolution for the entire year.

EXHIBIT 3
The Authorization Cycle from the Staff Perspective

(This exhibit, drawn from a conversation with a Senate staff person to the Armed Services Committee, traces the defense authorization bill cycle through bill passage. The comments might not hold for all committees or all years or all staffers, but it does provide an insight into a process that is not normally seen.)

The cycle starts with State of Union address. The first round of hearings are pretty cut and dried; the same witnesses appear before the committee each year: Secretary of Defense, the Chairman of the Joint Chiefs, the Secretaries of Army, Navy Air Force, etc.

The subcommittee hearings are different every year, dependent on issues. Staff work as facilitators, call 5 or 6 people, ask them what they would say if asked certain questions, then decide who to use, form panels of witnesses and script the hearings so that the issues are brought out and both sides aired. Staff suggest to members the questions to ask and what the answers should be so that expected issues get highlighted.

The hearings are valuable. They educate the Senator on a complicated issue; he learns when he gets truth, when he is being hoodwinked. The hearing builds a record to take new action. It is also used for oversight: has the agency done what it was asked to do last year? The hearing involves briefing books, statements by members and witnesses, questions, answers. Most of the time it is hard for staff to get ten minutes with the Senator so the briefing around the hearing is a two hour block of time to go over in detail what the issue is about, educate the Senator so that in mark-up he will remember this issue and be prepared to make a decision on it, or so that he can be put back into the picture by referring to the discussions at the hearing when the issue was first considered.

Markup follows hearings. This is usually in June, by subcommittee and by full committee. The subcommittees are given a number by the committee chairman that they have to attain. Staff sit where witnesses sat, answer questions, give advice. Members decide. It can take from 20 minutes to 4–5 hours. Staff have to agree on markups and what has been decided. Go late on Thursday night, put a report together, put a bill together, proof with members and staff, send to the Government Printing Office and file with Clerk of the Senate. Staff position is that bill is perfect when it comes out of committee and no amendments are needed, but amendments are always offered because Senators have to have a record for re-election.

Staff tries to fend off amendments, instead give them language in the report, or a sense of the Senate resolution, or promise to take it to conference. First couple of days serious amendments are offered, after that it is cats and dogs and the committee/staff tries to kill them. Staff talk around, try to find out who is going to offer an amendment, without giving them any ideas.

Floor debate on our bill is usually scheduled right before August recess; otherwise they would talk about defense issues all fall. Armed Services bill is a bill that will pass, so people try to add amendments. A Senator who gets an amendment accepted has a three-for: he gets to talk about it when it is accepted, again when the bill passes, and when it goes to conference with the House. He can talk about it three different times.

After floor passage, the bill goes to conference with the House. Members tell staff to negotiate a potential solution on 90% of issues, take them back to the member to be blessed. House are specialists, really tough task to prepare Senate member to go head to head with guy who is expert. When you get agreement, the staff member has to speak up and say "we understand the agreement is..." in order to make sure all agree on what has been agreed. Have to build in enough time in the conference process so people can talk, ventilate issues, but not too much time. At this point also the appropriations bill is right on the heels of the authorization bill, like passing notes through a hole in the wall between committees. If authorizers propose too much for a program according to appropriators, authorizers may change the shape of program a little to spend less.

Big ticket issues drive the conference. Most of the other issues (80–90%) can be settled by staff and blessed by members.

Precision in conference committee work is very important. When bill is in the hearing stage in committee, if errors are made they can be fixed on the floor (or if "bad" provisions inserted), floor mistakes can fixed in conference committee work with the House, but the product of the conference becomes law; has to be perfect,

> language has to be clear, precise, correct. To fix it requires passage of another law.
>
> Next the bill and the conference report go back to Senate. The Conference Report is not amendable and must be voted up or down.
>
> My job is to make the Senator look good: I might say "here are the pros and cons; I'll give you a recommendation if you ask me." As the Soviet threat vanished, the tendency to pork and earmarking seems to be increasing.
>
> The product of the Senate Armed Services Committee is the Defense Authorization bill. The sense here is that a getting a bill passed is a very significant achievement, like winning the Superbowl.

Congress also provides spending in "permanent" laws in addition to appropriation acts. These include provision of budget authority for paying interest on the national debt and most entitlement programs, like Social Security and Medicare. These do not need to be re-enacted each year. In fact, although much time and effort are spent on the annual budget process, most of the total spending authority available in any year is provided by permanent laws and budget authority created in previous years to be obligated in the current year. Consequently, most outlays in a year are not controlled through the appropriations process. For FY98, 32.8% of total spending was classified as discretionary. The Appropriations Committees have almost all of the discretionary spending, but they too have spending responsibility that comes from previously enacted budget appropriations. For FY98, $274.4 billion of the House Appropriations Committee total of $791.4 billion had been enacted in previous years (34.6%) and would be spent without any further action by the committee. None of this was entitlement authority.

Almost all taxes and other receipts result from permanent laws. Tax bills are initiated in the House. The House Ways and Means Committee and the Senate Finance Committee have jurisdiction over the tax laws. This includes programs financed by Social Security taxes. These facts make these two committees very powerful. Appropriators have sometimes complained that they get all the blame for budget deficits, yet much of what has caused deficits—the growth of entitlement payments and increased medical costs—is either outside their jurisdiction or outside the purview of the current budget process. Schick (1990a, p. 125) observes that for Congress, budgeting in the 1980s was a frustrating and unpleasant chore: "their misfortune has been to be blamed for both the spending cuts that the budget's dire finances force them to make and for the updrift in total spending that past commitments mandate."

The normal budget process runs from the President's budget to the Budget Resolution to the appropriation bills to the new fiscal year. Some programs (and entitlements) are governed by permanent law, while others must be authorized annually. The Department of Defense has an annual authorization, and it must annually present its programs before a substantive defense committee in each chamber, e.g., the Senate Armed Services Committee, and gain an authorization bill. This bill follows the same process as described above for an appropriations bill: hearings, markup, floor debate, amendment and passage, conference committee, vote on final passage and presentation to the President for approval.

In authorization bills, the issues involve the shape of the program; in Defense questions would be asked about strategic deterrence and nuclear weapons, how conventional forces should be assembled, how many tanks the Army should have, how many ships and what type should be bought and so forth. Authorizers see themselves as giving guidance to the appropriators (mainly the appropriations subcommittees which correspond to their authorization area), whom they see as concerned with issues of timing and pricing in the current year. Authorizers may create new programs and suggest a cap for funding for the program, but they do not provide the funding. In some years, the turmoil of the budget process has left dollars for programs in the appropriations bill that were not in the authorization bill. This is a problem for the agency; the money is appropriated but the program is not authorized. One year, in order to maintain good relationships with the authorizing committees, DOD leadership agreed not to spend about $5 billion that had been appropriated, but not authorized, until the authorizers could find a bill in which to authorize it.

The Budget Committees, the authorizing committees and the Appropriating Committees all look at the Defense function, each from a little bit different perspective, but some critics have argued that two sets of committees should be enough, since they all must basically review the same things to come to the decisions they reach. When the Budget Committees suggest a total for the Defense function, they do not do so by taking last year's budget and adding or subtracting 3%. Rather, they do much the same kind of review that the Appropriation Committees do. When the authorizers review defense programs and make suggestions, they are fully aware that there will be fiscal consequences, just as the appropriators are aware of the program consequences of fiscal decisions. Hence critics suggest that the process could be streamlined; others suggest the oversight role of the authorizing committees is so critical that, if the defense authorizing committees were abolished, the role would be assumed by other committees. Consequently this change is unlikely to happen soon.

The final step in the legislative process occurs when the President signs an appropriation bill into law. The President may veto a bill to which he objects and Congress may override the veto with a 2/3rds majority. As a practical matter, this size of majority is often hard to achieve, thus Presidential vetoes are rarely reversed. Even so, Presidents signal well in advance when and with what they are displeased. A veto is not costless to a President. While the act of vetoing may make him look like a strong leader, it also delays the start of whatever else was about to be funded and the next version of the bill may be only marginally better than the one he vetoed. If the veto is over a small amount in a large appropriation bill, the tendency is for the President to accept the bad with the good; members of Congress have counted upon this in the past and presented the President with "Christmas tree" bills laden with small items for specific purposes in their districts (pork) which might stand no chance of making it through the process on their own merits. Some bills become "veto-proof" due to grand political factors. In the fall of 1995, about to extend the Bosnian peace-keeping operation, President Clinton, unhappy with some additions to the Defense Appropriations bill, practically could not veto the bill for fear of the signals it would send within DOD and internationally to allies involved with the peacekeeping operation. During budget execution, Presidents can try to manage portions of a bill with which they have a problem.

Within a fiscal year, the President has power to withhold spending under certain limited circumstances—to provide for contingencies, to achieve savings made possible through changes in requirements or greater efficiency of operations, or as otherwise specifically provided in law. The Congressional Budget Act of 1974 specifies the procedures that must be followed if funds are withheld. *Deferrals*, which are temporary withholdings, take effect immediately unless overturned by an act of the Congress. In 1995, a total of $17.8 billion in deferrals was reported to Congress and none was overturned. Deferrals control the pace of spending and must be obligated by the end of the fiscal year. On the other hand, rescissions permanently cancel budget authority. They do not take effect unless Congress passes a law agreeing to rescind them. If such a law is not passed within 45 days of continuous session, the withheld funds must be made available for spending. From 1974 through 1993, Congress agreed with about one third of the rescissions proposed by the President, rescinding slightly less than a third of the total funds asked for. Patterns do vary according to the relations between Congress and the President; in 1981, President Reagan asked for 133 rescissions and Congress approved 101, rescinding almost $11 billion of the proposed $15.3 billion (Schick, 1994, p. 176). In other years, Presidents were much less successful (see Budget Concepts, 1996).

Table 1 traces five appropriation bills through the 2000 appropriation process (from the Library of Congress bill tracking web site). This was the last year of the Clinton era and very contentious. Some bills progressed rapidly through Congress. Agriculture was one of the first to be taken up,

Table 1.   Five Appropriations Bills and the Legislative Process

Bill No.	Subcommittee Approval		Committee Approval		House Passage	Senate Passage	Conf. Report	Conf. Report Approval		Public Law
	House	Senate	House	Senate				House	Senate	
Agriculture	5/4/00 (vv)	5/4/00 (vv)	5/10/00 (vv) H. Rept. 106-619	5/9/00 (vv) S. Rept. 106-288	7/11/00 (339–82)	7/20/00 (79–13)	10/6/00 H. Rept. 106-948	10/11/00 (340–75)	10/18/00 (86–8)	P.L. 106-387 10/28/00
H.R. 4461										
S. 2536										
Defense	5/11/00 (vv)	5/17/00 (vv)	5/25/00 (vv) H. Rept. 106-644	5/18/00 (28–0) S. Rept. 106-298	6/7/00 (367–58)	6/13/00 (95–3)	7/17/00 H. Rept. 106-754	7/19/00 (367–58)	7/27/00 (91–9)	P.L. 106-259 8/9/00
H.R. 4576										
S. 2593										
Energy and Water	6/12/00 (vv)	7/13/00 (vv)	6/20/00 9 H. Rept. 106-693	7/18/00 (28–0) S. Rept. 106-395	6/28/00 (407–19)	9/7/00 (93–1)	9/27/00 H. Rept. 106-907	9/28/00 301–118	10/2/00 (57–37)	10/7/00 Presidential Veto 10/11/00 - Overridden by House (315–98)
H.R. 4733										
H.R. 4635										
(See engrossed Senate amendment)										

Table 1.   Five Appropriations Bills and the Legislative Process (Cont.)

Bill No.	Subcommittee Approval		Committee Approval		House Passage	Senate Passage	Conf. Report	Conf. Report Approval		Public Law
	House	Senate	House	Senate				House	Senate	
Energy and Water	—	—	—	—	—	—	10/18/00	10/19/00	10/19/00	P.L. 106-377
Final Bill								(386–24)	(85–8)	10/27/00
H.R. 5483										
H.R. 4635										
Foreign Ops	6/20/00		6/27/00	5/9/00	7/13/00	7/18/00	10/25/00	10/25/00	10/25/00	P.L. 106-429
H.R.4811			(v v)	(v v)	(239–185)	(uc)6 Error! Bookmark not defined.	H.Rept. 106-997	(307–101)	(65–27)	11/6/00
S. 2522			H.Rept. 106-720	S.Rept. 106-291						
VA/HUD	5/23/00	9/13/00	6/7/00	9/13/00	6/21/00	10/12/00	10/18/00	10/19/00	10/19/00	P.L. 106-377
H.R. 5482	(v v)	(v v)	(v v)	(27–1)	(256–169)	(87–8)	H. Rept. 106-988	(386–24)	(85–8)	10/27/00
H.R. 4635			H. Rept. 106-674	S. Rept. 106-410						

Source. Adapted from: Library of Congress Web Page Tracking FY2001 Appropriations Bills Status.
Note. v v = voice vote; uc = unanimous consent. H. Rept or S. Rept = House or Senate Report. P.L. = public law number. H.R. or S. followed by a number is the bill number. These documents may be researched online or in the *Congressional Quarterly.*

in subcommittee in the House and the Senate, but it ended up being passed after the fiscal year had begun. The Defense Appropriation bill, usually one of the last due to its size, was passed and signed early in August. This is very unusual, but both parties had decided to add money to the defense budget. Other bills were much more controversial; five were vetoed for differing reasons. The Energy and Water bill was vetoed, and overridden in the House, but not the Senate. Thus the House had to draft a new Conference Report to gain the President's support as can be seen in the exhibit. The bills for Foreign Operations and Veterans' Administration and HUD were relatively noncontroversial, but nonetheless were passed after the fiscal year had begun.

In 2000, it took 21 Continuing Resolution Appropriations (CRA) before all appropriations bills were passed. The President vetoed three bills, Energy and Water, Legislative Branch, and Treasury. These three were brought together in an Omnibus Appropriation Bill, along with some other matters, and passed on December 21, as the last CRA expired. Supplemental Appropriations were also included in several bills for diverse matters where they would not normally appear, e.g., disaster relief appeared in the Military Construction Bill and counter-terrorism funding in the Transportation bill. It was not a normal budget year, but it was not all that far from the norm for the budgetary process. The closely contested Presidential election of 2000 had its impact as both parties tried to position themselves to "win" the election during the summer and early fall and some of the controversy around the CRA's had to do with waiting to see which candidate was finally going to be elected in the weeks that followed the election day.

Table 2 is another summary of the legislative process. This shows all the legislative products that affected the defense budget in 1981, President Ronald Reagan's first budget year. This year was interesting in several ways. First, Reagan won a big victory, his tax cut, with the reconciliation bill in July and August. However, as he continued to press for further domestic spending reductions, his power in Congress began to wane. There were three Continuing Resolution Appropriations, the last expiring on December 29. Even given a broad consensus to increase defense, the defense authorization, appropriation, and military construction bills were late. Notice also the two Budget Resolutions; although this was called for in the Congressional Budget Reform Act, 1981 was the last year this practice occurred in this form. The struggle to get the appropriations bills passed was simply too difficult to also consider passing a reconciling second Budget Resolution. Notice also the two supplemental bills, one for defense and one for non-defense matters. Usual practice in the last decade has been to do one supplemental for all matters, usually defense related unanticipated missions and natural disaster relief. The time period for these remains typ-

This table includes the dates each bill passed each milestone event and dollars appropriated. For example, the budget resolution was reported out of the House Budget Committee on April 9th, and passed by the House on May 7, for $764.55 billion. The Senate Budget Committee reported out of its version of the budget resolution on April 28th and passed it on May 12, for $775 billion. A conference committee was appointed out of members from both chambers. They met, resolved the differences and issued a report on May 14th. This report was voted on and passed the House on May 20 and the Senate on May 21st. At $770 billion it was slightly under what the President had originally requested ($772B), below what the House Budget Committee had recommended, and above what the full House gave ($764B). The numbers appear to indicate that the Senate and the House conferees split the difference in the conference report. The Defense Authorization bill falls under the jurisdiction of the Armed Services committees and the Appropriations and Military Construction bill are in the jurisdiction of the Appropriations committees. They each have their stories to tell. Part of it was driven by the fact that the Republicans controlled the Presidency and the Senate, but the Democrats controlled the House.

Table 2. The 1981 Budget Process

FY 1982 (BA) (in Billions $$)	Submit Date	House Cmte.	House Floor	Senate Cmte.	Senate Floor	Conf. Report Issued	Conf. Passed House	Conf. Passed Senate	President Signed	Public Law #
Budget Resolution[1]	10-Mar $772.40	9-Apr $787.65	7-May $764.55	28-Apr $775.00	12-May $775.90	14-May $770.90	20-May $770.90	21-May $770.90	N/A N/A	N/A
Budget Resolution[2]	24-Sep $753.70	8-Dec $787.65	10-Dec $764.55	24-Nov $775.00	8-Dec $775.90	9-Dec $770.90	10-Dec $770.90	9-Dec $770.90	N/A N/A	N/A
Defense Authorization	10-Mar $130.27	19-May $136.04	16-Jul $136.11	6-May $136.52	14-May $136.52	3-Nov $130.70	17-Nov $130.70	5-Nov $130.70	1-Dec $130.70	97-86 (S 815)
Defense Appropriation	10-Mar $200.88	6-Nov $196.60	18-Nov $197.44	17-Nov $208.50	4-Dec $208.68	15-Dec $199.69	15-Dec $199.69	15-Dec $199.69	29-Dec $199.69	97-114 (HR 4995)
MilCon Authorization	10-Mar $6.60	15-May $6.98	4-Jun $6.98	22-Jun $7.03	5-Nov $6.48	7-Dec $6.55	8-Dec $6.55	8-Dec $6.55	23-Dec $6.55	97-99 (HR 3455)

Table 2.   The 1981 Budget Process (Cont.)

FY 1982 (BA) (in Billions $$)	Submit Date	House Cmte.	House Floor	Senate Cmte.	Senate Floor	Conf. Report Issued	Conf. Passed House	Conf. Passed Senate	President Signed	Public Law #
MilCon Appropriation	10-Mar $7.30	23-Jul $6.88	16-Sep $6.88	12-Nov $7.28	4-Dec $7.31	11-Dec $7.06	15-Dec $7.06	15-Dec $7.06	23-Dec $7.06	97-106 (HR 4241)
Reconcilliation Bill	10-Mar $48.60	19-Jun $37.76	26-Jun $37.30	17-Jun $39.60	25-Jun $38.10	29-Jul $35.20	31-Jul $35.20	31-Jul $35.20	13-Aug $35.20	97-35 (HR 3982)
Omnibus Supplemental	1-May $8.40	4-May $6.40	13-May $6.80	14-May $6.60	21-May $6.60	2-Jun $6.60	4-Jun $6.60	4-Jun $6.60	5-Jun $6.60	97-12 (HR 3512)
Defense Supplemental	12-Mar $3.03	9-Apr $2.60	23-Jun $2.66	1-Apr $2.80	7-Apr $2.80	27-Jul $2.74	4-Aug $2.74	30-Jul $2.74	14-Aug $2.74	97-39 (S 694)
Continuing Resolution[1]		14-Sep	16-Sep	23-Sep	25-Sep	30-Sep	30-Sep	30-Sep	1-Oct	97-51 (HJ Res 325)
Continuing Resolution[2]		12-Nov	16-Nov	17-Nov	19-Nov	22-Nov	23-Nov	23-Nov	23-Nov	97-85 (HJ Res 368)
Continuing Resolution[3]		9-Dec	10-Dec	10-Dec	11-Dec				15-Dec	97-92 (HJ Res 370)

Notes:

[1] President's original March 1981 request for Defense authorization was $136.49B. This was later revised by the President in October 1981 to $130.27B.

[2] President's original March 1981 request for Defense appropriation was $222B, this was later revised by the President in October 1981 to $200B.

[3] Both Supplemental Bills are for FY1981 outlays.

Source: A composite from student presentations at the Naval Postgraduate School. Note that the numbers for the March 10th date are taken from the President's budget so that the difference may be more easily seen between what the President's budget requested and what Congress gave. Also note that in these years the Defense Authorization bill did not include dollars for personnel costs.

ical, with introduction later in the spring so as not to be confused with budget issues for the following year and passage early enough in the summer so that the dollars can be deployed and spent in the fourth quarter of the fiscal year.

Allen Schick has called the 1980s a time of improvisational budgeting, where the shape of the annual budget process could not be predicted and leaders in Congress and the Executive branches adopted whatever strategies and process steps they thought necessary to move the annual appropriation bills. Most bills were passed late; Continuing Resolution Appropriations were a common occurrence; some years were funded by omnibus continuing resolutions; off-site summit meetings were held between the key Presidential advisors and Congressional leaders with varying degrees of success and gimmicks pervaded the budgetary process and budget numbers. The two years displayed above illustrate this period and demonstrate that improvisational budgeting was still alive and well, in a time when the budget was in a surplus position.[10]

State Patterns

States vary in the power they give to Governors in the budget process. All governors except the Governor of North Carolina possess a veto power. In addition forty-three governors have an item veto power that allows them to void part of an appropriations bill. In theory, the item veto allows for the reduction of foolish spending, but Abney and Lauth (1989) have found that governors use line item vetoes for partisan and policy reasons. Moreover, the scope of the item veto differs. For example, in Illinois the Governor may amend or rewrite legislation as part of the veto process; in Wisconsin the Governor may change wording as long as the law remains workable and the changes do not alter the purpose of the bill. Governors also may reduce expenditures during budget execution if revenues fall short of estimates. In these circumstances, Governors in 40 states may cut budgets during the spending year without legislative approval. In seven of these states gubernatorial action is limited to across the board cuts; in the others the Governor may selectively reduce spending, save that seven states limit the percentage that budgets may be decreased without legislative involvement. The basis for this power is found in the requirement that states operate a balanced operating budget. In 43 states Governors are required to propose a balanced operating budget. In 36 states the budget enacted by the legislature must be in balance and 39 states require that the operating budget be executed so that it is balanced at the end of the fiscal year, although 11 of these may carry over a deficit into the next fiscal year. These requirements are found in the Constitutions of 35 states and by statute in 13. Balanced budgets are required in 80 of the 100 largest cities (Lauth, 1997, p. 270). Recent federal experience with the item veto did not make a compelling case for its merits. Then, too, it was declared unconstitutional. It seems clear that the item veto confers substantial additional legislative power upon the President.

BUDGET ROLES AND INCREMENTALISM

Whatever the legal framework of the budget process, it is the institutional procedures and the people who operate them that are critical to success in the budget process. American budget processes in all but the smallest jurisdictions are embedded in an executive budget system. This means that information is packaged and decisions about the budget are made by the executive and then presented to the legislature for approval. Analyzing this pattern, Ira Sharkansky noted that a "...favorable recommendation from the Governor seems essential for agency budget success in the legislature" (Sharkansky, 1968, p. 1230). Sharkansky also noted that those agencies that asked for more received more, a pattern supported in a study of the Department of Agriculture by LeLoup and Moreland (1972). Duncombe and Kinney asked state budget officials about budget success and reported a complex picture where agency officials were reluctant to use percentage increases as a measure of success. Instead they tended to think in terms of "satisficing" or getting enough to meet agency needs and maintain programs at current levels with, perhaps, a few improvements. They also believed in maintaining good relationships with legislators; this included maintaining credibility with legislators so that when an increase is really needed, the agency would be able to articulate that need and convince the legislature to fund it.

Aaron Wildavsky noted in his classic study of the federal budget process the necessity of gaining other participants' confidence and maintaining a reputation for "playing it straight"(Wildavsky, 1984, pp. 76–79). Duncombe and Kinney also suggest that agency staff had to maintain good relationships with the governor and the budget staff, keeping their executive budget analyst informed of new developments, being honest in budget presentation, and by being a team player (by not trying to get the legislature to add back cuts). Wildavsky had provided much the same portrait for the federal level (Wildavsky, 1988, p. 94). It is clear that in this complex process of information gathering, distribution, and decision making, participants strategize about how to play in the process. A variety of tactics have been identified which some players use to justify resource increases, and others adopt to retard budget growth (Anthony & Young, 1984; Jones & Euske, 1991; Meyers, 1994; Pfeffer & Salancik 1974; Wildavsky, 1964).

William Niskanen has suggested that administrators seek to maximize agency budgets out of a perception that as their budgets grow, so will their own personal rewards, both in terms of remuneration and prestige (Niskanen, 1971). Conversely, Lee Siglelman surveyed state budget administrators and found that "only" three or four of every ten called for increases greater than 15%; Sigleman (1986) did not perceive this as unbridled budget aggression.

During the last two decades with revenues growing more slowly than the demand for services, especially for the elderly and for health care, automatic cost of living adjustments as well as agency advocacy have led to an upward drift in spending despite reduction attempts (Schick, 1990b, ch. 4). Charles Levine (1978b) provided a conceptual template for assessing cutback management in terms or resisting or acceding to cuts that led to a significant body of literature on cutback management. For example, Peter Aucoin (1995) reported that central agency executives in industrialized democracies used a variety of techniques to limit agency growth; these included capping total spending, freezing hiring, and tightening eligibility requirements. Despite some dissent (Behn, 1980), the task of cutting budgets back tends to mirror the routines of incremental growth; down to a certain level, programs are cut incrementally. Leadership strategies tend to concentrate on ensuring equity (all suffer equally) and ensuring that only the most deserving programs get some money back. At some point, across-the-board cuts (horizontal cuts) may turn into total program cuts (vertical cuts) as a jurisdiction tries to hold on to the ability to do some things well as opposed to doing all things poorly. Nevertheless, as explained in Chapter I, the most common pattern whether cutting or growing is one of incremental adjustment.

Incrementalism includes a reliance on the budget base and a focus on the increment of change. The base is what was enacted last year and what may be expected to be reenacted with little difficulty. The focus of effort in this process is the increment of change. In this incremental world, the budget process remains one where agencies ask and reviewers cut and the best predictor of next year's budget is last year's (Wildavsky, 1984, p. 13). This means that the process is stable and outcomes are fairly predictable and in the aggregate certain percentage outcomes can be anticipated. In Wildavsky's original study, more than half of the increases were within 10% of the base (Wildavsky, 1964, p. 14) and LeLoup and Moreland found an average outcome year over year of 11% for the Department of Agriculture over 25 years of observations. Precisely what number should be considered incremental has been debated with different authors calling different increases incremental (Bailey & O'Conner, 1978) and research into individual agency patterns has shown great variation (Natchez & Bupp, 1973); for example, LeLoup and Moreland (1978) found some agencies asked for more than a 100% increase while others asked for less than they had the previous year.

Meyers (1994, p. 4) charges that incrementalism mischaracterizes present day budget strategies in almost every respect; for Meyers the budget process features actors who often make complex, rather than simple, calculations about budget decisions and roles that are unstable rather than clearly defined by institutional position (e.g., reviewers do not always cut). Meyers is particularly hard on those who used federal budget figures to measure increments of change. He suggests that the assumption that government reported data is reliable is open to challenge. After examining the Farmers Home Administration spending patterns, Meyers concluded that appropriations, budget authority and outlays were not good measures of how much money FmHA received or spent (Meyers, 1994, p. 37). For example, Meyers notes, "From the Johnson to the Carter administration, RHIF (The Rural Housing Insurance Fund) obligated increasing amounts on program activities without corresponding increases in outlays, budget authority or appropriation" (Meyers, 1994, p. 31). Most of this was financed by borrowing from the treasury and from the public directly. Meyers argues for a brand of incrementalism based on a more sophisticated knowledge of budget structure.

One illustration of the value of such a structural-analytic approach is an analysis of the report of an advisory panel proposal to increase embassy security in 1986: the Panel recommended an independent Property Board to own and operate embassies. The Board would take fees from the sale of visas, add borrowing from the Treasury and deposit the funds in an uncontrolled revolving trust fund and use the funds to build new embassies (Meyers, 1994, p. 60). The complexity of this mechanism combining sale of visas, borrowing, a revolving fund, and an independent board would have put almost all the operations of this entity beyond analysis and control. Lacking any appropriation, this Board probably never would have shown up in an incremental review of agency appropriations. As credit activities were put on budget, its loan activities might have been discovered. Meyers suggests that a theory of incrementalism based on budget structure should include the recognition that each program has its own method of accounting, decision procedure, policy design that guides how it may acquire and spend funds for different purposes, and commonly perceived effects of spending (Meyers, 1994, p. 50). Allen Schick (1994, p. 4; Cogan, Muris, & Schick, 1994) also argues for the study of micro-budgeting, emphasizing that totals must be understood in terms of the parts upon which they are built. Totals (total revenue, spending, deficit) remain significant as a quick scorecard, but the real work of analysis rests in the details of the budgets. Schick suggested that deficit control would be effective only when the budget's totals were understood in terms of the parts on which they were built:

managing the totals meant tracking and managing the parts (Schick, 1994, p. 6). Meyers and Schick push the frontier of incremental decision analysis into much more complicated territory and away from simpleminded analysis of percent change in appropriations.[11]

As noted in Chapter I, incrementalism, for Wildavsky, was also a decision strategy; budget review would be parceled out and experts would review their parts, examining intensely the items of change. This allowed for focusing of time and analytic skills and avoided comprehensive calculation and conflict over major priority shifts. Here, too, research into actual procedures has indicated a more complex pattern where reviewers do examine the base (see Gist, 1977; Kamlet & Mowery, 1980; Lauth, 1987), but the concept of base and increment of change remains a powerful summarizing tool for characterization of the budget process, even in an era where rising expectations outrun resources.[12] However, some things *have* changed. Far from disappearing, the base has become even more potent at the federal level with the use of baselines that not only keep last year's appropriation "safe," but project it into the future so that a claim is staked against future resources. To work, incremental decision making relies on feedback mechanisms to evaluate when a "bad" decision has been made, and assumes corrective action can be taken. When entitlements take up budget space in the current year and, with the current services budget and baselines, in the future, the concept of feedback and correction is attenuated. Nevertheless, despite its flaws, no concept has replaced incrementalism as an organizing concept for understanding the budget process.

BUDGET PATTERNS

While there are legal foundations to the budget process there are also informal budget patterns that are relatively stable and may be documented over time. For example, at the U.S. national level, agencies appeared to be advocates who ask for more and reviewers in the parent Department, OMB and Congress tend to cut those requests. The period from the end of World War II until the early 1970s is sometimes referred to as the classic period in American budgeting. There was a recognizable budget process, conflict over the budget among budget process participants was routinized and diminished by informal understandings between participants. These "informal understandings" included a balanced budget norm, even though budgets were never balanced and usually in a small deficit position. There was agreement on the general outline of public policy. The economic climate exhibited sustained growth and this growth resulted in growing budgets and the sense that government could and should attack and solve many of society's problems. This ethos was particularly strong during the early 1960s. Thus, budgetary growth became part of the political culture; budget claimants assumed that the next budget would be larger than the current budget and that the focus of budget discussion would be on the increment of change, not the absolute size of the budget, nor on a complete and thorough review of every program starting from zero.

Theorists argued that it was rational to analyze budgets in increments and not rational to attempt to do comprehensive analysis of the total budget in each cycle; they argued that aggrieved parties would announce when something was done wrong and that this could be fixed either in the next budget process or by amendments to the current budget. In the main, the budget was made by experts, and most of budgeting was done in various venues in agencies, in the parent departments, in committees and subcommittees in Congress, all out of the public spotlight. Some observers argued that since budgets cast up decisions as just a matter of dollars, and not fundamental principals, compromise was easier to achieve and the result was generally a stable and predictable budget process.

LeLoup and Moreland (1980) captured the essence of this period in an article describing the Department of Agriculture (DOA) budget process from 1946 to 1971. Their focus was on the hidden politics of budgeting that takes place within the executive branch between the agencies in Agriculture, the Agriculture departmental budget office, OMB, and in Congress. To do this, they examined what agencies within the department asked for, how these requests were treated by the Department budget office, what the Office of Management and Budget did to the Department recommendation and then what Congress gave and how this compared to the current appropriation. Budget changes are computed over the budget base (the appropriation for the current year): if an agency has an appropriation of $100 million and asks for an appropriation (budget) of $110 million, it is asking for a 10% increase over the base. If the department recommends $107 million (a cut, but still an increase of 7%) and OMB suggests $104 (a cut, but still an increase of 4%) and the final appropriation given by Congress for the budget year is $103 million, this means that all reviewers cut the agency request, but compared to the current budget, the agency received an increase of 3% over its base. For LeLoup and Moreland (1980, p. 185), each of these steps would constitute a measurement point or an observation. In this study, the authors evaluated 498 observations for 36 agencies over 25 years of budget history for the Department of Agriculture. Table 3 is adapted from their study.[13]

Table 3.   Agency, OMB, and Congressional Review Patterns

Agency change in Request	Instances	Percent of Total	Dept. Change %	OMB Change %	Congress Change %	Final Appropriation
decrease	60	12.05%	25.5	−6.5	2.4	−21%
up: 0 to 9.9%	99	19.88%	−2	−3	−0.3	0%
up 10–24.9%	121	24.30%	1.3	−8	−0.5	1.30%
up: 25 to 99.9%	182	36.55%	−10.9	−9.4	−0.7	6.20%
up: 100%+	36	7.23%	−20.2	−16.2	−10.5	130%
total (1946–71)	498		−4	−9	−2	11%
total (1980–89	228		−3.05	−6.11	5.90	17.41%

Source: Adapted from LeLoup and Moreland (1980). The last row is added by the authors.

The last row in Table 3 (1980–89) is calculated by the authors with selected discretionary accounts only. During this period of time Congress "protected" the Department of Agriculture from Reagan administration downsizing efforts, as we shall discuss later. In our discretionary account data set, we, too had instances of agencies asking for less than the current year appropriation (25 of 228, or 10.9%, and agencies who sought to double their appropriation (4 or 1.7%). Agriculture agencies were generally less aggressive; 159 of 228 or 69.7% sought increases between zero and 24.9%, as opposed to the 44% in the earlier study. However, if the agencies were less aggressive and the Administration attempted more control, Congress was substantially more generous with this group of discretionary agencies. Otherwise the patterns were similar, with the department balancing the extremes and OMB tending to always cut.

While the article illustrated how complex the budget process was, the reader is also struck by the regularity of the process. LeLoup and Moreland found that:

1.   The average outcome for all agencies was incremental; that is to say that the growth from one year to the next in the agency budget appropriation averaged 11%.
2.   Reviewers—the Department Budget Office, OMB, Congress—tended to cut budget requests. On average, the Department cut 4%; OMB cut 9% more and Congress cut an additional 2%, but the final appropriations averaged an increase of 11% over previous appropriations over the whole period.
3.   OMB always cut and cut the most, averaging 9%.
4.   Those agencies asking for the most, got the most, but also were cut the most. Those asking for greater than 100% (36 instances) were cut 20.2% by the Department, 16.2% by OMB and 10.5% by Con-

gress; however, for this group as a whole, their appropriations increased an average of 130%.

5. During this period, Congress was a marginal modifier: on average, it cut 2% from requests, and it cut less than 1% in 65% of the cases.

6. Agencies were varied in what they asked for. Some agencies asked for more than double their current year's budget (36 cases out of 498); others asked for less than they had in the current year (60 cases).

7. Those who asked for less than they had in the current year got cut; if these agencies thought being frugal would cause others to give them money they were in error. When asked about this profile, an OMB analyst volunteered "we are a 'kick them when they are down' agency; if they do not ask for money we sure are not going to give it to them. We have too many other places that need money."

8. The Department budget office appeared to balance the extremes; it cut a lot from those who asked for a lot, and it added money to those who asked for less than their current year appropriation. It is easy to picture the harried departmental budget officer trying to rein in his more aggressive agencies and encourage his less aggressive agencies, knowing full well that if they do not ask for enough money it will probably be up to the departmental budget office to find it for them during the budget year, hence the adding back of money by the department budget office. Nonetheless, those agencies who asked for less, received a cut of 21% in their appropriations and those who asked for a lot were cut a lot but were rewarded with increased appropriations averaging 130%.

While the average of all outcomes was incremental (11%), 37% of the agencies requested more than a 25% increase and another 24% asked for increases of 10 to 25%. The fact that final outcomes were increases for these two groups of 6.2% and 1.3% testifies to the effectiveness on budget reviewers in controlling demands for more. While these outcomes are moderate, it is clear that the agencies did not intend to be so moderate. Allen Schick's (1990b) analysis of the ability of controllers to hold down budget growth during this period would seem to be supported by this analysis, despite the aggressive behavior of agency administrators. Growth was slowed because of the reviewers who guarded the power of the purse during this period, including the departmental budget office, the Budget Bureau (OMB) and Congress.

RECURRENT PROCEDURES AND ISSUES

According to Senator Pete Domenici (R-NM) (1996), Chair of the Senate Budget Committee, by the 1980s the Department of Agriculture had become a potpourri of programs, ranging from direct provision of scientific information and advice about agriculture, to crop forecasts, to price stabilization programs, to direct spending on welfare programs, to a variety of credit programs. A majority of its budget (76%) consisted of what is called direct spending (because it is money that is sent directly to those who qualify and not used by the department to provide services), either mandated by entitlement programs or driven by changes in the economy that subsequently cause credit programs and price stabilization programs to change.

In general, administrators have little discretionary control over these programs; they cannot ask for a lot to get a lot, and neither can they ask for decreases and let the programs die out. These entitlement programs are embedded in law and what happens to them is a product of what happens in the economy. Good budget analysis in these cases does not involve asking questions about administrative travel patterns, personnel attrition rates, or the schedule of planned equipment purchases and their necessity; instead it involves estimating and forecasting what the economy is going to do and how this effects the number of people who will claim benefits. By the end of the decade these non-discretionary accounts had grown to 81% of the Agriculture budget.[14] What is striking is how closely the budget recommendations cluster around the final appropriation compared to the discretionary accounts. They do this because the agency, the department, OMB, and even Congress have little room to cut or add money; the key variables here are estimates of how many people will be entitled and how much they will be entitled to get. Normally, the decision closest to the time the budget is executed would be the most accurate; this would mean that Congress should be the most accurate (using numbers from the Congressional Budget Office) and the agency should be the least accurate because it must begin the budget process first and is farthest away in time. For fiscal years 1983 and 1985, the agencies were low in their forecasts, but for fiscal years 1981, 1984, and 1989 they were very close to the final appropriation. Over the ten-year period, the Agency and Department estimates for these four entitlement programs were identical just over half the time (on 22 out of 40 occasions). This probably indicates how difficult the estimation process is, although it may also indicate a policy preference to reduce or increase programs.

The discretionary budget accounts have room for value judgments at every step in the process and participants can add or cut depending upon what they believe the program is worth and their estimate of the politics of getting support for their position by others in the budget process. Entitle-

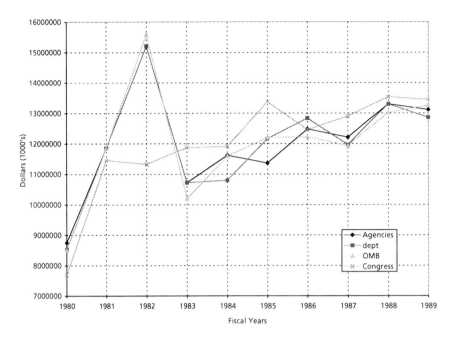

Graph 1.   Four Entitlement Programs FY80-89.

ments are different and this difference appears in Graph 1. There should be little disagreement over these program estimates because what each participant is obligated by law to do is to try to estimate what the economy is going to do and how many claimants will be entitled to claim benefits or want to participate in a program. In other words, outcomes in these programs are not up to the discretion of administrators, budget analysts, or committee members and Congress, but rather driven by who has the best estimate. There is little discretion in these programs; the differences are due to differences in estimation or forecasting. Changing an entitlement program first requires changes in substantive law guiding who gets what benefits; in the 1980s changes to taxes and entitlement programs were sometimes accomplished by passing a separate legislative vehicle called a reconciliation bill.

There is another trend in this profile that is interesting. To some extent, by the 1980s farm programs were counter-cyclical programs. They cost more during times of economic stress, when more people depend more heavily on them; in the 1980s these programs ranged from food stamps to child nutrition programs to increased subsidies for price supports, to credit programs, to crop insurance. When the economy gets better, the dependence of people on programs like these decreases and the programs cost less. For the four entitlement programs in Graph 1, this increase in dependence can be seen for fiscal years 1980 to 1981, 1984 to 1985, and 1987 to 1988 by examining the final appropriation trend line (Congress). The decrease in need can be seen for fiscal years 1981 to 1982 and 1985 to 1986. When need is increasing rapidly, mistakes are made; for example the huge increase in request by the agency, department and OMB between fiscal years 1981 and 1982 was a result of a mis-estimation of the cost of the food stamp program in a period when inflation and unemployment were rising rapidly.

Schick has argued that the old agency-centered routines of OMB, and for that matter the department budget offices, are no longer as relevant as they once were; that average paygrade of employees, or attrition rates, or spending on office supplies or exorbitant travel profiles now mean less to budget analysts than do changes in GDP, inflation and unemployment rates in the economy (Schick, 1990a, pp. 86–87). Shifts in these numbers drive changes in two thirds of the federal budget that is now considered mandatory (payment on the national debt, other federal credit obligations, entitlements, contracts). Thus, discretionary judgments and administrative expertise are no longer so important in budgeting as are the abilities to estimate growth and change in the economy and the number of clients or claimants who will be eligible for benefits and can make claims on the treasury. When these estimates are projected over three to seven year time periods, they are called baselines. In some years budget baselines have become very controversial and budget reviewers have argued about who has the most accurate baseline.

Budgetary politics are not absent from entitlement accounts. Sometimes it is a politics of rhetoric whose purpose is to gain electoral advantage by, in effect, confusing observers over what has been done to the budget. Schick calls this practice baseline alchemy. When there is an increase over the base (current year appropriation), but below the baseline forecast for the program adjusted for newly eligible claimants or inflation, supporters of the program can call the new number a cut (it is a cut from the baseline forecast) and opponents can call it an increase (it is an increase from the appropriation, but below what it will take to deliver the same program to all who are eligible) (Schick, 1990a, pp. 95–101).

Sometimes the politics of entitlements gets even more confusing when budgets are sent to Congress that anticipate that substantive changes will be made in entitlement programs in laws to be passed later in the legislative session. For example, in 1982, the Administration, supported by the House, proposed funding for food stamps, child nutrition, and the Women, Infants and Children (WIC) programs that were so low that funds would have run out before the end of the fiscal year. This meant the child nutrition program would have been funded for 10.5 months, WIC for 7.5

months and food stamps for 9.5 months. The food stamp program would have been $2.2 billion short in 1983. This was a way to reduce funding in these programs without first changing the substantive law which guided the programs. Advocates of this position suggested the substantive changes legitimizing these levels would be made later, and if they were not, then a supplemental bill could always be passed to make up the full annual funding for these programs.

The Senate stood firm for full funding of the programs in FY83. In December, the Administration gave in and sent the required budget changes to Congress, and House and Senate conferees agreed on funding the programs for the full year. This turbulence can be seen in the entitlement accounts for FY1983 on graph one. Here the administration did not make a mistake in estimating what it would take to fund these programs; rather, it incorporated policy changes in its budget requests for the programs which it assumed would be passed into law later in the year (*Congressional Quarterly Almanac*, 1982, pp. 258–261), notwithstanding that it knew there was fierce opposition to these changes in the Senate.

Had the Senate acceded to this budget strategy, but refused to pass legislation changing the substantive entitlement legislation (because it did not want to reduce these programs) and counted on passing a supplemental appropriation later in 1983 to fully fund these programs, it is highly likely that the House would have blocked the supplemental appropriation (because it wanted the programs reduced) and the programs would have remained partially funded despite the fact that there had been no change in the substantive legislation establishing entitlement criteria for these programs. In this case, aggrieved claimants could have sued after the money had run out, but redress of grievances through the Courts is normally far too late to effect events within a given fiscal year. In sum, what appears to be a technical area where all that counts is the right formula or computer model turns out to be filled with subtle political rhetoric and actions. This is also an object lesson in political strategies; the Administration took the initiative by suggesting budget amounts that reduced entitlements without the necessary entitlement law changes. The Senate held firm to a blocking position that was critical; it held its power. Had it given in, it would have been in the position of having to get a supplemental bill through the House. The outcome was that the Senate forced full funding, and in so doing, compliance with the current entitlement statutes governing these programs.

Agriculture Discretionary Expenditures

Department of Agriculture budget documents also allowed for analysis of some of the discretionary accounts during the 1980–1990 decade.

(LeLoup and Moreland did not divide their study into mandatory and discretionary accounts.) These accounts represented budget lines ranging from the Office of the Secretary, to various libraries and statistical services, to animal, plant, and grain inspection services and to the agricultural extension service. Some 19 accounts were followed over the eleven-year period, from the agency through the departmental budget office, through OMB and through Congress; this provided some 228 observations.[15] While these comprise almost two-thirds of the accounts in the Department of Agriculture budget structure during this period, they represent only about 19% of the funds. For example, according to the Congressional Budget Office summer 1991 baseline, mandatory expenditures amounted to 81.3% of the Department of Agriculture budget. Nonetheless, the accounts collected and pictured in Graph 2 illustrate the hidden politics of budgeting as it existed in the 1980s for discretionary accounts, those accounts agency administrators, departmental budget analysts, OMB, and Congress had discretionary control over in the budget process.

In general, the profile for these discretionary accounts resembles the profile suggested by LeLoup and Moreland only to the extent that in most years these agencies asked for more than they were given. The year 1982 might be considered typical for the LeLoup-Moreland era: agencies asked for a lot, were cut a lot by the Department budget office, were cut some more by OMB and were cut substantially in the final appropriation. The years 1980 and 1981 show evidence of great agreement among reviewers (Department, OMB, Congress) about what these agencies should get; naturally it was a lot less than they asked for.

The interesting aspect of this period lies in how different it was from the classic period. LeLoup and Moreland would have recognized 1982; here the agency request was greater than the departmental recommendation, OMB's mark and the Congressional outcome. However, the subsequent years were normal only in the sense that the agency request was greater than the final appropriation. Indeed, in five of the eleven years the final appropriation was closer to the Agency request than it was to either the Departmental budget office or OMB recommendation.

Part of the history of Agricultural policy in this decade was an effort in cost containment by the President; this can be seen in the OMB recommendation in 1983 and the Departmental recommendation in 1984; both suggested large cuts that were basically ignored by Congress. In 1983, OMB tried to cut rural water disposal grants by 40% and the supplemental food program by 100%; OMB suggested reductions in the Office of the Secretary of Agriculture of 12%, departmental administration of 17.8%, office of legislative liaison of 21%, cooperative state research service of 12%, animal and plant inspection of 13%; and in the agriculture cooperative service of 14%. In addition to departmental budget office cuts, the office of legisla-

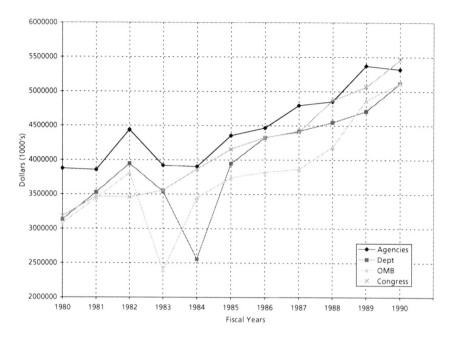

Graph 2.   Some Discretionary Accounts FY1980–90.

tive liaison would have been reduced by 54%, the cooperative state research service by 24% and the soil conservation service by 33%. In 1984, the Department budget office made the most effort to cut programs, suggesting, for example that the extension service be cut by 12%, rural water grants by 25%, the soil conservation service by 15% and the supplemental food program by 100%. These were intentional efforts to decrease the size of the discretionary accounts within the Department; they were generally rejected by Congress and suggested a battleground that would be played out the rest of the decade.

For most of the rest of the decade, Congress protected these discretionary agencies within the Department of Agriculture against the budget reduction efforts from both OMB and the Departmental budget office. When the President wants to reduce spending in a department or policy area, he can work through OMB or he can work through the head of the department, who is appointed by the President, and the department budget staff, who are responsible to that appointee. Graph two seems to suggest that both these approaches were attempted from 1983 on, but that support for the agencies within Agriculture was strong in Congress. Far from being a marginal modifier, Congress was an important supporter of these programs throughout most of the 1980s.

Some agencies asked for a decrease from their current year's base, just as they had in the previous study, and with almost the same frequency. Part of the negative baggage of incrementalism was the implication that agencies always asked for more and that budgets always went up. The LeLoup and Moreland study was interesting because it seemed to suggest that there were instances (about 12% of the cases) where bureaucrats would ask for less than they had in the current budget. The difficulty with putting too much emphasis on this argument in the LeLoup and Moreland study was that these constituted such a small percentage of cases that over a quarter of a century they might well have represented instances of bureaus ratcheting down as their clienteles disappeared, of mandatory expenditures that declined, or of bureaus that were simply closed as budget lines only to appear as a component of some other function. This still may be true for that period.

In the 1980–90 study of discretionary accounts, seven agencies asked for a decrease in a single year and five agencies asked for decreases in multiple years (24 instances total). For example, Animal and Plant Health Inspection requested a decrease from 1983 through 1986; the Agricultural Cooperative Service requested a decrease from 1983 through 1987 and the Agricultural Marketing Service requested decreases in 1983 through 1985 and 1990. Administrators do sometimes ask for less.

In these cases, the Department budget office did not change the requests of the agencies in twelve instances. In six instances the Department budget office further decreased the request, but in another six instances it increased or gave money back. This could be seen as the Department budget office balancing the extremes, just as it had done in the earlier period. OMB cut in 22 cases, but added money to two, more than the agency asked for and more than what the department recommended. This is a somewhat different profile for OMB from the LeLoup and Moreland study where OMB appeared to always cut. Congress for its part added money to all but four of these requests, but just as in the earlier period, the final outcome was still below the current year budget in the majority of cases (19 of 24 instances).

While Congress supported these agencies, it did not do so with blind enthusiasm; it seemed to know what it wanted and sent budgetary signals until the agency got it right. In 1988, Advisory Committees requested a decrease from the base of 6% and received exactly what they had in the current year from Congress (i.e., Congress restored the cut). Evidently taking this as a signal, Advisory committees became wildly aggressive and asked for increases of 74% and 68% the next two years and received increases of 14% and zero respectively. Asking for a lot did not get them a lot. In fact, over the three-year period, this account grew 14% and all in 1989. In 1983 the Office of Public Affairs requested an increase of 99%

over the previous year only to receive its current year's budget (no increase). The next year it requested a decrease below the base, but was restored to the current year budget (no decrease). This would seem to indicate that Congress had an idea of the size of the budget it wanted public affairs to have and maintained its idea of that size despite the agency's efforts first to grow a lot and then to let things slide.

The 1980s were a turbulent period in budget history, marked by disagreement over policy, deficit reduction politics, continuing resolutions, appropriations passed well into the fiscal year and for the latter part of the decade rather violent disagreement between Congress and the President over budget directions for the agriculture programs. It was also an era of divided government with the Republicans holding the White House and Democrats holding at least one house in Congress. This further complicated the budget process. Allen Schick suggests that the 1980s were a period of improvisational budget procedures where budget makers had to deal with intense policy preferences and a budget process that did not work as it should (Schick, 1990a, Ch. 6, pp. 159–196). Some of this turbulence can be seen in OMB's effort to reduce Agriculture's discretionary accounts only to have them restored by Congress. Moreover, while the hidden politics of budgeting still exists, for Agriculture, at least, most of the budget comprised entitlements and credit programs where what matters is not what Agriculture managers, OMB, and Congress think about a program but what the law says and what the economy does and careful budget analysis is less important than accurate estimation for programs whose structure is fixed in law, at least in theory. In practice, subtle and powerful political strategies are also employed in the entitlement programs.

The Budget Work of OMB and CBO

Perhaps the key players in the budget process are the budget analysts who review and recommend budget positions. At all levels of government, chief executives rarely spend much time on the minutiae of budgets. These are delegated to professional budget analysts led by a director of the budget agency. During budget preparation, analysts are responsible for conveying budget directions and policy guidance and assisting agencies in constructing their budget, even to including which schedules to fill out. During budget review, budget analysts indicate where cuts should be made and allow the agencies to respond to their proposals. They then help compile the executive budget and transmit it to the legislature for approval. During the budget execution phase of the budget process, budget analysts learn about their agency and its programs, knowledge that will serve them in good stead when they have to review program increase requests, and program performance and budget needs. Lehan argues that budgeting is a craft-like activity that involves analyses and judgments about the worth of things. The tools of this craft are, "…the reflective values of evidence and logic" (Lehan, 1981, p. 4). While budget analysis always has a cutting perspective, the total perspective of the budget analyst has broadened from accounting and accountability to performance and management. Thurmaier (1992; see also Thurmaier, 1995) calls budgeting a special type of policy analysis that is particularly concerned with how different resource allocations will affect the content of policies and programs. While budget analyst positions exist at all levels of government and in agencies and in the legislature as well as organized as staff to the chief executive, perhaps the two preeminent models for budget analysis exist in the Office of Management and Budget and the Congressional Budget Office.

The Office of Management and Budget (OMB) was created as the Bureau of the Budget by the Budget and Accounting Act of 1921 and renamed OMB in the late 1960s. This landmark piece of legislation created an executive budget system for the federal government, authorizing the President to compile and pass on to Congress a budget proposal. While the original director of the bureau minimized the policy role of the organization, it was clear the bureau had a policy direction; it was economy and efficiency. In the words of the first Director of the Bureau of the Budget, General Dawes: "…the Bureau … is concerned only with the humbler and routine business of government. Unlike cabinet officers, it is concerned with no questions of policy, save that of economy and efficiency … No cabinet officer on the bridge with the President … advising as to what direction the ship of state shall sail will properly serve … if he resents the call of the Director of the Budget from the stoke hole, put there to see that coal is not wasted" (Burkhead, 1959, p. 289).[16] Subsequent reorganization and expansion of the role of the federal government meant the steady increase in importance of the budget bureau with the growth of federal responsibilities during the Great Depression of the 1930s and World War II and its aftermath.

By the 1950s the Bureau had gained an impressive reputation for neutral competence and a professionalism that sought the most efficient way to get things done. However, the expanding role of the federal government steadily created a need for more emphasis on management as well as a bureau that would be more politically responsive to the desires of the President. In 1970 the Bureau was reorganized to enable the President to emphasize management and to be more responsive to the political demands of the President by placing a new layer of political appointees, called "program associate directors," in supervisory positions between the career budget examiners and the budget director.

In the 1980s, OMB began to focus more on what happened to the President's budget in Congress, creating an information system and a group of analysts whose focus was on keeping track of and interpreting what Congress was doing with the President's budget. This effort involved tracking the potential impact of a host of bills and resolutions that have budgetary impact and organizing testimony and rebuttal efforts for those which run counter to the President's program. This meant tracking efforts focused on subcommittees, committees and floor actions in each chamber and on the work of conference committees. This tracking effort allowed OMB and the President and his political staff to focus persuasive efforts at any appropriate step in the budget process in Congress to help advance the President's program. This is a different task than the post WWII role of BOB with its focus on neutral competence, (a term derived from the British system of a permanent civil service with great expertise who served to the best of their ability whatever political party held the reins of government) and presentation of the correct numbers and an array of alternatives which allow political decision makers to make policy choices.

These new tasks of tracking legislation and negotiating with Congress and Congressional staff have imposed a heavy workload on budget examiners when it is added to the ongoing routine of reviewing agency budget requests and preparing the President's budget. Given the makeup of the federal budget, with its increased emphasis on entitlements and programs with inflation linked baselines, the focus on what Congress is doing to shape programs seems appropriate. It is not without its dangers, however. For example, Schick (1990a, p. 162) suggests the President's budget has lost its authoritative status and come to be seen as an opening bid in the budget process,[17] and James Pfiffner (1991) has suggested that the movement of OMB from neutral competence to personal staff, the tracking effort and its public visibility and advocacy in Congress has meant a loss of credibility for career staff and their primary output: the President's budget.

The Congressional Budget Reform Act of 1974 substantially modified the congressional budget process, creating new Budget Committees in each chamber charged with preparing and presenting an annual budget resolution which would set overall targets for the federal budget and targets by functional area and enforce these targets by keeping score during the budget process. The budget calendar was revised and a new staff unit, called the Congressional Budget Office (CBO), was created to support the new Budget Committees. CBO was tasked with a hierarchy of missions, first to support the Budget Committees, then the appropriations and tax committees and then Congress as a whole, by providing economic estimates and budgetary information. With CBO, Congress would no longer have to depend on the economic and program forecasts of the executive branch.

CBO makes economic forecasts and projections for the major economic variables in the budget, such as GDP, unemployment, inflation and interest rates. These are released in two reports, in January and in August (e.g., The Economic and Budget Outlook). CBO also provides two baseline budget projections every year that are especially useful in indicating the trend in spending for entitlement programs. CBO is also responsible for doing a five-year cost estimate of any bill reported by an authorizing committee. Cost estimates are also prepared for many draft proposals, floor amendments, and conference agreements. In recent years CBO has prepared from 500 to 900 cost estimates a year. Schick (1990a, p. 99) has called the calculation of budget baselines the true separator of the budget insider and outsider, "…a dense barrier separating budget insiders, who know what the numbers mean from outsiders, including seasoned budget observers, who cannot figure out what is being done unless they uncover the assumptions behind the numbers." Unable to tell what the elements of the calculation are, the outsider cannot readily critique the resulting numbers. OMB Director Stockman's magic asterisk indicating dollars to be found later and confession that he bent a forecasting model to produce the numbers he wanted re-enforce this point.[18] Sensitive to these sorts of criticisms, CBO tends to fully describe how it makes its estimates. It may gather data from private sector economists as well as public sources, including program managers who administer the program in question. CBO generally provides a point estimate, indicates what the range may be and includes information about how sensitive the estimate is to changes in assumptions or methodologies.

Each February CBO analyzes the President's budget, substituting CBO's economic projections and assumptions for the President's. This allows Congress to compare Presidential policies to the Congressional baseline. CBO also issues other studies and reports on a variety of subjects, ranging from how to reduce the deficit to defense spending alternatives. In general, CBO does not make recommendations in these reports, rather it lays out alternatives so that members of Congress can see the consequences of their and the President's actions. Under the leadership of its first director Alice Rivlin (1975–1983), CBO quickly gained great credibility for outstanding staff work. This reputation was enhanced subsequently by the Directors who followed her and by the professional performance of CBO staffers. CBO's total staff number about 220. While they do not have civil service protection and can be fired immediately, they have built up a reputation for neutral competence and staff turnover has been relatively low. According to 1990 data, about 70% of the professional staff had completed advanced degrees. The majority of staff members were trained as economists with a substantial minority receiving training in public administration and policy.

Director Rivlin created an organization that was chartered to do both longer range program analysis as well as support the budget process. She set up the organization to separate these functions because she feared the short-run questions in support of the budget process would drive out longer term evaluations. In the ensuing years, the formal shape of the organization she created has changed relatively little. CBO is sometimes criticized for having too much power in the scorekeeping process and for being somewhat unwilling to make estimates of major program changes due to the lack of good information, and for being somewhat less accurate on long range forecasts because it is unwilling to forecast a recession, but it has been more accurate than the administration on short term forecasts and its work is almost universally respected in Washington. Whatever the success of other parts of the Budget Reform Act of 1974 (the fiscal year change, for example), the creation of the Congressional Budget Office has been an unqualified success.

CONCLUSIONS

Schick (1990a, pp. 10–11) has suggested that budgeting has three major components; generating, claiming, and rationing resources. The budget process is about how, when, and by whom claims are made and resources rationed. Schick observes that the rationing function is the heart of the budget process. Budgeting would not be necessary if all claims could be satisfied and it would be a waste of effort if few claims could be satisfied. Governments must have resources to allocate. Someone must generate claims and those claims must exceed available resources before a true budgeting process is invoked. Roy Meyers (1994, p. 15) has argued that budget participants may be classified on the basis of their goals for spending into either advocates or spenders; he also concludes that there are more advocates than controllers (1994, p. 201). He suggests that increased understanding of the effects of spending, a longer term view of the effects of governmental financial transactions as opposed to concentration on annual deficits or surpluses, and clearer rules for budgetary procedures like scorekeeping are needed (Meyers, 1994, pp. 199–201). Nonetheless, advocates are likely to continue generating claims that exceed resources and deciding which of those claims to augment may continue to be quite complex.

If the past is prolog, then the budget process will continue to be both complex and disorderly. For example, the federal budget process for FY1996, that should have been concluded in September of 1995 was not completed until April of 1996; in all, from 1948 through 2001, the federal budget process was completed on time only in a handful of years including 1948, 1976, 1988, 1992, 1994, and 1996. Nonetheless, as confused as budget processes sometimes seem to be, they do set priorities and they do provide the funding to attain those priorities. Moreover, as Allen Schick concludes, big, active governments would be unthinkable without the discipline and regularities of the budget process. As arguments over the size of government continue in the current years, there is little doubt that the government size that most Americans would support, even if substantially reduced from the current size, would still be very large and quite active. Americans expect government to act; the catalog over the last decade of what supplemental appropriations have been used for indicates the scope of this desire and includes, floods, fires, earthquakes, hurricanes, drought, civil unrest, economic relief, and various defense activities. These are all for tasks unforeseen in the current year budget. While they argue about the size and efficiency of the budget, it is clear that Americans will continue to insist on an agile and effective government of a very considerable size. Without the budget process, funding such a government would be unthinkable.

NOTES

1.   This chapter draws from *A Citizens Guide to the Budget FY97 to FY2002; Analytical Perspectives, Budget of the United States* (1996, esp. Ch. 25, pp. 311–315); Schick, Keith, and Davis (1991); Berner and Daggett (1993); and Schick (1994).

2.   For example the basic administrative expenses (salaries and supporting expenses) for the Farmer's Home Administration were only 3% outlays in 1985.

3.   For an excellent description of New Zealand initiatives, see Office of the Auditor General of Canada. Ottawa, Canada (1995).

4.   For an excellent discussion of the complexities of baseline issues, see Muris (1994, pp. 41–78); also see Schick (1990a, pp. 95–101) on "baseline alchemy."

5.   For more information on baseline assumptions see *Analytical Perspectives, Budget of the United States* (1997, Ch. 15).

6.   This work does not discuss the sequestration process. Under Gramm-Rudman-Hollings, sequestration, an across the board cut of a flat percentage, was applied to all non-exempt budget categories if the deficit target was breached. Such a sequester was done in 1986. Subsequent sequestration actions were initiated and then refunded in 1990. With the Budget Enforcement Act of 1990, the President had the ability to move deficit targets up when economic conditions warrant, thus avoiding major sequestrations. President Clinton adjusted targets upward for both FY94 and FY95. Positive actions by the President and Congress in spending constraints and tax increases, and an improving economy have made sequestration unnecessary, although the process for doing it still exits in law. From 1992–1994 only two "tiny" sequestrations have been applied to the discretionary accounts. In 1990 with its fixed deficit targets, meeting the deficit target would have required almost a 30% reduction in the Department of Navy budget, an almost impossible task that would have fallen heavily on readiness and personnel accounts. For more discussion of sequestration, see Schick (1995, pp. 40–41).

7.   Roy Meyers (1994, pp. 130–132) provides some examples of how baselines were used to increase the defense buildup in the early 1980s and to attempt to prevent deeper cuts in defense and agriculture from the mid-1980s on by using higher baselines.

8.   In 1992, the census of governments found 31,555 special districts, with 69% of the single function districts falling into three categories: water (water, sewage, flood, irrigation) 39%; fire protection 18.1%; community development 12 %. These were funded through a variety of revenue sources, including the property tax, user fees, grants, and other taxes. See U.S. Bureau of the Census (1994, Table 19)

9.   While reconciliation bills generally reduce spending, there are examples where savvy budget players were able to squeeze additional money for programs into reconciliation bills and make the increases stick because their votes were needed to pass the bill. In 1987 a three year increase for Medicaid was worked into the Reconciliation bill by Representative Henry Waxman and in 1990 Senator Wendell Ford attempted to preserve 1500 federal jobs in his home state (see Meyers, 1994, pp. 120–121).

10.   For more on improvisational budgeting, see Schick (1990a, pp. 159–196).

11.   To some extent incrementalism fell victim to the rise of computers and the information age. Appropriations constituted discrete numbers available over a series of years and with the new computing power available to them and the development of statistics in the social sciences, researchers simply went looking for statistical distribution patterns like percent of increase and correlation of spending with other factors, like population density, area, and a variety of population characteristics. With these techniques, useful insights could be gained without substantial knowledge of the budget process or the details that make up account structures. This was especially true when more complicated programs—like loan and loan guarantee—programs were analyzed. Meyers describes such a case where the wrong conclusions were drawn in an otherwise sophisticated study because appropriations constituted only a small part of the agency spending totals (Meyers, 1994, p. 37).

12.   In proposing an approach based on an understanding of budgetary structure, Roy Meyers notes that although incrementalism "mischaracterizes current-day budgetary strategies in almost every respect, an alternative understanding of budgetary strategy has not emerged" (Meyers, 1994, p. 4).

13.   Additional data is supplied from our own research.

14.   These programs included the child nutrition program, the special milk program, the food stamp program, and the food donations program.

15.   These were mainly accounts that carried out the administrative work of the Department; others included some information and inspection programs, some grant programs, and the supplemental food program. They included the Office of the Secretary, Departmental Administration, Legislative Liaison, the Inspector General, the Office of General Counsel, the Agricultural Research Service, the Cooperative State Research Service, the Extension Service, the World Agriculture Outlook Board, Animal and Plant Inspection Services, Food Safety and Inspection, Federal Grain Inspection, the Agricultural Cooperative Service, the Agriculture Marketing Service, the Rural Water Disposal Grant Program, the Soil Conservation Service, the Supplemental Food Program and the Foreign Agriculture Services program.

16.   Burkhead notes that the Annual Report of the Bureau for 1924 takes credit for focusing on pencils: "Only one pencil at a time is now issued to any one and he is expected to turn in the unused portion of the last one received. The results justify the practice. Our item of expense for pencils is materially less" (p. 290). While

that concentration may seem severe by modern standards, the Bureau quickly gained stature in the executive branch and Congress. The Chairman of the Senate appropriations committee praised the bureau in 1923 saying it had demonstrated its worth: "It helps separate the chaff from the grain. It gives accuracy as well as integrity to estimates ... Under the old system, congressional committees were obliged to spend a great amount of time on extravagant and questionable estimates" (Burkhead, 1959, p. 291).

17.   For more on OMB see Heclo (1975, pp. 80–98); Berman (1979). Berman gives President Nixon the credit for having politicized OMB and taken it away from neutral competence. Schick and others have argued that that the old Bureau of the Budget went out of existence because it did not meet the needs of the modern presidency. (see Schick, 1970, pp. 518–539)

18.   For more on Stockman, see Greider (1981). Stockman also used a higher baseline in order to claim greater savings. (see Schick, 1990a, p. 98). Meyers notes that beyond 1982 Stockman became a proponent of honesty in budgeting and the result was an increase in the deficit as many of the gimmicks were removed from the budget "...many of the deficit increases were technical because we were backing out of gimmicks" (Meyers, 1994, p. 37).

CHAPTER IV

BUDGET EXECUTION

INTRODUCTION

While budget preparation is a planning process, budget execution is a management process. Budget preparation involves planning for policy accomplishment, while budget execution involves managing the budget plan for policy implementation. Bernard Pitsvada explains that budget execution is, "...that phase of the budget cycle in which agencies actually obligate or commit funds in pursuit of accomplishing programmatic goals" (Pitsvada, 1983, p. 87). Following plans made in the budget preparation cycle, employees or contractors are engaged, materials and supplies purchased, contracts let and capital equipment purchased. Thus are undertaken all the minutiae of administration which are necessary to implement the programs, plans, and activities proposed and then approved in the budget process. While much can be observed in budget making as a result of the openness of the legislative budget process with its hearings, debates, and votes based on executive budget documents and various legislative analyses, only parts of the budget execution process are observable to outsiders. At the federal level, actions that require legislative approval or notification are observable. Impoundments, rescissions and deferrals, reprogrammings and fund transfers may be identified and studied. Gross breaches in propriety, program inefficiency, and even fraud, waste and misuse of funds may be discovered from audits, General Accounting Office studies, and Inspector General reports, reported in Congressional Hearings, or unearthed as items of interest by the news media.

However, the ordinary routines of budget execution are usually carried out far from the spotlight of media and public attention and the daily political crises that draw so much attention. Account administrators and program managers are slowly buried under an accumulating mass of detail about routine events and the arrival of new crises as the fiscal year and execution begins. At the end of the year, the administrator has survived another challenging year, but may be unable to remember the exact shape of any particular crisis or determine which was the worst. In retrospect, few execution problems provide enjoyment and they all take time and effort to resolve. Moreover, in all probability, few if any execution decisions change the course of history. Even program officials within an agency see little of the budget execution process as it unfolds, except when it affects their own program. It is assumed that the budget will be executed as planned once it is approved. It is also assumed that this is a relatively simple task compared to preparing and passing the budget. However, budget administrators know that the reality of administrative life is quite different. A substantial portion of their time is spent rescuing carefully laid plans from unforeseen events, emergencies and non-forecastable contingencies. Many of these events may involve relatively small amounts of money, but require the expenditure of disproportionately large amounts of time and effort to resolve. At the end of the year, in the aggregate and on average, budget execution may appear to have been a matter of uninteresting routine constrained by obscure and arcane rules and procedures and dominated by financial control mechanisms, clever cash management and accounting creativity. It is unlikely to have appeared so uneventful to the department budget officer and his staff or the manager charged with carrying out the program. However the saving grace to this situation is that most budget administrators are fully confident of their ability to solve these kinds of problems. They have seen most of them before and generally know what must be done. Moreover, if the old routines do not quite apply, they know where to go for help when they need it—what rules, regulations, and people to consult.

Despite the continuing attention to budget execution forced on practitioners by environmental uncertainties, the academic literature is still largely focused on budget preparation. However, there is a substantial body of literature developing on budget execution under other titles.[1] Textbooks now describe cash management and investment, debt administration, and tax administration, pension funds and risk management, capital budgeting and debt strategy, and property management as well as budget preparation (see Lynch, 1995; Mikesell, 1986). In this chapter, we extend the study of budget execution to a more detailed examination from the perspectives of departmental budget manager or comptroller. First, we examine the legal basis of budget execution. Then we describe some accommodating behaviors budget managers adopt to deal with budget execution. We next consider strategies to deal with end of year spending patterns, using examples drawn from the experience of the Department of

Defense (DOD). The chapter concludes in examining the discretion available to administrators at different levels in departments and agencies to adopt contingent and adaptive behaviors to meet budget execution crises. Our intent is to show the turbulence that exists in budget execution, while illustrating some of the rules and constraints federal managers must cope with in budget execution.

THE LEGAL FRAMEWORK OF BUDGET EXECUTION

All systems have set rules and procedures to help guide the jurisdiction through budget execution. In the federal government, once an appropriation is passed, the Treasury issues a warrant for the amount of money to be spent during the year. OMB apportions this amount to each agency. Each agency head then uses allotments to delegate to subordinates the authority to incur a specific amount of obligations. These allotments may be further subdivided into allocations by lower administrative levels. Following these allotments and allocations, obligations can be incurred (e.g., contracts let) and outlays can be paid when the work or service is completed or the equipment delivered. The apportionment, allotment, and allocation processes constitute the planning process for when funds will be spent, by quarter or month, by administrative level, and by category of expenditure.[2] These plans are guided by a well-defined set of laws and rules. Exhibit 1 describes the legal basis for budget execution in the United States Department of Energy. All except number 11 would apply to all agencies and any other agency is likely to have its own rule authorizing fund transfers. The scope of the list is also indicative of the complexity of budget execution.

EXHIBIT 1
Legal Bases for Budget Execution1

1. Article 1, Section 9, of the Constitution of the United States, which states that, "No money shall be drawn from the Treasury, but in Consequence of Appropriations made by Law" and upon which the apportionment and Treasury warrant process is based.

2. Title 31, United States Code (U.S.C.), Section 1301, "Application of Appropriations," which restricts the expenditure of funds to the purposes for which they are appropriated.

3. Title 31, U.S.C., Sections 1341, 1342, "The Anti-Deficiency Act," which states that no Federal officer or employee may authorize Government obligations or expenditures in advance of or in

excess of an appropriation, unless otherwise authorized by law, and that no Federal officer or employee may accept voluntary services except as authorized by law.

4. Title 31, U.S.C., Section 1512, "Apportionment and Reserves," which, provides the legislative basis for the apportionment process by requiring, except as otherwise provided, that all appropriations and funds available for obligation be apportioned.

5. Title 31, U.S.C., Section 1514, "Administrative Division of Apportionments," which requires establishment of administrative control of funds designed to restrict obligations against an appropriation or fund to the amount of the apportionment or reapportionment, and that the agency head be able to fix responsibility for the creation of any obligation in excess of an apportionment or reapportionment.

6. Title 31, U.S.C., Section 1517, "Prohibited Obligations and Expenditures," which prohibits making or authorizing expenditures or obligations in excess of available apportioned funds, or amount permitted by regulations under Section 1514, and requires the reporting of violations of this section to the President and the Congress.

7. "The Budget and Accounting Procedures Act of 1950," which defines the legal basis for the issuance of appropriation warrants by the Secretary of the Treasury, who is responsible for the system of central accounting and financial reporting for the Government as a whole.

8. "Congressional Budget and Impoundment Control Act of 1974," that establishes the fiscal year to commence on 10-1 (Title 31, U.S.C., Section 1102), and prescribes the rescission and deferral process (Title 2, U.S.C., Sections 681- 688).

9. Title 31, U.S.C., Section 1535, "Agency Agreements," (commonly referred to as the "Economy Act") which authorizes a Federal agency to place reimbursable agreements for work or services with other Federal agencies.

10. Section 111 of the Energy Reorganization Act of 1974, as amended, Public Law 93-438, which cites provisions and limitations applicable to the use of operating expenses, expenditures for facilities and capital equipment, new project starts, and the merger of funds.

11. Section 659 of the Department of Energy Organization Act of 1977, Public Law 95-91, which allows the Secretary, when authorized in an appropriation act for any fiscal year, to transfer funds from one appropriation to another, providing that

> no appropriation is either increased or decreased by more than 5 percent for that fiscal year.
>
> 12. Annual authorization and appropriation acts, which may contain specific guidance on Department funding as well as limitations on reprogramming, restructuring, and appropriation transfer actions.
> 13. OMB Circular No. A-34, "Instructions on Budget Execution," of 10-18-94, which provides instructions on budget execution including apportionments, reapportionments, deferrals, proposed and enacted rescissions, systems for administrative control of funds, allotments, and reports on budget execution.
> 14. Treasury Fiscal Requirements Manual, Volume I, Section 2040, which prescribes the procedures to be followed in the issuance of Treasury appropriation warrants.
> 15. "Government Accounting Office Policy and Procedures Manual For Guidance of Federal Agencies," Title 7, Fiscal Procedures, of 5-18-93, that provides guidance related to agency fiscal processes and financial systems.
>
> *Note:* The source for this exhibit is the Department of Energy, Budget Execution Manual . DOE M 135.1-1. Office of the Chief Financial Officer, Budget Execution Branch, CR-131. Budget Execution Manual (1996).

In his classic text on budgeting, Burkhead (1959, p. 340) states that budget execution is an executive responsibility. However, he observes that in the United States, history is replete with instances in which the legislative body has intervened in execution to modify decisions it has previously made, to influence administrative actions, and to interpose independent checks on specific transactions.[3] Burkhead divides techniques for budget execution into two groups, financial and administrative. Financial controls are directed at the various accounts used to record government transactions, for both receipts and expenditures. Administrative controls refer to the normal events of budget execution as they are experienced in the daily lives of most administrators and have to do with executing and adjusting the budget plan that was developed and refined in the executive branch and reviewed and approved in the legislative branch. Burkhead suggests that the goals of budget execution involve preserving legislative intent, observing financial limitations and maintaining flexibility at all levels of administration (Burkhead, 1959, p. 342).

These themes were reflected in research reported in 1983 by Pitsvada who examined the flexibility federal agencies have in budget execution in terms of object classification, appropriation structure, contingency appropriations, emergency provisions, and reprogramming authority (Pitsvada, 1983). Pitsvada suggested that object classification serves accounting and control purposes, but that planning and management purposes are not well served by object classification. He observed that no agency in the federal government prepared a budget solely in object format, but that object data was provided to Congress with programmatic budget data in order to support agency requests because Congressmen found it easier to understand. Pitsvada further suggests that in budget execution, object classification generally leaves agencies with great flexibility to shift funds around to meet needs within or between categories. Pitsvada states that funds can be shifted from personnel salaries to purchase supplies and equipment if there is a surplus in the personnel account and funds can be shifted from the utility account to communications if, for example, "a successful energy conservation campaign reduces the original requirement for utilities" (Pitsvada, 1983, p. 85). Pitsvada states that these transfers among various objects of expenditure occur at thresholds below which Congress would have to be notified. Pitsvada adds that, in general, Congress intercedes with specific constraints only if an agency has "performed in a manner that displeases Congress" (p. 86). Pitsvada concludes that the paradox of budget execution involves agencies, who feel they must have more flexibility to meet changing needs, and Congress, which feels that, unless it exercises meaningful control over execution, it is not performing its most vital constitutional power, the power of the purse.

The tension over the correct amount of control and flexibility in budget execution remains. Recently observers have suggested that too much control and controls of the wrong kind, impair program efficiency (see Jones & Thompson, 1994, Ch. 6), but with the growth in size of the federal budget converting small percentage errors into large dollar errors, the necessity for controls which ensure fiscal propriety contains powerful practical and symbolic value. Where managers might prefer more flexibility, the public insists that public monies be safeguarded, even if this results in more control than might be strictly necessary. Pitsvada (1983) believes budget execution is of fundamental importance because it is "...the entire reason that agencies prepare and justify budgets and Congress enacts them" (p. 100). He laments that budget execution remains the most neglected area of budget research and that this "paucity of research has existed for many decades" (p. 84), because budget execution is a "diverse complicated field that is filled with complex details" (p. 100). Nevertheless there are some patterns in budget execution that may be extracted for study.

BUDGET EXECUTION: PATTERNS OF ACCOMMODATION

Budget administrators have developed ways to cope with the uncertainty they face in budget execution. These are not patterns of optimization, but accommodation involving best estimate approximations that will provide for sub-optimal solutions and allow for continuing corrections over time, as opposed to rationalistic, optimized solutions based on perfect information, rational decision mechanisms, and a once and for all solution. Accommodating solutions may be seen in allotment and fund transfer patterns. Once the legislature has passed a budget or appropriation bill and the executive has signed it, decisions must be made about how to spend the money. Usually this is a fairly simple task, highly dependent on historical patterns. Most departments are forced to plan for the expenditure of their budget over the course of the fiscal year. This is usually done on a quarterly basis, although some departments might need to fine-tune this to a monthly pattern. In almost all instances, the allotment pattern follows the logic of budget construction and the numbers used to build the budget may be used to make out the allotment. This does not hold true for a budget where the administrator knows how much effort is required over the course of a fiscal year but does not know precisely when the work will be done in the fiscal year. The budget preparation process normally does not force stipulation of what quarters or months the money will be obligated in, but the budget execution process does. Thus, for simple functions, if the administrator knows the number of incoming units of work by quarter and the number of persons it takes to handle each case, he or she can then derive an allotment pattern. For example, suppose the unit doing temporary document processing expects to receive 100,000 units of work over the year, with 25,000 arriving in each quarter. Suppose it takes one clerk to handle each 5,000 units per quarter (This relationship may be derived from the unit's own history or history in comparable units). The unit will need (25,000 divided by 5,000) five clerks per quarter. If this is the only personnel requirement for this unit, the personnel budget can be estimated by multiplying the number of clerks per quarter times the correct salary rate (e.g., $18,000). Suppose for this function supporting expenses (paper and pencils, widgets), runs about 10% of the personnel costs, again derived from the unit's own experience or from an overall average. The allotment scheme for this simple program would be as follows:

Table 1. Allotment Example

Expense	Q1	Q2	Q3	Q4	Total
Pers Serv	$90,000	$90,000	$90,000	$90,000	$360,000
Support	$9,000	$9,000	$9,000	$9,000	$36,000
Totals	$99,000	$99,000	$99,000	$99,000	$396,000

This allotment then becomes a control document for reviewers within the unit and in the budget office. In the profile above, the allotment is spread equally over the four quarters; budgeteers often refer to this pattern as flat or level. Most units employing temporary employees have a skewed workload pattern, with different amounts of work occurring in each quarter. For example, an income tax processing unit might have 30% of its work coming in the January to March quarter (second quarter of the fiscal year) and 50% in the April to June quarter (third quarter) with the remainder equally divided between the first and last quarters. It is useful to note that the allotment process forces an administrator to incorporate a notion of within year time to budgetary calculations. This is not always easy to do. Sometimes administrators hedge their bets a little by allotting more money earlier than they expect the work to arrive. Thus if they need to they can gear up to meet a contingency without seeking approval from anyone else. In the example above, the height of the tax-filing season occurs in March and April, overlapping two quarters.

To avoid the possibility of a busy March filled with expectant refund filers and too few personnel, the administrator might allocate 40% to the January to March quarter and 40% to the April to June quarter, with any surplus from the quarter ending in March carrying into the quarter beginning in April. This "over-allotting" for the January to March quarter (allotted 40% of the budget for 30% of the work year) gives the administrator funds to meet unanticipated surprises in the workload environment, while carrying money not spent into the next quarter. If the jurisdiction will not allow surpluses to carry from quarter to quarter, this strategy does not work. Most jurisdictions allow for this kind of strategizing, except in times of severe fiscal constraint.

The allotment is also a means of controlling the budget expenditure pace. For example, if the fifth month of the budget year passes and personnel expenditures have already passed 50% of the personnel total on a flat function (spending should be 5/12ths or 42%), the administrator will have to take action to reduce the pace of spending for the rest of the fiscal year. The departmental budget execution people are likely to spot this pattern first. The allotment is also useful in warding off false alarms. Suppose, for example, that one is supplied with nothing but the budget for the income tax unit and its expenditure totals. After three quarters, this will show the unit spent 90% of its money with a full quarter yet to go (minus the time elapsed for the report to be generated). This could cause much panic and many desperate measures, unless the allotment plan for the unit was supplied and it indicated that a 90% expenditure rate was precisely where the unit intended to be after three quarters. Thus the allotment is a control document that also allows for variations from simple expectations about budget outlays.

During the execution phase of the budget, circumstances often change in ways that encourage administrators to modify their budget plans. All jurisdictions have set rules for these procedures. These can be quite complex and confusing to the uninitiated. At the federal level some transfers may be made by the agency without external notification, other transfers require notification and still others require approval. This is usually determined by the size of the amount to be transferred. However, Congress may insert special provisions in legislation to prohibit transfers into or out of a program or category in which it has a particular interest. For example, Congress may not want a program to get larger or smaller or it may not want the agency to add to or diminish the shape of the program it has created.

Sometimes emergency situations occur and funding is provided for them in vehicles called supplemental appropriations. These bills adjust current year funding levels. They may provide for natural disaster aid to states, regions and directly to people for blizzards, floods, drought, fires, and hurricanes. Supplementals helped out in the Mount St. Helens eruption in 1980 and the Loma Prieta earthquake in 1989 and the Northridge earthquake in 1994 and as part of an Urban Aid package after the riots in Los Angeles in 1992. No budget system could predict such events. Supplementals are also used for emergent military missions not foreseen in the DOD budget. When the President decides to evacuate embassy staff or rescue American citizens or deploy troops in an emergent peacekeeping action, these are emergency situations where the need happens almost overnight. DOD is authorized to carry out the mission. It does this by borrowing from the fourth quarter of its supporting expense budget, the operations and maintenance account, and then waiting for the supplemental appropriation to be passed to pay the account back so that its scheduled expenditures may be made. In the 26 years from 1974 through 1999, sixty-one supplemental appropriations were enacted, totaling more than 430 billion dollars. This is an average of $7 billion per year. The largest emergency supplemental was for the Persian Gulf War in 1991 and totaled $42.6 billion. In 1974 a supplemental was passed for $4.75 million. Twenty supplementals were passed from 1974 through 1979. In 1978 five were passed. More recent practice due to the discipline of the deficit and perhaps fewer natural disasters has seen fewer bills passed each year; only one supplemental was passed in 1995, 1996, 1997, and 1999. Over the 26-year period, the defense portion of supplementals averaged 19% and 6.5% if the Gulf War supplemental is set aside. Typically then, supplemental appropriations should be seen as a way for the President and Congress use to send immediate aid to a region, state or city and the individuals affected as a result of some natural disaster. Supplementals exist outside the scope of the budget preparation and execution processes. Nothing about them is predictable, except that Congress handles them expeditiously, in most cases introducing and passing them within a three-month period (Godek, 2000).

Agencies, conversely, need to have some discretion to take care of the more routine emergent events that happen within the scope of their own programs and budgets. Congress has officially recognized the need for agency discretion in budget execution since the growth of federal expenditures after World War II. Jones and Bixler (1992, pp. 58–60) suggest that the 1956 Defense Appropriations bill expressed Congressional policy on reprogramming that still remains in force. The report attached to the bill stated that there would always be some unforeseen changes in operating conditions and circumstances in the interval between building and presenting the budget and executing it. These might include changes in operating conditions, revisions in price estimates, wage rate adjustments and so on. Consequently, rigid adherence to the original budget might prevent the effective accomplishment of the planned program. The report cautions that it is not the intention of Congress to give the military departments unrestrained freedom to reprogram or shift funds from one category or purpose to another without prior notification and consent from the committee. Since 1959, Congress has emphasized prior approval before implementation of certain transfers, certain threshold requirements, and periodic reporting on issues of special interest to Congress. In 1974 Congress added a restriction that prohibited DOD from transferring funds to restore budget items specifically denied by Congress.

Jones and Bixler (1992) found that the Department of Defense classified reprogramming actions into four types.

1. *Prior Approval Reprogramming.* This occurs when DOD wants to increase the quantity of a purchase regardless of the dollar amount (e.g., increases in the number of missiles or aircraft purchased).

2. *Congressional Notification Reprogramming.* DOD notifies Congress when proposed reprogramming surpasses certain dollar thresholds or when it is for new programs or line items that may result in significant follow-on costs.

3. *Internal Reprogramming.* This includes changes within or between appropriation accounts but does not involve changes in programmatic use approved by Congress during the annual budget process.

4. *Below Threshold Reprogramming.* Reprogramming which occurs below the threshold set by Congress. This is coordinated by the military departments and a semiannual report is provided to Congress.[4]

Congressional interest can lead to complex guidance. In 1997, Congress imposed more restrictive guidelines upon DOD reprogramming. This meant for the Department of Navy that the prior notification threshold was lowered from $20 million to $15 million for ship, aircraft, or intermediate maintenance changes and $15 million was set as the threshold above which the Department would have to get approval to move money out of flying hours, ship operating tempo and real property maintenance categories. These thresholds vary over the years, sometimes as a product of the trust relationship between a department and the Congress; in the 1980s they were set at $10 million and advanced to $20 million in the 1990s after a period of harmonious relations between the department and Congress.

In the mid-1990s they were changed again to protect certain accounts from being bill-payers for others. These were expressions of Congressional interest and were attempts to control those accounts so that, for example, the Department of Navy would not move money out of these accounts to pay other bills without giving Congress a chance to approve the move prior to its execution. In practice, this meant any Department of Navy change would be first have to be approved at the Department of Defense level, then in OMB, and then by the House and Senate Appropriations and Authorization Committees. If some aspect of the transfer touched intelligence matters, then the House and Senate committees on intelligence matters would also have to approve the transfer. All it takes to block such a transfer is a no vote from one committee. Within the department, creating these more restrictive thresholds for prior approval meant that internal control systems had to be more closely monitored. For example, when two or three units are spending flying hour money and managing it to meet changing demands, their changes each may be below the threshold, but above the threshold when summed together.

In summary, there are reprogrammings that require specific written approval of the Secretary of Defense or his designee, others that require prior approval or timely notification of one or more Congressional Committees and still others that may be undertaken with Congress to be notified later in a semiannual report. The complexity of this process may make it seem as if a large share of the defense budget is reprogrammed. This is not so. Jones and Bixler note that a relatively low percentage of the defense budget is reprogrammed annually. From 1980 to 1990 the percent change in outlays reprogrammed averaged less than 1% of the Defense budget (.8%), ranging from a high of 1.2% in 1988 to .5% in 1981 and 1986 (Jones & Bixler, 1992, p. 60). Jones and Bixler speculate this is because the process is unwieldy due to the multiple levels of review and coordination and because congressional staffers seize upon reprogramming as an important micromanagement tool, hence the Defense Department (which they studied) and other departments and agencies avoid using reprogramming as a major policy vehicle. The requirement for semiannual reporting of below threshold reprogramming also provides a check on inappropriate use of reprogramming of funds.

Nonetheless, under Congressional thresholds, the agency has a great deal of flexibility in moving small amounts of money around to meet emergencies and to manage programs efficiently. These are generally called "below threshold reprogramming" and do not require prior submission to Congress or to the Secretary of Defense; they may be made at the discretion of the military department (Department of Army, Navy, or Air Force). For example, annually the report that accompanies the Department of Defense Appropriations Act contains language that grants to the Secretary of Defense authority, with the Office of Management and Budget, to transfer funds between appropriations and funds in the current fiscal year, upon determination that such action is necessary and in the national interest. These transfers are based on "unforeseen military requirements" and for "higher priority items than originally" appropriated. In no case are they to be for items specifically denied by Congress in the budget process. A dollar amount of transfer authority is usually set as a "not to exceed" target for the fiscal year. Once these transfers have been made, the Secretary of Defense must notify Congress of all transfers.[5]

In general the guiding principle of below threshold reprogramming involves staying true to legislative intent by not using (or creating and using) temporary surpluses to create long-term obligations. For example, suppose an agency has budgeted for a substantial capital outlay item (central office remodeling). Suddenly an emergency occurs in safety inspection, one that cannot be satisfied by overtime, and more personnel are needed. The agency determines it can get through this year and maybe next without the capital outlay item, thus it asks to transfer money from capital equipment to personnel. How should the budget analyst look at this request? What the agency is asking to do is to convert a one-time outlay into an every year outlay. If the request is approved, the new position or positions will go into the personnel base and have to be funded in subsequent years, thus creating a substantial continuing cost greater than the cost in this year and one that will continue to grow as the person (or persons) is given merit increases and promotions. Budget analysts call this "the camel's nose" and it is the type of expenditure that they delight in finding, exposing, and denying, if they can. It may be that the move has great political appeal (i.e., health and safety needs are often treated more kindly by the legislature than administrative systems improvements); if so it might be unstoppable, although the budget analyst would ask why this could not be put into the next year's budget. In this example, the agency risks losing the money for remodeling for a long time. After all, the reprogramming means that the remodeling was not really that high a priority to the agency and it will be some time before the agency can again present it to reviewers and expect them to fund it.

Out of this emerges a hierarchy of transfers, which says that transferring continuing money into one-time expenditures is acceptable, but the reverse is not. Creating long-term obligations for the agency budget is something that should be blessed by the legislature and not hidden away in the day-to-day operation of budget execution. In the following table, it is assumed there is a surplus in the first category and the manager has asked to transfer funds to cover a shortfall in the second. The second column considers long-term considerations and the third column indicates a judgment to approve or disapprove the transfer.

Table 2.   Transfer Consequences

Proposed transfer (from/to):	Long-term consequences	Approve or deny
Personnel to buy desks	Negligible	Approve
Personnel to office supplies	Negligible	Approve
Travel to personnel	Yes	Deny
Telephone services to office supplies	Negligible	Approve
Office supplies to local phones	Yes	Deny
Personnel to computer repair	Yes (if not done)	Approve
Personnel to buy computer system	Yes	Deny
Travel to long distance calls	?	?
Office supplies to temporary labor	?	?

In the last two cases in Table 2, some further analysis is necessary. For example, it could be that a transfer from the travel budget would allow for accomplishment of the mission in this instance by making long distance calls rather than on site visits. Thus, this may be a superior substitute to what is being done now, and cheaper. The same may be true of the transfer of money from office supplies to temporary labor. It may allow for hiring personnel on a temporary basis to meet a need in the current year while avoiding a long-term burden on the unit's personnel budget. This assumes either that the office supply budget has some slack in it or that the agency can control that portion of its budget to create that slack. If budgets were perfect, there would be little slack and, if the world were predictable, fiscal emergencies would not occur. Given the world as it is, there must be a continuous traffic in budget adjustments, of differing sizes and impacts and with differing levels of review mandated.

Even transferring funds within the same category can have implications that affect budget execution in future years. For example, as of this writing, Congress allowed departments to reprogram up to $10 million within the same procurement appropriation, without prior approval. Thus, if the negotiations for a contract scheduled to be awarded in the 4th quarter have not been completed on time, the money earmarked for that contract could be reprogrammed into another program with a funding shortfall. Until the start of the next fiscal year, both programs would then be able to continue. However, the donor program will eventually need the money when the contract negotiations have been completed. That will require either a restructuring of the program to accommodate the reduced funding or reprogramming money from another program. Therefore, even though the rules allow it, money is available, and there is a need, the long-term perturbations may dictate against approval.

Not all budget adjustments are the result of internal actions and not all budget increases are beneficial. Congress frequently adds "special interest" items to the department budgets. To the uninitiated, these additions often appear to be a real boon for the department. Nowhere is this so apparent as in the Department of Defense. For example, for a number of years Congress added money for the Air Force to purchase additional C-130 transport aircraft despite the fact that the Air Force did not request the aircraft and had no requirement for them within their current inventory. In 1997, $142.2 million was added for the procurement of three additional C-130J aircraft to the Air Force budget request for four. The Senate Authorization Committee Report language acknowledged that the Air Force had no requirement, yet the money was added for political reasons. Congress did not, however, add $142.2 million to the Defense Budget to pay for the additional aircraft. Instead DOD was directed to find the money in its current budget. This meant that one or more programs that DOD had requested and had a bona fide need for were either not funded or under funded. Additionally, there is a logistics tail associated with each of the aircraft that includes support equipment, maintenance personnel, fuel and oil, and flight crews. None of these items was funded, which meant that even more programs would be under funded. The service life of each of the aircraft is 20 to 30 years. Thus, the $142 million "gift" in 1997 will result in budget perturbations within DOD for the life of these aircraft.

One last point of interest is the ability of Congress, and the President's Office of Management and Budget for that matter, to structure the control points for the organization. Budgets are passed at different levels of detail, but they are almost always more detailed than the final numbers that appear in appropriations bills. What is assumed is that the budget will be administered in the way it was built. If the budget number was arrived at by computing the cost of five new employees and their supporting expenses, then what is assumed is that the agency will use the appropriated money to execute that plan, minus whatever amounts reviewers have pared off. What usually happens is that the central budget office reports back any changes in the agency's request made in its legislative passage. As it administers its program the agency has some latitude to set what the barrier points are for its subdivisions. For example, central authorities may only require that the agency control the totals for personnel and supporting expenses. But the agency itself may choose to require subordinate managers to report in more detail, for example in terms of line items that go to make up its major expense categories (e.g., personnel, travel, computer supplies, computer maintenance, office supplies, utility costs, rent, and capital outlay).

This provides managers with the necessary information to build budgets by providing them with cost data and leaves them with a template to execute the budget according to the way it was built. Because the agency's control is set at the total number, it then has flexibility to shift money between line items and between subprograms, while still keeping within the total dollar amount for personnel and supporting expenses. Table 3 supposes an agency with two programs, each with three subprograms, and each subprogram with a budget for objects of expenditure.

Table 3. Execution Template Example

Program	Subprogram	Object of Expenditure
Income tax	Processing	personnel, supporting expenses
	Filing	personnel, supporting expenses
	Auditing	personnel, supporting expenses
Sales tax	Processing	personnel, supporting expenses
	Filing	personnel, supporting expenses
	Auditing	personnel, supporting expenses

If controls are set at the subprogram level, then the agency may transfer money from its sales tax auditing function to its sales tax processing function (as may the income tax unit), but it may not transfer anything from sales tax to income tax. The same rules as discussed above would apply between transfers from one category to another: transfers from personnel to supporting expenses are favored more than from supporting expenses to personnel. If the control is set at the departmental level, then it may transfer money among programs. Controls may also be set at the object of expenditure level, with programs being the subordinate category. Here transfers may be done horizontally, but not vertically.

If controls are set at the object of expenditure level, then the department may have the flexibility to transfer among personnel in income and sales tax or in the travel account between income and sales tax, but not between the personnel and travel accounts. Nonetheless, the department may still make the income and sales tax administrators operate as if they were on separate budgets. Usually these structures are negotiated between the central budget office and the agency for it is a responsibility of the central budget office to oversee budget execution at the appropriate level.

Table 4.   Crosswalk Showing Program Resources by Object of Expenditure (Line Item)

Item	Income tax	Sales tax	Total
Personnel	100000	50000	150000
Travel	10000	5000	15000
Computer	1000	1000	2000
Office supplies	4000	3000	7000
Rent	10000	5000	15000
Utilities	2000	1000	3000
Total	127000	65000	192000

In the federal government departments may also choose at what level they wish to set responsibility for anti-deficiency violations. The higher the level, the more flexibility an administrator has to move money around. When an administrator knows a unit is in for a difficult year, he may set the anti-deficiency responsibility one level higher in the organization, thus giving him the ability to move money into that unit from others in case of a shortfall, exempting the unit from a legal charge of overspending the budget. The control is still on within the agency, so the budget number will not be overspent, but some relief is offered the lower level manager. Conversely, an administrator may wish to punish or force a careful spending pattern on an administrator; he can do this by pressing the anti-deficiency responsibility down in the organization, by placing it on the administrator he wished to control. Any shortfalls then become legal matters and the hope is that the threat of legal sanctions will create a more prudent manager. If the manger does not have control over a turbulent environment, then this strategy will not work. That legal frameworks do not always supply the anticipated behavior may be found in the federal government's constant battle to fend off a "spend it up" mentality in the fourth quarter, indeed the last month, of the fiscal year. In the next section, we turn to the fourth quarter phenomenon.

BUDGET EXECUTION PATTERNS

In their introduction to *Reinventing Government,* Osborne and Gaebler (1992) state that the federal budget system encourages managers to waste money:

> If they don't spend their entire budget by the end of the fiscal year, three things happen: they lose the money they have saved; they get less next year; and the budget director scolds them for requesting too much last year. Hence the time honored rush to spend all funds by the end of the fiscal year. (p. 3)

Federal budget managers participate in this rush. They must obligate their money before the end of the fiscal year or else they lose it. Table 5 shows the obligation rate of the defense department Operations and Maintenance (O&M) account. This account is analogous to the supporting expense category in most other budgets; it funds everything from steaming hours to flying hours, from yellow tablets to yellow paint. It does not fund military personnel, weapon systems procurement or research and development. This account is closely watched, for it is a major contributor to training and readiness and to the ability of DOD to go places and do things. It is also closely watched when new missions emerge or budget reductions are necessary. To assume a new, unbudgeted, mission in the national interest within a fiscal year often means finding money in the O&M accounts and spending it, with the reimbursement coming later. When quick budget reductions are needed, the O&M account is often the first target, because it is usually spent out in one year and a dollar reduction means a dollar of saving in the particular year, while the ship procurement account may require $20 of reductions in program over the life of the item to get one dollar of reduction in the current year, because ship construction is a multiple year account. In sum, the O&M account, which averages more than 35% of the DOD appropriation (Perry, 1996, p. B-1), is a sensitive and important account that funds much of the daily business of DOD. By the same token, it requires close and skillful management.

Kozar studied the DOD O&M account over 14 fiscal years (FY1977 through FY1990) and found O&M account managers obligating more than 99% of their funds before the appropriation expired at the end of the year (Kozar, 1993, p. 73). This is a remarkable performance by these fund managers, given legal constraints and penalties against overspending.[6] However, within this orderly pattern of commitment of resources, there were quarterly variations and monthly variations, and variations among the Military Departments.

Table 5.   Average DOD O&M Monthly Obligation Rates With High-Low Ranges (Percent) 1977–1990

Month	Average	High	Low
October**	11.235	12.30	9.83
November	8.018	9.73	7.03
December	7.346	8.18	6.47
January*	10.048	11.42	8.11
February	7.165	8.35	6.10
March	7.223	7.96	5.65
April*	9.083	10.61	8.30

Table 5.   Average DOD O&M Monthly Obligation Rates With High-Low Ranges (Percent) 1977–1990 (Cont.)

Month	Average	High	Low
May	6.708	7.61	6.09
June	6.726	7.49	5.89
July*	8.778	10.57	7.43
August	6.887	7.39	6.17
September	10.616	12.05	9.78
Total	99.833		

Note: High = highest October and low = lowest October in 14 year period, ** = start of fiscal year; * = first month of quarter.
Source: Kozar, "O&M Total Obligations" (pp. 132–133).

In general, the *first and last* months of the fiscal year are the highest spending months. October generally surges as a result of new contracts being let. The summer is low as year-end positioning takes place and then September is high as managers rush to spend their funds on what had been planned for and those new needs that have arisen. October shows the highest rate of commitment of funds and the first two months show a higher rate than any other two months of the year. September illustrates the end of year spending surge; it was the second highest individual month and the rate of change from the preceding month to it (53.6%) exceeded any other pair of months. The fact that August is the lowest month of the year helps create this relationship. There is also evidence of a quarterly trend. The months that start quarters (January, April, and July) are the third, fourth and fifth highest months, behind only October and September (October has a double bonus; it starts both the fiscal year and a quarter). The first month of any quarter is high and the next two months low. Thus, there is a substantial change from the last month of a quarter to the first month of a new quarter. This would seem to indicate the existence of quarterly allotment patterns, or at least that new money has become available with the opening of each quarter. The quarterly pattern would seem to indicate that each quarter has pressing needs that are met in the first month of the quarter. Interestingly the surge does not take place from one fiscal year to another; the change from September to October is only 5.6%. This is primarily due to the surge in September. Therefore, there is more variation within the year than there is from one year to the next for DOD as a whole. This changes for the individual Military Departments. The Army actually decreases from September to October, perhaps indicating that it fills many fall needs with September spending, while Air Force increases dramatically from September to October, perhaps indicating that it really needs the new fiscal year money. It is the average of these fluctuations that make it appear that there is little intra-departmental turbulence around the close of the fiscal year and the start of a new one.

The data in Table 6 are presented in a monthly format for DOD and the Military Departments.[7] Not only are there quarterly and monthly variations, but obligation rates also vary by Military Department, particularly in the first month of the fiscal year.

Table 6.   O&M Monthly Obligation (Percent) 1977–1990

Month	DOD	Air Force	Army	Navy
October**	11.235	14.192	9.188	11.690
November	8.018	8.520	8.059	7.736
December	7.346	6.815	7.968	7.212
January*	10.048	10.526	9.117	10.814
February	7.165	6.224	7.851	7.429
March	7.223	6.251	7.979	7.166
April*	9.083	9.399	8.209	9.690
May	6.708	6.159	7.046	6.445
June	6.726	5.881	7.141	6.490
July*	8.778	9.324	8.113	8.525
August	6.887	6.173	7.276	6.670
September	10.616	10.662	12.473	9.319
Total	99.833	100.130	100.420	99.186

Note: Percentages exceed 100 due to rounding; ** = start of fiscal year; * = first month of quarter.

Graphs 1 and 2 clearly demonstrate the cyclical nature of those obligations. October, the first month of the fiscal year is the highest. Then the first month of the next three quarters are high, but lower than October, with average obligation rates decreasing during the fiscal year, with September, the last month of the fiscal year, representing a significant surge, exhibiting an obligation rate only slightly lower than October. There are two legal bases for these patterns. The first may be found in the U.S. Code, Title 31 Section 1512, Apportionment and Reserves which states that an appropriation available for obligation for a definite period should be apportioned to prevent obligation or expenditure at a rate that would indicate a necessity for a supplemental or deficiency appropriation for the period. An appropriation subject to apportionment may be apportioned by months, calendar quarters, operating seasons, or other time periods.

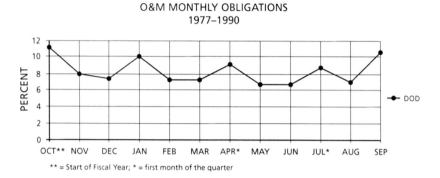

Graph 1.   Obligation rates.

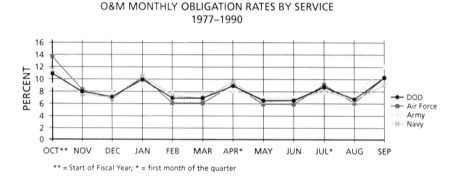

Graph 2.   O&M monthly obligation rates by service (1977–1990).

O&M appropriations are apportioned by calendar quarters by the Office of Management and Budget under the authority of Title 31 Section 1513. The apportionments, available on a cumulative basis unless reapportioned by OMB, are based on input from the Military Departments through the Secretary of Defense, as is the case for other department secretaries who receive information from their component agencies and bureaus. According to Title 31 Section 1514, the Department Secretaries are then responsible for enacting regulations to administratively control and divide the apportionment. The system is designed to limit obligations to the amount apportioned, to fix responsibility for violations of the apportionments, and to provide a simple way to administratively divide the appropriation between commands. Apportionments are an effective tool for preventing too rapid an obligation of total funds at any point in the fiscal year. However, because funds are available on a cumulative basis, apportionments are better able to prevent obligation surges at the beginning of the fiscal year than at the end of the fiscal year (Kozar & McCaffery, 1994, p. 3). The data in Graph 1 clearly show an end of year spending surge. When compared to the actual average obligation rate of the last month of each of the first three quarters (7.098%), September's rate of 10.616% is 49.6% higher.

The second legal basis for these patterns may be found in Title 31 Section 1502 of the United States Code which states that the balance of an appropriation or fund limited for obligation to a definite period is available only for payment of expenses properly incurred during the period of availability, or to complete contracts properly made within that period of availability and obligated consistent with Section 1501. A balance remaining in an appropriation account at the end of the period of availability must be returned to the general fund of the Treasury according to this section. This is reiterated annually in the general provisions of Appropriations Acts that typically state for DOD and other departments that, "...no part of any appropriation contained in this Act shall remain available for obligation beyond the current fiscal year, unless expressly so provided herein."

As a matter of practice, the budget execution box in which the funds administrator is forced to work is bounded by appropriation life, appropriation size, and the penalties associated with either over- or underspending. The first quarter surge reflects the award of annual service contracts that must be in place for the entire fiscal year but cannot be awarded until money is appropriated and allocated for a new fiscal year. The second and third quarters each start with a "surge" as quarterly allocations are received in the first month. However, overall spending is tempered by the realization that funds must last for the entire fiscal year. Some funding is held in reserve for unknown contingencies. That funding is held until the end of the fourth quarter when it is spent on those contingencies or, more likely, to cover requirements deferred from earlier in the year. In either case, the money *is* spent.

When the O&M appropriation expires at the end of the fiscal year, any unobligated funds, with few exceptions, are lost. This gives managers a very strong incentive to spend all available funds and explains the 99% obligation rate and the September surge. The obligation rate data indicate that DOD managers, as those in other departments, are highly skilled at obligating funds before the end of the fiscal year and are able to commit substantial funds quickly in September, despite numerous rules and provisions designed to forestall this process (e.g., to prevent abuses in commitments of funds). Federal funds managers must find valid current fiscal year needs to legally justify obligating the funds before the remaining obligational authority expires.

Undoubtedly, some of these September purchases help meet needs in the next fiscal year and thus by supporting purchases other than current fiscal year needs, funds can be freed up in the next fiscal year which is, in September, less than 30 days away.[8] Managers in the O&M accounts know they are managing a multiple year stream of resources. Replacing inventory or beginning a ship or aircraft overhaul are examples of obligations the manager may take at the end of the current fiscal year to meet fiscal burdens which he certainly would have had to meet in the next fiscal year. The O&M account is not a neat and orderly world. Prices and inflation rates change; commodity prices fluctuate; operating tempos change from what was anticipated and fund managers must adjust to these changes. This means that they pay the bills they must when they must, like service contracts that come due at the first of the year and in the first month of each quarter, and then hold back a little on other items that can be postponed until later in the year.

For example, although it is a small percentage of the total funds, the item for "Equipment" in the Department of Navy O&M appropriation shows a large peak in obligations near the end of the fiscal year.[9] This category includes items such as motor vehicles, furniture, machinery, ADP equipment, armaments, instruments, and appliances. Overall, an average of 41% of O&M Navy equipment obligations occurred during August and September (Kozar & McCaffery, 1994, p. 19).

This pattern is understandable from the point of view of budget managers. The equipment purchase category constitutes a source of flexibility. If a piece of equipment scheduled for replacement is still operational, the unit may be willing to delay replacing it until closer to the end of the fiscal year, then if no higher priority need appears, it may purchase the item or items previously budgeted. By accepting uncertainty and delaying certain purchases, the financial manager provides some slack that may help reduce the impact of unpredictable events upon him. Toward the end of one fiscal year, budget managers are also positioning themselves for the next fiscal year by examining actions they can take in this year which will help them meet the burdens of the following year.

EXECUTION PROCESSES AND PROBLEMS

The problems associated with budget execution are captured in the old saw, "Where you stand depends on where you sit."[10] The layers of management faced by a comptroller in the federal government can severely limit the options available to make the adjustments needed to correct an emergent problem. Typically, the higher the level, the more control an organization has over its own resources. Yet the nature and size of the problems also change with the various levels. For example, when departments receive the funds apportioned by OMB they, in turn, allocate those funds to the agencies within their jurisdiction. Typically, a portion of these funds is withheld to accommodate either known or potential problems. If funding for programs has been appropriated but not authorized, that money may be withheld pending negotiations with the authorizing committees. Similarly, those programs that received funding in excess of the President's budget request may have the additional funds withheld as a source of funding for contingencies. Those programs that anticipate additional funding have to proceed with the uncertainty associated with any rescission list, that is, will the list be submitted and if so, when, and will it be approved by Congress? At the very least, any actions must be delayed until the end of the process. If Congress does not approve the rescission, an already late allocation will be even later. If the rescission is approved, there will be no funding at all. Given that the Congress has 45 days to approve a rescission after the President proposes it, the funds will not be available for obligation, at the earliest, until one to two quarters into the fiscal year. When the President and OMB add an item to a rescission list, internal practice typically is to defer execution of spending until the outcome of the rescission action is known.

The following section analyzes some of the issues that are common to all levels of budget execution. However, while they are common, they affect each of the levels to a differing degree. Table 7 provides an indication of who is affected by what, and how much flexibility parties affected have to respond to problems at their level. Each of the issues is expanded upon subsequently in this chapter.

Table 7. Manageability of Budget Execution Issues

Issue (Problem)	Level		
	Local	Headquarters	Agency
Taxes (Administrative)	1	2	3
Timeliness	1	2	2
Discretionary Dollars	1	2	2–3
Color of Money	1	1	1–2
Politics	1	1	2
Flexibility	1	2	2
Management Information Systems	2	2	2

Table 7 assigns a number to each of the issues or problems noted to indicate their judgment of its manageability. That manageability typically varies with the level at which the problem is experienced. Manageability as it relates to the ability to control a problem at a certain level is scaled as follows: 1 = Little ability to control at this level; 2 = Some ability to control at this level; and 3 = A great deal of ability to control at this level.

Withholding Funds for Flexibility

At nearly every level of budget control, fund administrators have a tendency to save or set aside a "little off the top" of the funds they administer to accommodate either known or anticipated contingencies.[11] These "withholds" can range, for example, from those imposed by Congress such as the 2% reduction applied to all Department of the Navy procurement and research and development programs in FY 1997 to pay for a shortfall in the Defense Business Operations Fund; to a 1 to 2% withhold by the Department of the Navy to all Operations and Maintenance accounts; to a base Commanding Officer keeping a small percentage of his operating funds in reserve until toward the end of the fiscal year.[12] While each of these actions may be known early in the year, each requires an adjustment to the level of spending which had been justified in the budget-planning phase. Because budgeting for contingencies is not allowed officially in Appropriations Law and budget submissions are carefully examined to eliminate "excess" (poorly justified) funding proposals, a withhold, by definition, means that the money received at the lower levels is less than that requested or anticipated as a result of what was requested and then appropriated. Additionally, if the "contingency" does not materialize, money that had been set aside will likely be released late in the fiscal year, requiring additional perturbations to the revised plan under execution.

Timeliness

All budgets are premised on a spending plan that assumes receipt of funds at a certain time. In a perfect world, Congress would finish deliberations in time to pass authorization and appropriations bills by the first of October. Treasury would be ready to issue its warrants and OMB to apportion the money on the first day of the fiscal year, with the receiving agencies following closely behind. In that the first step rarely occurs on time, none of the follow up steps can be timely either.[13] This entails adjustments to the plans upon which the budgets were approved. In the case of a Continuing Resolution Authority (CRA), Congress typically specifies not only the level of spending but also imposes other restrictions (e.g., no spending on new program starts). Spending levels are normally limited to prior year rates or the lower of the House or Senate versions of the appropriations bill, assuming that a conference between the House and Senate has not yet taken place. For a program that is fairly new, reverting to a spending profile that matches that of the previous year may require laying off employees, postponing tests and delaying contract awards.

Over the course of the previous fiscal year, a new program typically will have hired additional people, started testing and increased the rate of spending in other areas. If the program must revert to a pre-expansion level of spending because of a CRA, inefficiencies, additional startup costs, and other costs will be the inevitable result, requiring program restructures and perhaps additional funding. Whenever funding is not received when it is anticipated, budget execution is affected.[14]

Discretionary Dollars

The greater the flexibility and control available to the manager over the dollars allocated to any entity or programs, the easier it is to execute a budget. The degree of control over the dollars allocated in federal organizations depends on the amount and the level of specificity tied to each dollar by Executive branch and congressional budget control agents. Obviously, if a certain number of employees must be paid a specific amount of dollars and these amounts are all that are available, there is little discretion for the budget manager. Unless employee attrition occurs, there is little flexibility to accommodate changes in work requirements or to pay for promotions, to give bonuses or commit to other spending actions. However, if a comptroller has access to additional funding, the ability to pay overtime or hire additional workers is present should the workload dictate such action. The availability of discretionary dollars typically is directly proportional to the strata of management in the organization. This is not surprising given the increase in the level of aggregation of funds at higher levels. If there are 1000 employees in a major organization, accommodating the departure and replacement of 25 employees across the organization is relatively simple. However, at a lower level, the replacement of 2 employees out of a 20-person workforce could cause major problems. Moreover, with no turnover, the smaller unit manager accrues no slack in the personnel account to use to meet unforeseen needs.

Specific Categories

Money is appropriated in specific categories identified in appropriation language or language written into reports that accompany spending legislation, each having specific rules and limitations. The categories of appropriations restrict the manner in which a budget can be executed. While all dollars are the same, restrictions make the use of these dollars so different they might as well be of different colors. For example, in the defense department the Operations and Maintenance appropriation has a one-year life and finances the cost of ongoing operations (e.g., base operations, civilian personnel salaries, maintenance of property, training) Aircraft Procurement has a three-year life and finances the procurement of aircraft and related supporting programs. Military Construction has a five-year life and finances the purchase of land and construction of facilities. The restrictions on each of these appropriations create legal boundaries that put the budget manager in a "box" with walls that are difficult to breach. The ability to move money from one account to another is normally beyond the control of lower level funds administrators. Should one account or sub-account have too little money and another too much, typically it is not a simple matter to shift money from one to the other. This can only be accomplished within the restrictions imposed by such mechanisms as reprogrammings, transfers, supplemental appropriations and concomitant glacial approval processes, first within the Executive branch and then, for some types of flexibility, within Congress.

Politics

While there is no question that the budget formulation and approval processes have political dimensions, it might be surprising to some to find out about the degree to which the budget execution process is politicized. In general terms, any congressional special interest items for "the folks back home" (i.e., "pork") have the potential to change a budget plan. Assuming a zero sum game, if Congress adds three C-130 aircraft to the President's Budget Request for the defense department, the C-130 program manager has to make changes to adjust for the additional aircraft in everything from the quantity of training materials to the amount of support equipment required. Additionally, some other portion of the budget must be reduced to pay for the additional aircraft and support, causing perturbations to programs unrelated to the C-130 program. This is the double-edged sword of special item additions or "plus-ups" in congressional language. Not only does such spending rearrange the spending and policy priorities of the agency, it creates new fiscal burdens to bear that are not funded and must be taken from the base of support for existing programs.

Oftentimes, decisions are made by Congress with respect to a preference for specific suppliers of services to government, both foreign and domestic, that have little or nothing to do with agency requirements, but are driven by political considerations. For example, in the past, nuclear submarines for the Navy have been constructed in two domestic shipyards ostensibly to maintain an "industrial base," even though a single shipyard has the capacity to build all the required submarines. Using two shipyards increases costs and delays contract awards, but it also ensures that workers from two states and many more congressional districts are employed. Buying products overseas to satisfy commitments to foreign governments certainly affects the execution process when congressional language specifies such things as currency exchange rates. Requirements to hire minority firms, to buy American, to ensure that facilities and equipment fit both men and women, all have political origins, some narrowly designed to reward special interests and some based on social equity concerns. Regardless of motive, all such restrictions affect budget execution. Additionally, agency program managers may adopt political strategies to enhance the life of their programs. For example, ensuring that contracts are let in as many congressional districts as possible may enhance the attractiveness of the program in Congress, but it also complicates the execution of the program by increasing the number of contracts and contractors.

Flexibility

Flexibility in the budget execution process means the ability to make adjustments within the resources that have been allocated. As noted with respect to discretion, the higher the level of management in the organization, generally the greater the degree of flexibility. However, at the local level, dollars for maintenance and repair are typically not tied to specific buildings or projects. The local manager can decide to use dollars to fix a leaking roof or paint a building. But there may not be the flexibility to do both. If money is appropriated to construct a new building, there is essentially no option other than to build that building, even if repairing another building would be more cost-effective. Thus the degree of flexibility depends on the amount of money available as well as the specificity with which it is authorized and appropriated. Even "common sense" decisions are sometimes restricted. For example, in 1988, a program manager for a missile program negotiated a contract that would have allowed him to procure eight more missiles for the same amount of money. However, he could not sign that contract without prior congressional approval because the missiles were line item appropriated with the quantity specified. While it seems to make sense to buy the additional assets under these conditions, some members of Congress may argue against it on the grounds that only the original number of missiles was necessary and any money saved should be put elsewhere.

In sum, Congressional approval of changes like this is neither quick nor certain. There are many additional examples of the restrictions on flexibility that might be cited here, but the basic point is simple—Congress and budget control agencies in the Executive attempt to restrict flexibility for reasons that are explained at the end of this chapter. However, it is also useful to note that experienced budget managers know how to gain additional flexibility in the systems within which they work. For every rule that reduces flexibility, there are probably three ways that experienced managers have learned to get around the restrictions without detection or violation of the Anti-deficiency Act or other parts of federal Appropriations Law. Budget officers often state, when they are confronted with the imposition of controls that create problems as the budget is formulated, debated and enacted that, "We will have to fix that in execution." And there are many ways in which this happens. (See Appendix B: Case Study of the Navy Flight Hour Program Cash Management Process.)

Management Information Systems

We do not claim that our list is exhaustive and covers all constraints on budget execution. Our effort is more to illustrate the types of constraints that are present. In this regard it is necessary to cite one final area of constraint. Budget comptrollers in the federal government are often at the mercy of their management information systems, particularly accounting systems, to provide specifics on funds available, funds obligated and funds expended, as well as for preparation of what often seems like an endless stream of special reports, some of which with very short deadlines (e.g., in a matter of hours or one or two days).

Manual ledger sheets are long gone (except in small offices where bookkeepers maintain parallel records to insure accuracy) with their labor-intensive and inflexible routines, but automated systems with their speed and versatility also have their problems. As with any system, the quality of the input directly affects the quality of the output. If account or sub-account category definitions are not accurate or understandable, and if staffs are not trained or motivated to record data at the source of transactions accurately, entry errors are inevitable. Budget officers may not know how to simplify and clarify data entry instructions. Typically, the budget comptroller has little or no control over inputs and insufficient resources for training accounting staff, many of which are employed at very low compensation levels. Data inputs may be made in distant field activities or in a contractor's facility, or worse, not at all. Some accounting systems inevitably are not compatible with the systems of other organizations or units which, in turn, means manual intervention with all its attendant risks of error, becomes necessary to compile data "creatively" drawing information from different systems.

In 1993, the Department of Defense had 270 financial management information systems. It also had $24 billion of unmatched disbursements (see Perry, 1996, p. 107). That is, bills had been paid but who had been paid and out of what accounts they had been paid could not be determined. Contractors were not demanding payments so it was logical to assume that they had been paid. Yet, how they had been paid and how much they had been paid was a mystery. Errors ranged from simple numerical transpositions (not surprising when strings of manually entered numbers and letters are 16 characters long or longer); to funds paid out of the wrong appropriations or the wrong years. Budget execution documentation and records at local levels often did not match those at the headquarters levels. Executing a budget without precisely knowing the status of funds and accounts, causes stress for even the most experienced budget comptrollers. Fear of Anti-deficiency Act violations and damaging audits is endemic in the budget offices of the federal government.

THE HIDDEN SIDE OF BUDGET EXECUTION

Financial managers must meet the challenges of a turbulent environment, but their discretion is circumscribed by custom, rules, Congressional intercessions and, fundamentally, by law. The Anti-deficiency Act, the common name for Title 31 Sections 1341, 1349, 1350, 1512-14, and 1517-19, prevents managers from obligating more funds than are available and from obligating funds before an appropriation is enacted unless provided for by a Continuing Resolution. Title 31 Section 1341 includes limits on the expenditure and obligation of funds and states that an officer or employee of the United States Government may not make or authorize an expenditure or obligation exceeding the amount available in an appropriation for the expenditure or obligation; or involve the government in a contract or obligation for the payment of money before an appropriation is made unless authorized by law.

Penalties for those who break this law can be substantial. Often, they can end careers. Penalties range from administrative discipline to criminal prosecution that can include suspension without pay, removal from office, fines up to $5,000, and imprisonment for two or more years.[15] The same penalties apply to officials who authorize exceeding apportionments, allotments, or operating budgets as to those who actually commit the errors. Penalties associated with a willful act are more severe than those associated with a violation caused by ignorance or negligence, yet violation punishment does not depend on intent. Typically, a willful act results from an attempt to circumvent statutory laws through creative bookkeeping involving a violation of Title 31, Section 1301 that restricts the expenditure of funds to the purposes for which they are appropriated.

As an example of the former, the comptroller of an agency de-obligated (removed) funds from valid and known obligations in September, understanding that the expenditures would not be recorded as of September 30 by the supporting accounting activity. The comptroller knew that there would be a 3 to 6 month delay in posting the expenditures against de-obligated, yet still valid, requirements. Those funds were then obligated for additional requirements in the fiscal year for which funding was not previously available. As a result, expenditures exceeded the authorization for that year. In this case a violation occurred through a willful attempt to manipulate the system. This type of transaction is common; some are detected but most are not, otherwise comptrollers would not engage in such questionable and risky behavior. Still, actions of this type are often the result of good intentions to put money where it is most needed and will be best used. However, this is not always the case. Where fraud and abuse occur, it should be detected and punished. However, given the size of the federal government and the amount of money spent every day, and especially given the drive to "spend it or lose it" at the end of the fiscal year, and where underfunding is endemic, strong incentives exist to cause some budget officials to try to bend the rules under good intentions.

In another case, a part costing $7,900 was ordered. The part was not in stock and was backordered. While awaiting delivery, a temporary repair was made using spares. The idea was to pay back the spares when the requisitioned part arrived. Unfortunately, the replacement part did not arrive for three years, and when it did arrive, the unit delivery price had risen to $57,000. Sufficient unobligated funding was not available to cover the difference from the original year appropriation in which the part had been ordered, resulting in a violation of the Anti-deficiency Act because of the lack of an adequate tracking system.

In yet another example, various items of equipment were purchased with specific account funds. These items could not function independently; however, when assembled with other items purchased or added to an existing system, they created a complete and functioning system. The aggregate cost of all the equipment items that had either created or become part of a system exceeded the expense/investment criteria in place during the fiscal year in which the funding was appropriated. Initially, a Sec. 1301 violation occurred because the items were purchased from the wrong appropriation. Then a Sec. 1517 violation resulted because there was insufficient funding in the "correct" appropriation account to pay for the items that had been received.

Some scholars have argued that the laws and rules that surround financial management substantially decrease mission performance, efficiency, and effectiveness. Jones and Thompson argue that controls on budget execution ought to be tailored to the type of good produced, with simple and homogeneous goods relying on after the fact controls (ex post) and complex and new goods relying on before the fact controls (ex ante). Differentiation would also occur by type of organization and degree of probable competition to produce the good. Ultimately, a more appropriate and effective, and less costly, set of controls would be developed.[16] Until this happens, federal financial managers will have to cope with a turbulent environment and the compendious constraints that inhibit entrepreneurial and often cost-effective behavior while punishing illegal actions that in some cases result from legitimate efforts to meet program requirements. Still, we should not lose sight of the fact that management and budget control is absolutely necessary for the proper functioning of all organizations. The trick is to balance the degree of control with flexibility and discretion, and to accept that some types of apparent errors expose correctable weaknesses or the inadequacy of control system design. After all, the purpose of management control systems is, ultimately, to motivate employees to make cost-effective decisions while maintaining proper safeguards over the expenditure of public funds.

CONCLUSIONS

The reality of daily life in any large bureaucracy is that some administrators spend a great deal of time managing the execution of budgets. The reasons for this differ but one principle is critical: budget planning cannot ever anticipate the numerous contingencies that emerge as spending occurs. The world of public policy and finance in the federal government, with its vast range of responsibilities and programs, is highly complex. Some tasks of government are simple and are simply executed. However, many seemingly simple tasks become complex in implementation—and budget execution is at the heart of policy implementation in government. Let us consider what can go wrong using a simple example.[17] We may suppose that as a budget request is being negotiated, the whole budget process becomes delayed and a new fiscal year begins without an enacted budget—a fairly common occurrence. The manager cannot start some programs, and when this becomes possible, they will begin during the fiscal year. If far enough into the year, the manager may have to double the labor component. Is there the necessary permission to hire twice the number of positions to make up for a work backlog? If not, the manager cannot implement the program. Many federal government systems are controlled both by dollars appropriated and number of positions. The manager may have the dollars available, but not the positions. How about overtime as a solution? This depends on how many dollars are available and the overtime rate. Will this mean weekend work at an even higher rate? How about a combination of permanent and temporary labor? Will this mean unequal pay for similar work, and if so, will this result in a grievance, complaint or strike? Is this an outdoor project? It could be that if it begins late, weather will interfere or make it more expensive (e.g., for heaters, delays, overtime on good days).

Alternatively, let us assume that the budget is passed on time. May it be assumed the project will be implemented as designed? What if the labor market has tightened and hiring people with appropriate skills is difficult or increased on the job training is necessary? What if the personnel office has to rewrite its examination for particular types of positions needed due to changing legal constraints? Both these could lead to late starts. What about materials? Normal administrative patterns may have been disrupted due to strikes at raw material producers in foreign countries, or by fire or other natural disasters that destroy a plant that produces a key product or ingredient. Or suppose all goes well but suddenly a new hazardous substance is found and the project cannot begin until an environmental impact analysis is done and a permit is gained? Suppose none of these happens, but the economy begins to slow, revenues begin to fall below projections and the chief executive decrees that there shall be a hiring freeze before new people have been put to work, and that there will be a freeze on purchase of equipment of the type needed to run the project. These are some of the types of problems that can and do happen to inhibit or prevent implementation of a program.

These are only a few examples; this does not constitute an exhaustive list. However, these examples indicate that budget execution as enacted cannot be taken for granted, neither for relatively simple nor for complex programs. What is certain is that the environment changes constantly for many service programs and budget controls, by their very nature, often inhibit adaptation to new conditions. Still, as noted, proper rules and enforcement must be in effect to prevent costly fraud, waste and abuse of public monies.

One final question must be asked in any review of federal budget execution. Why are funds so strictly controlled in the federal government? The general answer is absence of trust between the Congress and the Executive, and a legitimate desire to prevent fraud, waste and abuse of taxpayer money. However, as has been observed elsewhere (Jones & Bixler, 1992), the tendency of Congress is to control executive agencies related to achievement of political objectives, coupled with the fact that a number of members of Congress and their staffs have been or are lawyers. Lawyers prefer highly specific rules versus less specificity, or the use of other means of control, e.g., incentives that economists would favor, for example. In the Executive branch, control may be explained by a preference to avoid actions that might be sanctioned by Congress or its legal arm, the General

Accounting Office, or punishment that would result from violation of overly complex permanent federal Appropriation Law, and annual appropriation controls erected by Congress and OMB. The federal government appears, relative to other levels of government, to "manage to audit" to an excessive degree, irrespective of evidence that the costs of control often exceed the benefits (Jones & Thompson, 1985; Jones & Thompson, 1999).

NOTES

1. For example, recently *Public Budgeting and Finance* has carried articles on "Local Government Reserve Funds" (Tyer, 1993); "State and Corporate Cash Management" (Mattson, Hackbart, & Ramsey, 1990); "Surviving a Revenue Collapse" (Gould, 1990); "Federal Financial Management Control Systems" (Hildreth, 1993), and "The Impact of State Rainy Day Funds in Easing State Fiscal Crises During the 1990–1991 Recession" (Sobel &Holcombe, 1996).

2. For more detail on the federal budget execution process, see OMB circular A-34.

3. See Burkhead (1959, p. 341). Historically, Burkhead noted, there has been a strong decentralized component in the United States, particularly at state and local levels. Burkhead quotes A. E. Buck on the reason for this "...agencies were often arranged in a haphazard and disjointed fashion, their administrative officers, in many instances not being even remotely under executive control or supervision... Although the executive might prepare a satisfactory financial plan for the legislative body under these circumstances, he could not hope to be able to enforce the plan once it had been adopted" (Burkhead, 1959, p. 342).

4. Budget Manual, Department of Navy (Ch. 61, pp. 373, 374).

5. Department of Navy Budget Manual, Ch. 3.

6. For further discussion of these end of year patterns, see Kozar and McCaffery (1994).

7. The data in Table I are derived from Kozar, Appendix A, from the following tables: "O&M Total Obligations" pp. 132–133, "O&M Air Force" pp. 126–127, "O&M Army" pp. 120–121 and "O&M Navy" pp. 116–117. Fourteen years of monthly obligation data provided by the Defense Finance and Accounting Service for 11 Department of Defense O&M accounts were studied for the fiscal years 1977 through 1990.

8. By law, it is illegal to use current year money to meet next year's needs. The money must be obligated to meet needs which arise in the current year. The actual outlay of funds may happen in the following year. For example, in 1984 GAO found that DOD industrial funds illegally carried O&M funds over to the next fiscal year. Reporting to the Chairman of the House Appropriations Committee, GAO reported that the six DOD industrial fund activities carried over about $35.7 million from fiscal year 1982 to 1983 through the improper use of industrial funds, extending the life of one-year appropriations which would have otherwise expired. The primary causes for the improper carryover of funds were the lack of a legitimate current need for the good or service and the failure of the industrial activity to start the work before the end of the fiscal year. These actions violate Title 31 Section 1502 and the general provisions of the DOD Appropriation Acts. See "Improper Use of Industrial Funds by Defense Extended the Life of Appropria-

tions Which Otherwise Would have Expired." GAO Report AFMD-84-34 (Washington, DC: U.S. Government Printing Office, June 1984).

9.   Kozar and McCaffery (1994, p. 10). Although this is a small account, the profile is striking. In FY 89 50.8% of this account was spent in the last quarter and 41.3 in the last two months, FY90 saw 49.1 and 41.8, FY 91 saw 66.7 and 57.4 and FY92 saw 57.0 and 46.5 respectively. It seems clearly to have been used as an emergency bank.

10.   This is often called Miles Law, attributed to a famous Department of Agriculture budget officer, Jerry Miles, who supposedly defended conflicting statements by indicating that he had now assumed a different role.

11.   Legal authority to establish reserves rests in Title 31 Section 1512, Apportionments and Reserves. Section 1512 states that in apportioning or reapportioning an appropriation, a reserve may be established only (a) to provide for contingencies; (b) to achieve savings made possible through or by changes in requirements or greater efficiency of operations; and (c) as specifically provided by law. A reserve established under this subsection may be changed as necessary to carry out the scope and objectives of the appropriation concerned.

12.   Kozar and McCaffery found varying practices in the three Military Departments. In the early 1990s, it was customary for the Chief of Naval Operations to hold back a 2% reserve at the beginning of the year; the Army Chief of Staff had a similar contingency policy, holding back about .5% of his O&M funds or $100 million. Differing from Army and Navy practices, the Air Force Chief of Staff held back no reserve funds in this account. Normally these reserve funds would be given back to subordinate commands based on new needs during the middle of the year budget review. At the same time, commands that were underexecuting their budget might well have money taken from them to be given to others that were perceived as more needy; or they might be told to pick up the pace of execution (see Kozar & McCaffery, 1994, p 10).

13.   All appropriation bills have been passed on time in 1948,1976,1988, 1994, and 1996. During the period studied in Table I, DOD appropriations were passed on time in 1976, 1977, and 1988.

14.   Even a slightly delayed appropriation may have large consequences for a project: "If the weather during the winter and spring precludes work on an outside project, funding and subsequent contract delay in the first quarter of the fiscal year may force some projects to be delayed for considerably longer periods of time than one might have predicted, given the length of time covered by short term funding legislation." The same administrator commented that late appropriations were not a problem for other accounts and programs he had to administer, unless an increase in program scope was planned. Thus does he reflect the essence of the budget execution dilemma: some things roll on as planned, others do not (see Kozar & McCaffery, 1994, p. 12).

15.   The penalties are described in sections 1349 and 1350 of the Anti-Deficiency Act, Title 31.

16.   To pursue this argument see Jones and Thompson (1986, pp. 33–49; 1994, esp. Ch. 6); Jones and Bixler (1992).

17.   Pressman and Wildavsky (1973). *Implementation.* In this classic study, the authors calculated decision points in a seemingly simple urban redevelopment program and suggested that even for seemingly simple programs when one considered how many things could go wrong, it was a wonder that anything went right.

CHAPTER V

ENTITLEMENTS AND DIRECT SPENDING CONTROL

INTRODUCTION

Entitlements are permanent appropriations enacted by Congress, budgeted under the authority of congressional authorization committees, that provide benefits to citizens who meet qualifying eligibility criteria, e.g., age, income level, type of disability. The largest and best-known entitlement programs include Social Security, Medicare, Medicaid and various pension programs. However, there are hundreds of such programs that exist as permanent accounts administered by the Treasury. In most cases, payments from entitlement accounts are made directly by the federal government. However, some entitlement monies are transferred to state governments, for example, to support programs that are administered under the law by both federal and state governments, local governments or other entities.

Entitlements, as permanent commitments of financial support, have been enacted piecemeal over a long period of time (with the greatest growth in the 1930s and 1960s) largely out of concern for equity, social stability and compassion for citizens with special needs for support. As such, they bear what may be interpreted as the moral commitment and responsibility of government to fund them annually and to maintain them in a financial position that insures their short-term liquidity and long-term solvency.

Entitlements are paid from revenues raised in various ways (e.g., employee paycheck deductions, mandatory employer contributions, special taxes) dedicated for deposit to and expenditure from specific accounts (trust funds). From a cash flow perspective, the government is responsible for ensuring that there is sufficient money maintained in these accounts to pay current (annual) liabilities. Consequently, if revenues are not adequate to fund liabilities from dedicated sources, the Congress has to appropriate sufficient funds in the regular appropriation process (through action by revenue, budget, authorization and appropriation committees) to cover projected liabilities. Entitlements are such an important part of federal budgeting and fiscal policy because they comprise approximately 54% of annual federal spending. In Fiscal Year 2000, approximately $796 billion was spent from entitlement accounts. This does not include interest on the national debt, a mandatory payment, but not classified as an entitlement, or the administrative costs of administering entitlement payments, since these are carried in the discretionary accounts. Since entitlement funding is based upon formula written into the law, the amounts spent from these accounts depend not on annual decisions by Congress but on the numbers of people who qualify for payments and the size of payments relative to their eligibility. Consequently, expenditures from these accounts can and have risen rapidly since the 1970s, far outpacing increases in spending in any other portion of the federal budget. Medicare is one example of an entitlement that has grown rapidly as the population of the United States has aged. Table 1 indicates the actual payout of entitlements in 2000, and estimates to 2011. The last column compares CBO's estimates of the 2011 entitlement costs with an inflation adjustment computed by the authors, of 2.5% a year compounded over the 11-year period from the year 2000 actual amounts to the year 2011. What this illustrates is that entitlements may grow faster or slower than inflation and that there are other factors at work than inflation in determining how much money will be paid out. Medicare and Medicaid, for example, are estimated to grow much faster than an inflation rate of 2.5% a year.

The Budget in Brief for FY2002 helps illustrate the scope and importance of these entitlement accounts and what they were budgeted to do in FY2002:

- The largest Federal program is Social Security, which will provide monthly benefits to more than 46 million retired and disabled workers, their dependents, and survivors. It accounts for 23% of all Federal spending.
- Medicare will provide health care coverage for more than 40 million elderly Americans and people with disabilities. Since its creation in 1965, Medicare has accounted for an ever-growing share of spending. In 2002, it will comprise 12% of all Federal spending.
- Medicaid will provide health care services to a little more than 34 million Americans, including the poor, people with disabilities, and senior citizens in nursing homes. Unlike Medicare, the Federal Gov-

ernment shares the costs of Medicaid with the States, paying between 50 and 83% of the total (depending on each State's requirements). Federal and State costs are growing rapidly, although the rate of growth has fallen from the double-digit pace of the late 1980s and early 1990s. In 2002, Medicaid will account for 7% of the budget.

- Other means-tested entitlements provide benefits to people and families with incomes below certain minimum levels that vary from program to program. The major means-tested entitlements are Food Stamps, Supplemental Security Income, Child Nutrition, the Earned Income Tax Credit, and veterans' pensions. This category will account for an estimated 6% of the budget.[1]

Technically, the monies deposited, maintained, invested and paid from entitlement accounts do not belong to the federal government. The government is merely the fiduciary manager of these accounts on behalf of beneficiaries, present and future. Although entitlements are permanent appropriations, they can be modified or even eliminated by Congress. Initiatives to modify entitlement programs, eligibility criteria and standards, and amounts to be paid may be made by Congress through legislation that must originate in authorization committees, as noted. Entitlement programs often are relatively easy for Congress to enhance but, because of their moral and equity basis, they are difficult to reduce either in terms of eligibility criteria or levels of spending and payments to individuals. Since 1990, as a result of budget legislation, the attempt to exert entitlement spending control has been largely centered on the pay-as-you-go principle, i.e., that to add spending to an entitlement program, either new revenues must be enacted or spending from other areas within entitlement programs must be cut to pay for the increases proposed.

This chapter investigates the basis for entitlements, also referred to as direct spending, in the federal budget. No effort is made here to document the history of entitlements or the nature of specific programs. This is covered well in other texts (see, e.g., Wildavsky & Caiden, 2001). Then, because entitlements are frequently characterized as the "uncontrollable" part of the budget, we recommend a set of measures to the President and the leadership of the Congress to enhance budgetary balance and control over entitlements. These measures are intended to apply to federal initiatives to control annual spending and reduce the total federal debt over time. The individual measures recommended include (a) holding increases in entitlement expenditures at or below the rate of GDP growth, (b) establishing ceilings (envelopes) for major accounts, (c) placing all entitlements on a pay-as-you-go (PAYGO) basis *and enforcing this rule strictly*; (d) means testing of entitlements, (e) elimination of automatic entitlement indexing, (f) considering the option of marginal reductions in some entitlement programs, and

Table 1. Entitlement Programs and Payments from 2000 to 2011
CBO's Baseline Projections of Mandatory Spending (By fiscal year, in billions of dollars)

	Actual 2000	2001	2002	2003	2004	2005	2006	2007	2008	2009	2010	2011	2011 at 2.5%
Means-Tested Programs													
Medicaid	118	130	142	151	164	177	192	208	226	245	267	291	154.8
State Children's Health Insurance	1	4	4	4	5	4	4	5	5	5	5	5	1.3
Food Stamps	18	19	20	21	22	23	24	24	25	26	27	27	23.6
Supplemental Security Income	31	27	31	33	35	39	38	37	42	44	47	53	40.7
Family Support[a]	21	24	25	25	25	25	26	26	26	26	26	26	27.6
Veterans' Pensions	3	3	3	3	3	3	3	3	3	4	4	5	3.9
Child Nutrition	9	10	10	10	11	11	12	12	13	13	14	14	11.8
Earned Income and Child Tax Credits	27	27	27	27	28	28	28	28	29	29	29	29	35.4
Student Loans	1	-1	5	4	4	4	4	4	4	4	4	4	1.3
Foster Care	5	6	6	7	7	8	8	9	10	10	11	11	6.6
Total	236	248	273	287	303	324	340	356	382	406	432	466	309.7
Non-Means-Tested Programs													
Social Security	406	429	451	474	498	523	550	578	608	643	680	719	532.7
Medicare	216	238	253	270	290	315	333	362	391	422	456	501	283.4
Subtotal	622	668	704	744	787	839	883	940	999	1,065	1,136	1,220	816.1
Other Retirement and Disability													
Federal civilian[b]	50	53	56	59	62	65	68	72	75	78	82	85	65.6
Military	33	34	35	36	37	38	39	40	41	42	43	44	43.3
Other	5	5	5	5	5	5	5	5	5	5	5	6	6.6
Subtotal	88	92	96	100	104	108	113	117	121	126	130	135	115.5

Table 1. Entitlement Programs and Payments from 2000 to 2011
CBO's Baseline Projections of Mandatory Spending (By fiscal year, in billions of dollars) (Cont.)

	Actual 2000	2001	2002	2003	2004	2005	2006	2007	2008	2009	2010	2011	2011 at 2.5%
Unemployment Compensation	21	24	26	27	29	32	33	35	38	40	41	43	27.6
Other Programs													
Veterans' benefits^c	24	21	25	26	28	31	30	28	31	32	33	36	31.5
Commodity Credit Corporation Fund	30	17	11	10	10	9	8	7	6	5	5	5	6.6
Social services	5	5	5	5	5	5	5	5	5	5	5	5	
Credit liquidating accounts	-11	-7	-6	-6	-7	-7	-6	-6	-6	-6	-5	-5	
Universal Service Fund	4	5	6	6	12	13	13	13	13	13	13	13	5.2
Department of Defense health care	0	0	0	6	6	7	7	7	8	9	9	10	
Other	14	6	20	17	17	16	15	15	15	15	15	15	18.4
Subtotal	66	47	60	64	70	73	71	69	72	73	75	79	86.6
Total	796	831	886	935	991	1,051	1,100	1,161	1,229	1,303	1,383	1,477	1,044.4
Total													
All Mandatory Spending	1,032	1,080	1,159	1,222	1,294	1,375	1,440	1,518	1,611	1,710	1,815	1,942	1,354.1

Source: Congressional Budget Office. Summer 2001.

Notes: Spending for the benefit programs shown above generally excludes administrative costs, which are discretionary. Spending for Medicare also excludes premiums, which are considered offsetting receipts (such receipts are not included in this table).

^a Includes Temporary Assistance for Needy Families, Payments to States for Child Support Enforcement and Family Support, Child Care Entitlement to States, and Children's Research and Technical Assistance.

^b Includes Civil Service, Foreign Service, Coast Guard, and other small retirement programs and annuitants' health benefits.

^c Includes veterans' compensation, readjustment benefits, life insurance, and housing programs.

(g) voting on total federal budgets as single, omnibus packages. In our analysis of entitlement control, in some cases we draw upon the experience of other nations to illustrate or support our arguments.

ENTITLEMENTS AND SPENDING CONTROL

Various types of leverage can be used in attempting to control deficits and debt in entitlement spending through enactment of new measures to increase revenue and through controlling the growth of expenditures. Of course, as is always the case in budgeting, the key to balancing the budget is the summoning of the political will needed to bite the bullet and actually pass tax increases and cut spending. What is difficult is to reach political consensus on how to manage public finances to meet the control goals and criteria. The purpose of this chapter, as noted, is to provide advice on the types of policies that should be considered to meet the requirement to control the growth of entitlement program spending, including that for Social Security, Medicare, Medicaid and others as the fiscal demands placed on these accounts in the federal budget increase through the first half of the twenty-first century as the baby boom generation ages and becomes increasingly eligible for entitlement benefits. That such control is needed is indisputable. Social Security is projected to remain solvent for at least the next thirty years with some modification. However, Medicare is forecasted to be broke by 2010 if not repaired, and increasing demand on Medicaid assistance to states and for a myriad of other entitlement programs is projected to increase rapidly in the next three decades.

In budgeting as a part of fiscal policy (taxing and spending), and in life in general, the most general problems of social and economic decision making involve managing the divergence between individual and collective rationality. The essential problem is always to make doing the "right" thing from a policy perspective worthwhile for both the interested and the uninformed citizenry. The essential dilemma of budgeting is that it has to be worthwhile for everyone to sacrifice something to achieve expenditure control, for purposes of economic stability (e.g., to balance the budget) and perhaps efficiency, in order to benefit the long-term interests of all.

What usually happens in budget negotiation is that whoever offers to sacrifice their program, interest, and reputation finds that the expenditure cuts they have made are absorbed by other spending interests, thereby accomplishing two things at once: their reputations are ruined and the national interest is not served. To secure effective expenditure control it is necessary to create rules under which it is worthwhile for everyone to contribute to a common interest.

What is needed to accomplish this goal is a set of norms and rules of procedure that facilitate political convergence and agreement on mechanisms of control that will last over a considerable period of time. The first consideration, in our view, is that command and control methods, though minimally essential, cannot perform this task alone. It is not possible to imagine that the federal government use procedures that specify for each account the exact tax or expenditure policies to be implemented permanently. Controls must be contingent and responsive to economic circumstance.

Command and control approaches also violate an essential rule of our experience; central controllers are very far away and the spending departments are very close at hand, so that in a struggle over who knows the most about local conditions, the central controllers will lose. Therefore, while a reserve power should be retained to place sanctions on accounts that deviate from their responsibilities for deficit and debt limitation, if this tactic is overused it will fail, thus weakening the overall political will to exert control (i.e., the threat of imposition of controls is much better than the use of controls). Controls, while inevitable, must be approached carefully for political, social, economic, and budgetary reasons. Interference with entitlement accounts without regard to particular problems facing both administrators and beneficiaries must be avoided. Instead, there should be a series of norms and procedures that, if adopted and reinforced by mutual education as well as self-interest, would lead to desirable outcomes most of the time. Thus, the need for self-defeating central control measures would be obviated.

THE RATIONALE FOR BUDGET CONTROL AND EXPENDITURE CONSTRAINT

To make our case, it is necessary initially to explain that expenditure control is more important rather than the alternative—continuous revenue enhancement. For one thing, the smaller the number of items one tries to control, the greater the chances of success. If one places the control over budget balance rather than either revenue or expenditure, the difficulties multiply.[2] One has to control both expenditure and revenue when it is very difficult to control either. The possibilities for strategic misrepresentation, for end runs around every rule developed, (on the general proposition well attested to in human experience that people will find a way around almost any rule), suggest that one should seek to create, maintain, and educate people in the smallest number of rules possible. This will be much easier if either an expenditure or revenue limit is adopted.

The second reason is that for modern capitalist democracies, taxes and revenues are already quite high. Most social democracies have found high income tax rates self-defeating. As a result, rules are needed that will be effective in most nations now and will be necessary in all of them in the next twenty years. Further, the major impetus to unbalanced budgets has come from the rapid rise in expenditure, a rise exceeding the growth in national product, rather than shortfalls in revenue. If we accept the perspective that Federal activity keeps increasing as a proportion of GDP (we use GDP rather than GNP as our reference point throughout this chapter because it is a better, more measurable standard than GNP), which has been true for over a century with the partial exception of the 1980s, we may assume that, left to their own devices, governments will continue to grow and spend more. Moreover, we emphasize in this analysis that expenditure control is necessary because, if one looks at the rationales given for increasing Federal activity, they appear not to make sense.

Why have expenditures grown over the last hundred years? In the United States our answer is that because our country is so large we need considerable infrastructure. Other nations maintain that because they are so small, people hang all over each other and need many social workers to separate them. We say that expenditure is rising because our populations are growing old, and that has its logic. However, another view is that expenditure is growing because our population is very young. Previous work on the logic of public sector growth shows that all such explanations are contradicted by the exact obverse (Wildavsky, 1985). Among other things, this indicates a tremendous desire in social democracies to spend for egalitarian purposes, for unmet social needs. If there were not unfortunate effects of high levels of borrowing over time, a number of nations might all follow the high debt course taken by Belgium for example. Indeed, they might do more than Belgium. They would perhaps multiply their debt many times over based on the belief that it is so desirable to spend money on old and young people and big and small spaces. There is hardly any rationale for increasing spending that is not being used already. Indeed, progressivism, leftism, and egalitarianism basically all mean more spending for whatever is defined as in the interests of the larger social welfare, to which we now quite properly add environmental purposes. And, our populace is growing older, not younger.

These factors are much more powerful than a desire to tax citizens. Indeed, tax decisions are painful and generally lag behind spending decisions, which is one reason for high deficits. Do we believe that the problem for most nations is that for political reasons the government decides to tax too little or that, given the enormous rise in expenditures, governments find it difficult to raise revenues to keep programs going? Our position is that expenditure control is the way to control deficits. Our idea is to start with what exists, namely a criterion that deficits should not grow beyond 3% of GNP. We do not see any other norm that is obviously much better, accepting that specific percentages are adjustable and never final. This norm could perhaps be altered or replaced, but the view expressed in this chapter is that this criterion should be augmented by other measures, the benefits of which are explained in the following section.

MEASURES TO "INCENTIVATE" BUDGETARY CONTROL

It is unreasonable to expect budgetary behavior to change unless the incentive structure that motivates this behavior is altered. The verb we coin to capture what we believe is necessary is "incentivate," that is, to establish incentives that will motivate better, more responsible, budgetary policy decision making. This term, composed from a noun and a verb, will not be found in the dictionary, but we intend hereby to add it to the English language generally and to the already bizarre lexicon of political economy and budgeting (where else outside the world of budgeting do the terms "logrolling," "ear marking," "offsets," "end runs," or even "sequestration" mean much of anything?). What follows are the rules that, in combination, form the structure of an incentive system badly needed to preserve democratic decision making and fiscal stability in the United States and, by example, elsewhere.

Rule One: Expenditures Tied to GDP

To our overall 3% criterion, it appears desirable to add another, more specific rule to accomplish the purposes desired. This rule is that spending should not be allowed to grow at a rate higher than the growth of gross domestic product. This may be measured in a very straightforward way, or at least as straightforward as human ingenuity will allow. One takes last year's expenditures and multiplies by the percentage increase, or decrease, in the GDP.

The question may be raised whether a main defect of this norm would be that government could not therefore engage in counter-cyclical economic activity. The 3% criterion specifies that if there is a deficit above a specific percentage of GDP, governments must consider reducing that deficit as their primary economic goal. Where then is economic management? One may argue over the appropriateness and feasibility of counter-cyclical policy, but it is valuable at this point to pursue a tangent regarding counter-cyclical policy before continuing our overall statement of the rules needed to reorient budgeting and fiscal policy. This is appropriate because many nations often would like their governments to pursue a more ambitious counter-cyclical policy to assist their economies in recovery from a very serious bout of recession. As we demonstrate, there are other reasons to examine more thoroughly the evolution of thinking about the advisability of counter-cyclical government fiscal policy. Part of this review must consider the experience of various countries with such policy. In addition, there are other factors relevant to our overall argument in this chapter that will be served by this digression.

First of all, fiscal policy, in the sense of counter-cyclical activity, is becoming extremely rare. In the United States there has been a virtual abandonment of any idea of fiscal policy (see White & Wildavsky, 1990). When was the last time the government sized its deficits so as to manage the economy? Rather, governments are driven by their deficits. Monetary policies—interest-rate and money supply setting by central banks—have become the key instruments of economic policy.

The Keynesian approach has steadily declined in importance because, in our view, it is fundamentally fallacious. It is fallacious economically, which is controversial, but it is also fallacious politically, which is not at all controversial and is understood by virtually everyone. Therefore, we will take the easy part first. It is unfortunate that Keynesianism is wrong politically because it upsets the great budgetary norms of the past, which told us that deficits were bad and, therefore, high spending was bad. What did Lord Keynes tell us? Spending under certain circumstances is good. You should cut your taxes, you should raise your spending, you should increase your deficits, and that would help moderate economic swings. Keynes, who was an English Brahmin, thought that very clever people dedicated only to the public interest would decide these matters. On the basis of long experience in politics, we are still not clear why he assumed this would be the case. He believed that governments actually would follow his advice, that is, they would increase spending and lower taxes when the economy was slow, but when the economy was overheated, they would then cut spending and increase taxes. In the political arena, of course, this was greeted with immense cheer; at long last there were decision rules that politicians could understand and talk about as if they were knowledgeable.

There was a period when many talked about economics as if first, there was macroeconomic theory that worked to accurately predict, guide, and explain after the fact the performance of the economy, and second, as if they knew what they were doing in applying the theory to tune the economy. However, in practice they behaved in accordance with the first assumption (analysis was performed and advice given based upon theory), but rarely with the second, that is, when they ought to have increased spending only in the short term, they often increased it over the long term. However, when they ought to have cut spending, they only decreased the rate of growth over the short term or not at all. The result was greatly enhanced spending.

Now for one of the more controversial reasons for rejecting Keynesianism. It has been assumed in economics that there is something called the multiplier effect. When you tax people and put that money to work by the government, it has certain multiple positive economic spillover effects. This entire assumption may be questioned. The variations in government spending and tax policies do not have in our view the extensive effects that are credited to them, although on the margin there is some effect, no doubt.

In any event, we take it that the whole point of the 3% norm is to rule out counter-cyclical activities that push spending beyond a certain level of deficit. What our norm does is to provide a line of defense. The task is to defend that line so that governmental expenses will not grow beyond the rate of growth of the economy. However, the growth norm has to be backed up by a number of rules, without which it will be either ineffective or much less effective. A number of the mechanisms adopted in Denmark and Britain, for example, as well as in other countries are very close to what we suggest here. There is reason from experience for this convergence.

Rule Two: Expenditure Envelopes for Major Accounts

To recapitulate, the first rule is that the overall ceiling is determined by the previous year's spending multiplied by the percentage increase of the GDP. The second rule is that sub-ceilings on the above principal should be established on major, traditional spending accounts. The idea of sub-ceilings is absolutely critical. If you simply try to defend a national spending ceiling as such, you would never know who is responsible for what, and it would be impossible to observe discipline. Therefore, it is important to elucidate this consideration. If you have too many spending accounts to control you will fail. If you only have one you will fail; it is between these two that you need to go.[3] In the United States, there are traditionally thirteen major spending accounts, and it is these types of accounts that are recommended. Also, there are certain other warnings: do not invent new accounting rules. It is not that the existing ones are wonderful, or that we understand them, or that there might not be others that are better. Rather, it is best to find some series of accounts whose numbers are certified in various accounting decisions where there is as much certainty in them as possible, and as much tradition behind them as possible.[4]

Rule Three: Entitlement Growth Financed Only by Specific Revenue Increases

The third rule, related to the second, is the PAYGO rule, earlier known as the offset procedure. It has been followed in the United States Senate but, alas, not in the House of Representatives, and the differential consequences are extremely instructive. What the PAYGO rule says is that within your sub-account you may do whatever legislators can agree on within existing revenues. But, if you wish to exceed that amount, then you must either agree on a revenue increase of some kind or get some other account and its beneficiaries to cut their own spending and have the reduction reallocated to your account. Naturally, this is not easy to do, but at least everybody will understand that sacrifice is required.

What the PAYGO rule does, when taken together with sub-ceilings, is alter the fundamental rules of rationality in budgeting. It makes collective sacrifices worthwhile. It means that the administrators of one account and their beneficiaries cannot reach into other different accounts to fund whatever they want or need. Mutual consent and sacrifice are the order of the day. It is this combination of the first three rules that can restore rationality to expenditure budgets. By rationality we mean the doctrine of opportunity costs: that something is worth what you have to give up for it. This is, of course, budgeting, and budgeting is a political process, where the tradeoffs in the end are made by top-level political decision makers in processes of bargaining. By conducting the bargaining within these rules, we know that they either accept the allocations as they come out of the formula (the first rule proposed, i.e., that spending not grow faster than gross domestic product), or agree to explicit tradeoffs. This is as much rationality as one should expect from any form of government.

Moreover, this type of rationality should work to overcome one of the most unfortunate splits in society: the conflict between producers and the redistributors. One might well be interested in redistribution, whether among nations or within them, but one also has to be interested in where those resources will come from and therefore be interested in production. We foresee that if these budget rules were believed in and enforced over a period of years, different political coalitions would form.

In the relationship between the Treasury and a department in the United Kingdom, there is the rule that every minister defends his or her own corner, and many devices were tried to overcome this dynamic of self-interest. There were committees of non-spending ministers. There were morality sessions in which the Prime Minister gave lectures about the common good, but none of these prevailed. Under the rules that we are talking about here, however, it should become in the interest of those who care about redistribution to support means for achieving greater production.

To put it more forcefully, if it is recognized that the only way to get greater redistribution is through enhanced production, then there might emerge much more interesting dialogue leading to cooperation. We would hope to hear statements such as, "Why do you not make more economic decisions so that there can be greater tax revenues so that there can be greater redistribution to protect the environment, old people, and the homeless?" It is very important in our society that we encourage the comprehension of a connection between redistribution and economic productivity.

PAYGO also completely reverses the old idea of budgeting by addition. The interest groups and politicians who support these programs, which are largely entitlements authorized and funded permanently in the law, see themselves as supporting good things. They do not and have never seen themselves as supporting bad things like taking resources away from other needy people. However, in the United States Senate, the national defense interest is looking into the welfare budget, the welfare people are looking into the defense budget, etc. In other words, instead of every legislator defending only his or her corner, each is now looking into other people's dark corners. They know that this is the way for them to grow. Interest groups, particularly retired people's lobbies, complain bitterly that it is not right to do so, that it is immoral to have them come up to Congress and hunt for resources in this manner. Their constituents are worthy, blameless, needy, and they should not be sullied by the business of from where the money is going to come. The rules proposed here would force answers to such questions. Our basic point is that having the PAYGO rule is necessary, but that to be effective, it must be enforced strictly.

Rule Four: Means Test Entitlements and Eliminate Automatic Indexing

The fourth rule is composed of two parts. The first part is easy. All entitlement payments by government should be calibrated against the income and possibly the wealth levels of potential aid recipients. There is no economic logic to support sending payments to people who have sufficient income and/or wealth to provide for their own financial welfare. Two approaches might be used to define need: income or a combination of income and wealth. Income could be measured using the previous year's amount by individual, or an average over two or more years. A weighted, multi-year formula could be applied to give greatest weight to income level in the immediate past year and less to previous years. Another approach would be to combine the income criterion with some measure of wealth, for example, individual equity owned in stocks, bonds, and property. Data on income are available from tax filings. Data on wealth would have to be collected in most cases through a process similar to tax filing; individuals would have to submit to government statements of their wealth holdings. Technical valuation problems could be worked out just as similar problems have been resolved for income tax filing. The tax codes of most nations typically include instructions to manage high degrees of complexity in income measurement. Consequently, measurement and valuation problems are not sufficient reasons to reject the use of wealth as criterion to determine level of need for government assistance. The principle here is that assistance from the government should be based strictly upon financial need, and public resources should be used exclusively for the truly needy.

The second part is more controversial: no provision of an automatic inflation premium (indexing) for entitlement programs. Entitlement program spending ceilings for the coming year should be established strictly by prior year spending levels. The British at one time employed what was referred to as volume budgeting: spenders were promised whatever it took to carry out last year's policy at this year's prices. Why are we concerned about dragging up this bit of history? Because in the United States we are still doing what the British long ago abandoned and for good reason, we have something called the current service budget, which means that a program gets what it got last year times inflation. The idea is to provide the same volume of services.

The consequences of embracing inflation are problematic. The discussion should go quite differently. Is our problem that governments spend too little, or is it that they spend too much? If we think that they spend too much, then we do not wish the Congress to chase the spenders but the spenders to have to come to their elected representatives. We wish the Congress to indicate that if there is 3% inflation, explain to us why you have not achieved an efficiency to absorb this amount, rather than to have the Congress claw back what was given automatically by formula. This rule is not impartial. It is designed to help the central controllers. Therefore, we must explain why it is desirable to help central control.

For the last 100 years, with some partial exceptions in the 1980s, central controllers have generally lost out in the larger picture of spending control to the spenders. Controllers sometimes have won for a year or two, but over time they have lost. Why? One reason is that there are so few of them and so many more advocates on the spending side. They also lose because the spenders feel their gains much more powerfully than those who are taxed feel their losses. That is to say, almost any program can be financed by a few pennies of additional tax here and there. It is only when you add them together that they cause budget imbalance difficulties. When you look at the picture as a whole, spending interests are much more powerful than saving interests. Therefore, as noted, we have to seriously consider as political economists how we can alter the rules so as to restore some balance between spending and saving.

The idea embodied in the first four rules is to place spending interests into conflict. Rather than trying to increase the unilateral power of budget controllers, (which is generally not politically feasible beyond the control they already possess due to unwillingness of legislators to give controllers more fiscal policy leverage that might be used against the legislature), these proposals attempt to use some of the power spending interests have to offset the power of other spending interests. The interest in one spending category may be opposed to the interest of others, so that in order for one to get more for its side, it will have to generate the onus of raising taxes or get some other spending department to accept reductions.

One of the ways in which the preferences of our citizens are safeguarded is by entrusting them to governmental departments in some part, expecting that agriculture departments will defend their corners and labor departments theirs. If it were the case that every person should look out for everybody else's interest, about which they know very little, there would be such confusion in the world as to who wanted what, that governments would have to pass laws introducing selfishness to make the world work. It is not desirable for spending departments to pursue only their interest. On the one hand, it should be feasible for them to sacrifice when they feel that is either necessary or desirable. On the other hand, we want to make it obvious to them that they cannot have a great deal more than what they are getting without taking others into account.

Has this worked in the past? In the U.S. federal government in the 1950s, for example, there was agreement on major implicit budgetary norms. One was annularity but another was a respect for another program's base, and in the 1980s and 1990s, tradeoff budgeting became the norm in the United States under deficit control laws (Gramm-Rudman-Hollings Acts, Budget Acts of 1990 and 1993, and the Balanced Budget Act of 1997). It may be a long time before any country will choose a two-year budget cycle to give poor budget officers a little relief, but respect for the base generally prevails, and tradeoffs will occur, we believe, if the proper structural mechanisms for budgeting are established to "incentivate" it.

Another norm was protecting the base, which remains a serious problem in many places in the world. This norm may be attributed in part to state budget officers in the United States, and budget controllers in general, in their attempts to protect the general fund (see Thompson & Jones, 1986). In many governments in the past several decades, including the United States, this was not done, so there have been horrendous deficits. In addition to the norm of balancing, there was understanding that revenues would not rise very fast. Now if revenues did not rise very fast and people believed that terrible things would happen if the budget became unbalanced, if you busted the budget, or if your expenditures increased greatly in one area, then you would take it out of the hide of other departments. Therefore, among agencies there came to be a common interest in keeping down demands within an overall constraint. Keynesianism destroyed this whole understanding. So one could look at the rules and norms proposed here as an effort to replace by design what was built up by the accretion of understandings over long periods of time and then lost.

Rule Five: The Option for Marginal Reduction in Entitlement Spending

The fifth rule is that government is given authority to reduce entitlement spending 5 percent a year. The reason for this is that the burden of sacrifice between the citizen and the government has become unbalanced. We view government and society as immense centipedes—insects with enormous numbers of legs; the idea used to be that the government helps the citizen and the citizen helps sustain government. But now, if you look at the rules that have evolved over time, government sustains citizens, but citizens do not do very much to sustain government. Government upholds all those feet, but who upholds government? Let us review an example.

Referring to our discussion under Rule Four, forty years ago there were no cost-of-living increases written into Federal budget legislation in the United States. Because there was no or little inflation, it was unnecessary to have written entitlement provisions against inflation. However, in the 1970s when inflation resulted after the oil supply "crisis" of 1973, the value of entitlements for citizens eroded. Before indexing, the government had greater discretion in responding to inflation. Politicians could come back and argue for and vote in favor of tax increases to finance increases in entitlement spending to compensate for inflation and get public credit for doing so. Also, due to high inflation what we call "bracket creep" occurred, which meant that inflation pushed people into higher tax brackets while the value of what they could buy was diminished. Bracket creep increased tax rates for many citizens as their incomes rose. By the late 1970s and early 1980s in the United States, bracket creep gave the government about 1.6 times the amount of tax, revenue for every one percentage point increase in the price index.

The point here is that the rules of the game under traditional budgeting were established to protect the government. It received more revenue from inflation and it had less expenditures, but then we created entitlement indexing against inflation. Now in many countries like the United States we also have indexed tax brackets. The result has been to take away the budgetary flexibility from the government. Also, by automatically indexing entitlements, the opportunity of members of Congress to gain credit with the voting public through entitlement increase expenditure voting was greatly diminished.

The reason for giving special interest to this area of budgetary policy is due in part to our concern about the viability of much criticized democratic government in the Western world. Especially unfortunate is the criticism that suggests, sometimes accurately but often not, that civil servants and elected officials are beholden to "special interests." Of course, these interests are special to those who profit directly from them and to those in government who continue to have jobs by serving the beneficiaries of special-interest programs that in many cases are entitled (permanently authorized) in the law. Just as children are special to those who have them, every interest group is special to somebody.

Accusations of special interest are one way of challenging the programs of those against whom you compete for resources in the budgetary process. After all, there are always two perspectives available from which to view government programs and spending: the other side of the coin of special interest is provision of necessary services to citizens who vote in the district or state of a member of Congress. A selfish and undeserving special interest to one critic is a needy constituent and, not incidentally, a vote for reelection to another. However, the level of complaint through the media and elsewhere about the evils of government programs serving special interests has become immense. Another image is that politicians are like pool balls: the interest groups have big sticks and they knock the civil servants and the politicians into their pockets. Therefore, with the intent of serving democracy, it is necessary to think not only about how to hold elected officials responsible, but also about how to give them discretion so that their responsibility may be actualized.

With galloping incrementalism rapidly increasing the size of the budgetary base, and with entitlements threatening to squeeze out other concerns, politicians are often excoriated regardless of what they do; critics demand that the budget must be balanced, the beneficiaries and their sponsors in government bureaucracy demand that entitlement and other spending must continue to keep pace with inflation (at minimum), and the public will not accept any tax increases. Meeting all these demands is impossible in the first place, but elected officials no longer have the political leverage or resources available even to at least fail in attempting to try to satisfy them.

However, under the rule where there is no automatic inflation premium and another that permits up to a 5% cut in entitlement spending (unless a PAYGO revenue increase is accepted), governments have several percent more a year, perhaps 5 to 7%, to reallocate up or down. This is a lot of money and probably as much as the government would try to reallocate in any particular year anyway. Interest groups could not automatically dictate how to allocate this discretionary money. Only the government, through its committees and political process, can do so. We believe these rules would make government much more resistant to naked interest group pressure and, better still, make government appear more important and responsible to the public than interest groups in budgetary decision making.

Rule Six: Voting the Budget in Total

Finally, the last rule is simply the affirmation of governmental responsibility—the budget should be voted up or down as a whole. We do not want to burden the rules with various particularities, but the greater the control that the central authorities have over the budget, the better the chances are of achieving expenditure control. It is by no means certain that every government will be dedicated to expenditure control. However, if a central government is not so dedicated under circumstances of high and rising deficits and fiscal stress, it is unlikely that any set of rules, other than punishment at the polls, would be appropriate for this purpose.[5] Having the budget voted upon as a single, omnibus measure increases the visibility to the public of the achievements and compromises made in negotiations over budget priorities and the degree of fiscal responsibility evident in the proposed match between revenues and expenditures.

CONCLUSIONS

In conclusion, it must be stressed that the measures outlined here are meant to serve and assist members of Congress and the President as they make entitlement policy and fiscal decisions over the next decade. Because entitlement policy cannot at present meet all of the criteria, choices have to be made on how to deal with this dilemma in a way that provides flexibility but still preserves the integrity of the criteria and sustains the political will to accept the desirability of moving toward compliance. One choice, of course, when faced with criteria that cannot be met, is to change the standards, as was done with deficit-reduction targets in the United States for more than a decade prior to balancing the annual budget in FY2000. Another choice is to develop a plan to phase in compliance over a longer period of time according to some type of realistic schedule for hitting benchmark targets along the way. This also has been tried, and indeed some success is finally being achieved in this endeavor as the President and Congress agreed upon and actually met some of the deficit-reduction targets as early as passage of the Federal budget for Fiscal Year 1994.

The advice presented here assumes that elected officials and budget managers know more about their circumstances than we know. Therefore, they may want to amend, eliminate, or substitute certain rules for others proposed here. Still, if some incentives were established, especially the first that spending not grow faster than GDP, together with spending restrictions by envelope, a strictly enforced PAYGO principle, and entitlement controls, there is reason to expect that effective budget control would be achieved over considerable periods of time in those countries whose governments adopted them. Governments might come to believe in these measures, teach them to others and, therefore, some sense of professional pride in maintaining them would grow.

During the first years of the Reagan administration (1981–1984), the spending estimates of the President's Office of Management and Budget (OMB) were wildly off target. In a number of instances, the Congressional Budget Office (CBO), the House Budget Committee, and the House and Senate Appropriation Committees would greet OMB estimators and ask them what dreams they were putting down on paper in the President's budget instead of numbers. Of course, nobody wants to be thought of as a poor professional, especially when testifying before Congress. However, after the passage of the first serious measure by Congress to attempt to control spending, the Gramm-Rudman-Hollings Act of 1985 (GRH), an increasing professionalism was evident in OMB. In addition, a greater degree of agreement between OMB and the staff of the CBO over budget estimates was achieved in the fall of 1985 in negotiating how to apply GRH sequestration rules to cut the budget by nearly $12 billion. Agreements between OMB and CBO on how to share budget databases over time and how to count (score) expenditures in analysis of spending proposals under the constraint of deficit-reduction targets also emerged. A closer correspondence between OMB budget estimates and reality resulted. All of this cannot be attributed alone to the impact of GRH, but is there reason to doubt that some of it may be so explained?[26]

One final point should be emphasized. It may well be that instead of relying on five year expenditure estimates in the United States in the annual congressional Budget Resolution, we could have a more simple rule: spending estimates for the next fiscal year will be exactly what actually was spent the year before as closely as can be ascertained at the time that estimates for the upcoming budget year must be stated. This practice has been adopted in some years as OMB is asked to report on revenue and spending estimates in May each year, six months after the President's budget estimates are prepared for presentation to Congress. Such close to "real time" review of budget estimates might result in less strategic misrepresentation and gimmickry by the government, agencies, and legislators, less time wasted in preparation and presentation of unreliable estimates of future spending that can never sufficiently accommodate contingency, and greater fit between budgeted appropriations and actual spending. In summary, we note that the same advice argued in this chapter with respect to budget control applies equally to U.S. budget decision makers and officials as to those in other nations. If elected officials and budget professionals understand and begin to trust that some established norms and rules make sense and will work to control spending on the margin then, over time, such measures will have greater use and potency among both those who analyze and those who make budgetary decisions. Therefore, attempts to violate the rules will more likely be caught at the source and budget authorities, already overburdened and under attack, will not have to employ draconian and ad hoc controls as forcefully or as frequently. Greater budgetary control, to the extent that we may expect such discipline in democratic governments, will be achieved, and the sacrifices made to gain some measure of control will be distributed as they always are, through the political process.

NOTES

1. Source: Budget in Brief FY2002.
2. See Wildavsky (1980). See also Jones and Thompson (1986). We wish to acknowledge co-authorship of portions of this chapter by our colleague, the late Aaron Wildavsky.
3. For a more complete statement of the proposal for envelope budgeting for the U.S. government, see Jones and McCaffery (1989, Ch. 9).
4. These norms were initially described and analyzed in Wildavsky (1964). The difference between traditional budgeting and what has followed are detailed in Wildavsky (1992).
5. See the concluding chapter of Wildavsky (1992).
6. See Joyce (1993b, p. 45). Joyce cites four other studies that support his and our conclusions (see p. 48).

CHAPTER VI

BUDGET ANALYSIS AND ANALYSTS

INTRODUCTION

This chapter considers the role of the budget analyst and the skills demanded of the position.[1] Budgets are not natural phenomena; rather they are the result of long hours of work in creating and manipulating both words and numbers so that policy makers may review the choices confronting them and make decisions that will dispose of people, time, and money in ways that will best fit the needs of the particular jurisdiction. Schick has argued that with the bulk of the federal budget concentrated in mandatory expenditures, the old budget tools are no longer relevant to most of the federal budget. Historically, budget analysis focused on last year's base plus proposed changes, with limited review of the base, as dictated by incremental decision making, and fierce concentration on the items that were new or changed from one year to the next. In their reviews, budget analysts often invoked tried and true rules of thumb, like limiting personnel growth, slowing down purchases and other expenses, recommending study for complex and expensive new systems and in general attempting to sort out only those expenditures which were absolutely necessary for the coming year to accomplish the mission of the program or department (see Schick, 1990a, p. 86).

These rules applied to the discretionary side of the budget and the extent of their ferocity depended on estimates of the fiscal situation for the budget year, with a healthy economy and a productive tax base allowing for more generosity in budget review than a tight or depressed fiscal environment. On the mandatory side, about two-thirds of the federal budget, budget analysis is different. Here the analytic focus is on changes in the economy, growth rates, inflation and unemployment rates, number of beneficiaries and levels of benefit estimation. Mandatory programs do not allow for denial of benefits, or slowing down of payment of benefits and the cost to administer the programs where the old techniques could be used is minuscule, and often not legal. If people qualified, they got the money and the old budget tools could not, should not, stop this from happening. However, that still leaves one-third or almost $700 billion in the federal budget where these rules may be applied. State and local governments also have their discretionary or general government accounts. Here too, the rules for discretionary budget analysis apply. This chapter examines the nature of work in a budget office and as a budget analyst.

THE BUDGET PROCESS AND THE ROLES OF BUDGET ANALYSTS

In the executive budget process, budgets are submitted and reviewed at different levels within the agency and between the agency and the central budget office where budget analysts review budgets for and in the name of the chief executive. The agency budget process produces the budget; the central budget office reviews it for conformance with directives of the chief executive issued at the start of the budget process and subsequent changes to those directives. Budget analysts at the agency level and in the central budget office tend to ask many of the same questions, but they also have differing concerns. An agency analyst may be more concerned that budget makers have presented an executable budget and included all the costs it will take to carry out a program within the fiscal year. The central budget analyst may be more concerned with the overall impact of the program and its relation to other programs carried out by other departments or to overall policy goals of the chief executive.

Over the long run, both sets of analysts focus on reviewing agency budgets for policy and numerical integrity. This includes checking the budget for basic calculations and projections, for efficient use of current resources and for effective deployment of new resources against the major problems facing the agency and the jurisdiction. The bulk of this work is accomplished by budget analysts who are generally adept with numbers and prose, may possess a master's degree in business, economics, or public administration (or English for that matter) and are quick studies with a skeptical turn of mind which leads to a questioning attitude. They must be good communicators, able to understand complex issues and communicate them to others with the appropriate level of complexity when decisions are being reached. Barry White suggests that four principles underlie budget analysis. They are:

1. Resources are finite.
2. Tradeoffs must be made, even though data is rarely comparable.
3. The budget base must be examined.
4. Budget analysis begins with an unbiased analysis of the evidence.

White (1999, pp. 468–469) suggests the two central questions budget analysis seek to answer are why a particular program should be funded and if funded, at what level?

To help answer these questions, the budget analyst has to work issues that extend along a continuum from simple numerical accuracy to questions that involve basic reasons for adopting such a policy. Thus, his questions may be on the one hand, "Why do it? Does it make good public policy? Who gets what? Who benefits? Who pays for those benefits? Is there collateral damage elsewhere because some other problem is not attacked while this one is? How bad is that damage?" On the other hand, the analyst has to assure that the numbers are accurate. Computers do most of the brute computational work, but the old lesson of garbage in-garbage out still applies and analysts have to make sure the right numbers were put into the right starting places. Dick Zody (1998b) suggests that budgeting depends upon both very sophisticated analytical concepts such as benefit-cost analysis and a set of everyday common sense tools, which may depend upon intuition, focusing on both what is said and not said in a presentation, using percentage displays rather than just raw numbers to help analyze data, using graphic displays to present and summarize data, and choosing comparison to different, but relevant, sets of information to help decision makers see problems clearly. Zody warns that the tendency to see anything a computer prints as correct should be resisted. If data entered is wrong, or if a formula is misspecified, then whatever the output is will be wrong too, notwithstanding that it has been computed correctly. As complex as budget schedules are and as prone to err as humans are, errors are inescapable. Everyone knows this, but no one likes it when it happens. Errors always carry the extra freight that there may be more errors somewhere in the presentation that were not caught. Thus watching for numerical integrity is still important, if more complicated, now that computers have taken over so much of the budget processing.

For most analysts, the middle range questions are the ones that take the most effort. These concern what is to be done, how it is to be done, how many units will be produced, what the cost will be, when it will be done, what staff will be needed, including their rank and appropriate classification and the extent to which there are hidden costs or benefits in the proposed changes. Lastly the analyst might consider how a specified change might affect other programs with similar functions or services: if approved, will this change set a precedent for other agencies to also ask for increases?

Numbers are critical in this process. White quotes Paul O'Neill, a former Deputy Director of OMB, as saying: "Numbers are the keys to the doors of everything. Spending for the arts, the sciences … everything … and reve-nues from every source … are reflected, recorded, and battled over in numbers … If it matters, there are numbers that define it" (White, 1999, p. 463). It is hard to be more eloquent about the main thrust of a budget ana-lyst's task. However, the process is about more than numbers. Jacqueline Rogers and Marita Brown state that all budget making is political, at all lev-els, and that the process is "agenda against agenda, wit against wit, guile against guile, bludgeon against bludgeon" (1999, p. 442). In this game, the wiliest advocate with the best hand triumphs. Rogers and Brown note that not all agencies are created equal, that those with external constituencies are more powerful than internal agencies who exist to service other agen-cies. They note that there were 85,006 official units of government in the United States, that they all have a budget process, and that the budget pro-cess is probably the least standardized of the primary government fiscal functions, including budgeting, finance and accounting (Rogers & Brown, 1999, p. 441). Nonetheless, Rogers and Brown continue by painting a gen-eralized but realistic picture of agency budget concerns where the agency budget office has to mediate between the top level desires of its own lead-ership and the central budget office and the down the line internal needs of lower level agency managers who do not know or care where the money comes from, so long as they get enough of it to carry out their programs and services. The agency budget office is a key mediator and gatekeeper in this process (Rogers & Brown, 1999, p. 447).

The central budget office has its concerns too. During both budget preparation and execution, the central budget office is flooded with spend-ing requests from agencies. The central budget office and the budget ana-lysts within it function, as Wildavsky taught us, as control agents or gatekeepers. Thurmaier notes, "The chief executive (and the legislature) count on the CBB (central budget office) to hold back the spending flood by denying the bulk of the new funding requests. This may seem self-evi-dent at the national level, but it also holds true to a great extent at the state and local levels, too." Their proximity to the action gives them, "…formal responsibility for a much larger set of specific decisions than the other actors in the budgetary process" (Thurmaier, 1998, p. 233).

As gatekeepers communicating decisions both up and down the organi-zation and from the political executive to the administrative branch, cen-tral budget bureau analysts are important players in the budget process. They help their agency understand not only which forms are required, but also what kinds of items and issues others might look upon favorably in the budget review process. They test new ideas proposed in budgets and are particularly sensitive to those that have a steep future year growth curve. A budget analyst may also shield agencies from capricious or unreasonable demands passed down the organization. As an expert in an area, the budget analyst is seen to have great power, some in his own right, and some in the name of others, because the agency cannot always tell who is speaking when the budget analyst speaks. If they do not like what he says, they are far more likely to appeal it if they think it is only his idea, than if they think that it might possibly be something voiced by the chief executive. Which it is, is not always clear. Agencies can challenge the decisions of their budget analyst, but as a practical matter they cannot challenge all of them. Even experienced agency budget officers must rely on the central budget bureau analyst to help set the calendar of events between the agency and the central budget bureau and indicate which items are hot items this year. When an agency budget staff is new or thin, the central budget analyst can seem a godsend ... or a nightmare.

Agency budget analysts are also gatekeepers and they, too, have great power in their position as communicator, but probably not as much latitude as the central budget bureau analyst. In both the agency and central budget bureau, budget analyst tasks are manageable because basically someone else produces the data. The responsibility of the budget analyst is to review that data. To accomplish this, most experienced analysts develop decision routines that they employ. For example, they may challenge all new programs, try to avoid increasing personnel complements, scrutinize closely capital outlay items and try to reduce rising trend lines or budget requests that jump above the historical rate of increase. Reversion to the mean is an article of faith for budget analysts, hence a budget request with a big increase or decrease is immediately suspect. When agencies talk about future spending increases, budget analysts busily scrutinize actual expenditures for last year and the probable actual for this year against the budget to see what the size of the increase would be and to compare actual to budgeted expenditures. It is a bad sign to a budget analyst when an agency asks for more without fully executing or spending its entire current budget. When requests in the new budget are below actuals (last year's actual expenditure or the estimate for the current year actual expenditure), and thus constitute a decreased budget request, budget analysts do not necessarily applaud the agency for its frugality. Instead, they tend to worry that the agency has not done the numbers correctly or has left out some significant component of the program that may have important policy consequences. When this happens, they ask questions until they get enough data to be reassured.

THE LEGISLATIVE CONTEXT OF THE BUDGET ANALYST

Budget analysts are also found in the legislative branch of government, acting as committee staff or housed in central review agencies including the Congressional Budget Office or the Office of the Legislative Analyst in California. Analysts serving the legislature tend to have roles that are more broadly based in policy. Often their primary interest is in general policy questions, and like CBO they may provide analysis of the chief executive's budget proposals or independent estimates of revenues, spending, and national or state economic conditions. While they also have interests in individual departments and policy areas, they rarely delve into the details of administration as deeply as their administrative counterparts. When they serve a committee or committee chairperson, his concerns are their concerns. If the legislator is fixed on an issue that has great relevance to her state or district, then the legislative analyst may be immersed in the details of the issue at levels even deeper than the agency analyst as the job focuses around a single issue for that legislative session.

A legislator with a military base or a defense contractor in his district may also have perennial concerns about what happens to this important constituent in every budget session and hence his staff will also become experts in this area and adept at scrutinizing budgets for items that affect this prized constituent. It goes without saying that all legislators have prized constituents. An important part of the job of his staff is to track budgets to ensure that no great harm is done his constituents, especially those who may have facilitated his last campaign. To find out about the degree of harm, the legislative staff must ask budget analyst type questions in the right places. And, of course, the legislative context for budget analysis is highly charged politically, as members (and staffs) from different parties, and with different interests relative to their constituent bases, compete vigorously for limited funds. Legislative political intrigue is often Machiavellian, and the analyst is caught up right in the middle of the fray.

Budgetary technology has changed since Wildavsky's original *Politics of the Budgetary Process* (1964) was written. Currently, much of the work for budget hearings is based on computers and the printouts and spreadsheets sometimes pile half a foot high on the tables and desks. However, computers do not solve any problems other than basic manipulation of data, valuable enough in itself, but all of the decision making surrounding budget schedules and their review is a human process done by experts in their areas, some to propose a budget, others to review those proposals. What is illustrated time and again is that even experts do not know everything, because expertise is compartmentalized and because issues grow and change over time and present themselves in different ways in different years. Moreover, even subject matter experts have to be coached to make the best case for themselves in the budget process.

Budget analysts do not have the same level of control over all issues. They have enormous power over the small items, but their power over major issues is weaker, because these decisions are often resolved by political agreements reached later in the budget process. Still the budget analyst is often able to come to decisions that will be respected and affirmed later in the decision process because he is able to craft a solution to a decision that follows budget guidelines while also anticipating how the political system within and without the agency will react to the proposal (see Thurmaier, 1998, p. 236). For the most part, it appears that the budget analyst is asking an annoying set of "little" questions whose purpose is unclear, but the total effect of these questions structures the agenda so that decision making may proceed with a clear focus on more important issues. We now turn to a consideration of the budget analyst and what it takes to be one.

ATTITUDES OF BUDGET ANALYST

A budget analyst provided us with the draft letter reproduced below. It is a proposed standard reply from the budget analyst's perspective to most or all complaint letters directed to a state Governor. This proposed form letter would be prepared for the Governor's signature. We have included it here to show the bias and unsympathetic narrow-mindedness that is often typical of the view of the seasoned career budget analyst. Needless to say, this letter would never actually be sent.

Dear Sir:

Since taking office, one of the many wasteful practices I have eliminated is the preparation of individual responses to letters from constituents. While the personal nature of an individual response yields a great deal of political mileage it costs a great deal more than the taxpayers can really afford. In addition, the entire practice is a big fraud anyway. I neither read these letters nor do I prepare the response and I seldom read the ones prepared with my signature. In fact, I didn't even write this letter and probably would never sign anything like this with any knowledge of what was in it. However, regardless of what you may think, I am not indifferent to you problems. I am just a very busy man. In any case this all points to the fact we all know to be true. Government is run and even controlled to a great extent by people not visible to you—whom you might regard as the "faceless bureaucracy." But is this so bad? While this practice of sending you an impersonal letter is less polite than the old system, let's face it. It is cheaper. And isn't that what you wrote to complain about to begin with? So in the long run it is better, right? You will get over your initial outrage, we will save you money on letter writing, and your complaint will be duly registered with the invisible (to you) bureaucrat responsible for the program that upsets you. This is a pretty good deal when you think about it. Please do.

Sincerely yours,

Governor Smith

What kind of people would think of drafting blunt letters like this? Budget analysts working in a municipal, state or federal budget offices might wish to write it. They comprise an elite group of bright, sometimes brash (as the draft letter indicates), highly trained, typically overworked folks who are crucial to the functioning of the budgetary apparatus. They are an elite group and know it. They take a certain pride in producing quality work under the pressure of deadlines. With this goes a certain style, one manifestation of which may be seen in this hypothetical response to a complaint letter.

As an organization, generically a budget bureau may by viewed to serve at least five functions. These include:

1. Oversight of budget preparation.
2. Oversight of budget execution.
3. Legislative clearance.
4. Management review.
5. Information gathering.

The mission statement for OMB puts these complex tasks into a cohesive statement of Purpose:

> The Office of Management and Budget serves the President by preparing the annual United States Budget and carrying out other statutory requirements, developing integrated fiscal, budget, program and management policies, leading government-wide coordination in policy making, and ensuring, through management oversight, government-wide effectiveness and consistency in policy implementation, in accordance with Presidential priorities. (Mission Statement, 2000)

While this statement is specific to the OMB, state and local government budget offices often are tasked with similar functions, and the larger, more complex jurisdictions often model their executive budget office role on OMB. The OMB strategic plan notes that OMB works for the President and occupies a unique position at the center of government. Given its comprehensive view of program priorities and strategic interests, the mission statement adds that "OMB has a hand in the development and resolution of budget, policy, program management, legislative, regulatory, information, procurement, financial management and associated issues on behalf of the President." With these responsibilities and its crucial location at the center of government and next to the President, OMB is in the middle of policy making and resource allocation tradeoffs as it strives to maintain coherence and consistency among the President's priorities and government programs.

OMB's responsibilities include:

1. Preparation of the President's budget;
2. Oversight of financial management, federal procurement and information technology;
3. Review and clearance of proposed legislation, regulations, and executive orders;
4. Oversight of program management;
5. Implementing of other statutory responsibilities;
6. Ensuring continuity of these functions during the transition to new Presidential administrations (Mission Statement, 2000).

The plan adds that OMB's strength is its central placement and unique government-wide perspective and warns that few of the major policy issues with which a modern President must contend fit neatly into the confines of a single department, but rather require coordinated analysis and action across many Executive Branch agencies. The plan also advises that OMB operates in a "fast paced environment, dealing with complex issues on a daily basis." This is true for OMB, and to a lesser extent for state and local budget offices also. The position next to the chief executive at the center of government is crucial. State and local problems too rarely are solvable within a single department and as the government gets smaller the problems often loom larger with no consequent increase in analytic talent to solve them. If anything, the central budget office may become even more important at sub-national levels of government.

Whoever directs the central budget office has a complex job. An article describing the OMB Director noted that he had the responsibility to craft a budget proposal early in the year and then make sure that the final outcome in the fall when Congress is done comes as close to the original proposal as possible (Schlesinger, 2001, pp. 1, 7). This means that preparation is virtually a year around task, given the spring preview, the fall agency submittal, the winter decision making, compilation, and presentation to Congress and then the tracking and negotiating to keep the President's program on track. Since budget execution is more routine, it is usually handled at lower levels within OMB, but any single issue can require the Director's attention. Clearance of agency legislative proposals is also handled routinely, but it too can see issues raised to the highest levels when the

President and Congress reach an impasse or when the President threatens a veto. In the summer of 2001, Director Daniels tried to keep the lid on a farm aid bill and was largely successful. At one point when the Senate was threatening to raise the bill total to $7.5 billion, Daniels convinced the President to threaten a veto. When the Senate Agriculture Committee Chairman approached Daniels looking for a last minute compromise, Daniels apparently won the day by suggesting that if "Congress didn't pass the smaller bill right away ... the cash infusion would be delayed well past the fall." The Democrat-controlled Senate gave in and sent President Bush the $5.5 billion farm bill he wanted (Schlesinger, 2001, p. 7). This is a fascinating display of the interplay of power, the threat of a veto, and the threat that even if the veto were overridden, the payments would be very late, and the Democrats in the Senate would be blamed for their lateness. It also illustrates the interweaving of process between the two branches of government. The executive branch does not hand the budget over to Congress and wait for it to pass bills back to it to be signed or vetoed; it actively works to gain desired outcomes. Conversely, Congressional hearings on the budget currently under consideration cannot help but influence agency budget construction of the next fiscal year budget.

In this interweaving of policy and process between the executive and legislative branches of government and within the executive branch, the budget bureau is a key player. As an institution the bureau pursues presidential or gubernatorial desires, but it also has program preferences of its own. Agencies can never be quite sure for whom the budget analyst is speaking. He may be speaking for the chief executive or for the budget bureau itself, or he even may be speaking for himself—the budget analyst. The budget analyst may deliberately manipulate that ambiguity to increase the perception of his or her role. Then, when the analyst suggests a cut in a sensitive item, the agency will be more likely to accept it. The budget analyst usually presents himself to the agency to make it appear that everything he or she says is from the Governor or the President and is spoken with the weight of the Governor or the President behind it, when, in reality, it might only be the opinion of the budget analyst.

In the budget process, the virtue of the budget bureau is that it reduces an enormous amount of paperwork and a variety of complicated and complex forms to comprehensible and manageable numbers. Barry White has called it "frozen policy," speaking of the budget OMB produces that the President sends to Congress. White notes that the President's budget sets out in one place and for one moment in time for all the world to see what he would spend and why, and how he would tax and why in order to provide for every single activity of the federal government. White suggests that this document is unique and all the bills and reports that Congress considers and passes do not produce a document quite like the executive budget.

White suggests this document remains the most complete benchmark of the budget process that everyone uses in one way or another, even in years when most of the President's policy changes are called "dead on arrival" (White, 1999). At state and local levels, budget bureaus also typically turn out a budget book representing the chief executive's proposed budget. Behind that book stand literally shelves of other documents all of which have been summarized into that budget book. In the process of budgeting, the budget bureau sets the agenda for the legislative branch by the way it prepares and submits budgets to the legislative branch, by the way it highlights certain changes, or by the way it attempts to cut certain functions and embellish or enhance other functions. Thus, even though the legislature is an independent and equally powerful branch of government, knowledge management gives the executive branch an edge—things that the budget bureau does structure how a legislature looks at the budget. This edge is much more pronounced at the state level where the legislature tends to be understaffed, at least compared to Congress.

Wildavsky (1964) suggested that the agency's perception of the budget bureau was that it could hurt the agency, but not help it much. The measure of hurt or help was the addition of dollars to the budget. In those years, the budget bureau was known for cutting, not for adding money to the budget, thus Wildavsky's observation was a logical extension of the budget bureau's primary responsibility, cutting budgets. Agencies with solid support in Congress had a different perspective on the budget bureau. If it were to cut them too deeply, they could ask their "friends in Congress" to restore the cut, as our reporting of Department of Agriculture patterns illustrates. At state and local levels, most observers see the budget bureau as a critical element; it can hurt, but it can also help a lot.

Wildavsky noted that Congress' perception of the budget bureau and of budget analysts was that of technicians who tried to set policy and usurp the role of Congress: "Nobody elected them to anything." This view is often expressed by legislators at all levels of government. The budget analyst's perception of Congress or of Congressmen is as a group of self-interested and somewhat parochial individuals who do not understand what the national interest demands, or for that matter the Governor or Mayor's plan. Budget analysts know that their executive represents a national constituency, and, by extension, so do they. The agency knows that the outcomes of the budget process are going to be some sort of compromise between what the agency requests and the budget bureau recommends, modified by congressional interests. The budget bureau knows that Congress is going to be interested in the total figure proposed in the budget as well as those figures proposed for an individual Congressman's district. Budget analysts have to be able to function in an environment where the stakes are high, information plentiful but little is certain.

For the first 30 years after the passage of the Budget and Accounting Act of 1921, popular perception of the BOB was that it was an agency designed to control spending—to say no to requests. This role changed in the 1950s, as an OMB official noted:

> As government grew ... the bureau has acquired a programming role that it did not have at least to the same extent before. The problem of choice among the programs is increasingly important and perhaps to some extent the negative role of the bureau has been less important.

The importance of this insight should not be overlooked; it means that the Bureau began to turn to program advocacy in the late 1950s, at least a decade before the Nixon reforms that created OMB and gave it a clear political mission. He continues "...our initial answer was to be no. And everybody would have been surprised if we had said yes the first time around." However, with programs where there was Presidential interest, the bureau changed to positive program emphases,

> And so we have increasingly tried to give consideration to how to do something rather than lining up a long list of reasons why they should not be done.[2]

The shift, then, in the perspective was from always saying no and thus cutting down budget costs to sometimes saying yes, "because the President wants it." What that means is that the budget bureau was no longer a neutral analytic tool. Rationally, if all the budget bureau ever did was say no to everything; certainly agencies would adopt strategies to counter a continuously negative role from it. It is probable that the bureau has always had this inclination, but until recently budgeting was such an inside affair that it would have been hard to discover. Moreover, the bureau does retain a cutting bias, as do all budget bureaus, because demand for spending always outruns supply and the bureau is the most powerful gatekeeper. The statement from Dawes, the first director of the budget bureau that, "...we are just down in a stokehold of the ship making sure that the fires don't go out" (Burkhead, 1959, p. 289) is picturesque, but hardly believable. However, it was a sensible thing for him to say, for cultivating the image of the neutral technician is a way to mask real power and the exercise of policy preferences.

Different administrations may require different styles by the budget director. It has been noted that OMB's goals in the Clinton years often had more to do with getting specific programs funded than with preventing spending, (thanks to political opposition from the other party in Congress) while in 2001 the first Bush budget session was marked by a goal of keeping a lid on outlays, by first holding discretionary spending to a 4% growth rate in the spring and then allowing for a 7% increase in the summer. Mitchell Daniels, OMB Director for President Bush, was the man on the spot. As is usual with Budget Directors, Daniels was portrayed as an economizer; in his personal style he was said to "make a good poster boy for thriftiness." As an indication of this, former aides said that he edited their memo's to one third of their original length. It was further observed that he spoke in a clipped style, ended meetings ahead of time, and lived in a "one-bedroom apartment with bare walls." Mr. Bush had nicknamed him "the blade" which prompted Daniels to decorate his office mantelpiece with an "authentic samurai sword" (Schlesinger, 2001, pp. 1, 7). These symbolic trappings and behaviors are meant to give Daniels the aura of a budget cutter; the mystique helped him say no to agency budget requests and increases the likelihood that agencies accept cuts as legitimate. This is not an easy role, particularly in a year with a big budget surplus; even with the tax cut, the budget surplus in 2001 was the second largest in history at $160 billion, behind only the surplus in the year 2000. An indication that this environment made for tough going for the budget cutter could be seen from President Bush's support of Daniels. The President urged his cabinet members to cooperate with Daniels, saying in early August "I know Mitch often displeases you, but cooperate with him" (Schlesinger, 2001, p. 7). This may also have marked the time when Daniels began to move toward increases of 7%. Long time observers note that when the President has to start publicly supporting his budget director, trouble is usually brewing for him.

The role of the budget analyst is a complex role. The budget analyst basically has three major responsibilities at the state level. (1) To assist the Governor in the legislature and in determination of appropriate budget and program goals. (2) To ensure that the agency works within legislative intent, and that the tools and techniques that it chooses to carry out that intent are consistent with good management practice. (3) To gather, review, and transmit information to the Governor, legislature, and interested committees on a wide range of legislative, policy, and organizational matters. At the federal level, agency budget analysts control more dollars, but at state and local levels budget analysts are closer to the people who make policy and may see more and influence more of the policy making process.

Budget analysts are facilitators. They are in unique places to acquire information. This is especially true of state and local government analysts. By transmitting certain kinds of information from one place to another budget analysts can facilitate changes and can either enhance or diminish the power of other participants. There are structured times when a budget analyst manipulates power and information as during the budget session, in preparation or execution of a budget. There are nonstructured times when budget analysts may do special studies and find innovations in one department worth communicating to other departments. Or a budget ana-

lyst in talking with his peers in the budget bureau may hear of some innovation worth suggesting to his agencies. As a communicator and facilitator
the budget analyst can make a great impact on agencies and programs.

A budget analyst may have one part of a major agency or he might have
five or six small agencies, but whatever budget analysts work with, there will
be a certain number of functions that he or she can impact. One analyst in
his first years as a budget analyst was proudest of abolishing ten of the agencies he was given. They were all very small nonfunctional boards and commissions, but it was an achievement, nonetheless, particularly since they had
standing in state law, which had to be changed to permit their abolition. The
bottom line is that the budget analyst, by virtue of his mobility in the system
and his closeness to information and to policy making powers, has great
leverage that he or she can use to communicate information about policy
and management across departmental lines. Recognizing that power, an
operating agency normally tends to be somewhat wary of the budget analyst.

Conversations with state budget analysts lead to some interesting points.
Most budget analysts tend to stay only for two or three budget cycles. The
work pressures are very high, the hours long, but the opportunity to make
major achievements is great. White suggests that the same phenomenon
occurs to OMB analysts; some do not like the pressures of the job, but others thrive on it and thanks to the contacts that they make, move out into
better positions in the bureau or in the line agencies. White notes that in
OMB stretches of ten to twelve hour days for weeks on end are not uncom-
mon, but with this workload also comes the opportunity to have an impact
on programs at the highest level including, on rare occasions, briefing the
President (White, 1999, p. 465). White suggests that the seasoned analysts
who enjoy the attractions of the job try not to get too high or too low but to
treat it like a 162 game baseball season, to go the distance. White says, "For
those who can handle it, few career government positions rival the satisfaction of budget examining" (White, 1999, p. 465).

Agencies tend to see these budget analysts as "kids." When agencies look
at these young, innovative "kids" they wonder what this budget analyst is
going to do to them. This leads to certain tensions; "The budget analyst is
generally a young man with a minimum of experience and practical knowledge and a great deal of authority and responsibility." Agencies suspect this
to be a bad combination; they expect to pay dues in unreasonable deadlines, minimally useful reports, and an inundation of trivial check-backs on
paperwork while the new budget analyst acquires experience. Most agencies hope that this happens in the off-budget season, because it can really
hurt them to have a new analyst assigned to them during the budget season
when time is critical and the right word here and there may be the difference between good budget outcomes and bad budget outcomes. The experienced budget analyst is expected to know these words and when to say

them. He is expected to manage his own workload and let the agency manage its without putting unnecessary information strains upon it. After all, the normal budget preparation requirements impose a heavy enough burden. What else does the experienced budget analyst have to show? "The burden on that analyst is to prove that he has a genuine interest in the programs, goals, and problems of the agency. And that he will not act arbitrarily or capriciously." One state-level budget analyst commented that one of the other budget analysts in the bureau delighted in asking agencies to submit voluminous reports. "He would ask them on a Friday afternoon and tell them they had till Monday morning to get it done." What is interesting is that the agencies would do it. This is unusual; the agency also has power and could use it to "punish" the budget analyst by going to his superior, but in this case the agency chose not to challenge the analyst's behavior. This may be a case of being able to live with a known evil in order to avoid a greater evil. In terms of budget analyst behavior, asking for unnecessary reports with unrealistic deadlines is irresponsible, but it happens and not only at the state level. Occasionally, the press of business is such in Washington that agencies get requests for information from their budget bureau or OMB the day before Thanksgiving or around Christmas and they sometimes end up working the holidays. This happens often enough that no one talks about it as extraordinary, although it would certainly seem a little extreme to the non-budgeteer.

Generally, the experienced budget analyst has to assure the agency that he is not going to act capriciously or arbitrarily. This does not mean, however, that the analyst is a rubber stamp for the agency, but it does mean that he assists the agency in setting and achieving desirable goals. One supervisor remarked, "This is done by introducing ideas, thoroughly testing any proposals made by the agency, and alerting the agency to new trends and developments. This means giving the benefit of a doubt to the agency where there are no substantial reasons for dispute."

He felt that, "The ideal analyst agency relationship is one of mutual trust, respect, and understanding. This relationship is supported by knowledge of the agency's programs, goals and personnel, of management tools and techniques and of the budget bureau's role and responsibility. It is maintained by open lines of communication between the analyst and the agency." This relationship is built during the year and during the overtime hours of the budget cycle. The analyst gets to know what the budget bureau's goals are as well as the goals of the agencies with which he works. He will also get to know what his agencies do—the people, their programs, their tendencies. Track records are important because they allow for short cuts in decision making. If an administrator is known to be a pinchpenny, his routine budget requests may be passed unchallenged and the non-routine may be lent undue credibility. If another is known to be a big spender, everything he sends to the budget bureau in preparation or execution may be closely examined. His non-routine requests may require extraordinary amounts of justification, no matter how meritorious the request.

The experienced analyst keeps the lines of communication open. This is not an easy task. One budget supervisor remarked: "The good analyst recognizes that he is a babe in the woods" at first and therefore must spend a good amount of time reading about the agency and talking to these key people. There isn't too much to read about agencies. There are memos and files, but the best thing a budget analyst can do is meet people. The agency in turn recognizes an informed analyst will be better equipped to interpret the agency's budget and management requests. And therefore the agency will intentionally seek out the analyst to explain any new directions it is considering, any problems it is having, and any help that it may need."

One analyst compared this process to "running a trapline," commenting that there were certain people he had to talk with on a regular basis if he wanted to remain an effective player in the budget process, and some of the important ones were not in his immediate decision hierarchy, but were placed where they had a good view of what might be going to happen to his program and his money. In another example of this, one regional administrator explained that he called around to the other regions to see what they were going to ask for. Then he could either ask for what they asked for and enjoy group support, or he could ask for something different, betting that he could get what he wanted because his request would be unique and small and he might also get what the others were all asking for as part of a Department-wide package. He also confessed that once he told the others who called him that asking for item A was certain to fail, thus discouraging them, while he then asked for it himself. When asked by a peer, he said, "The boss wanted it, what could I do?" This is generally believed to be a one-time only stratagem; if word gets out that your word is not to be trusted, no one will call on you and your budget analyst is likely to challenge most of your requests. Only the press of work prevents him from challenging them all.

The experienced analyst tries to be selective in the items chosen to challenge. The budget analyst is always overworked. His in-basket is always full. Requests to purchase a typewriter, requests to certify a reclassification from a clerk 2 to clerk 3, a request to buy a $5 million helicopter, he cannot challenge all of them. He cannot go back and make people recalculate basic data on all of them. Some of them he simply must take on trust. And so perhaps the budget analyst looks at the name of the person who generates the request and says, "Good man. I will approve this one." For others he may say, "Oh, no. Not again." And he will have to check back on that request even though the dollar amount is minor. White suggests that there is never time for a budget analyst to do all the analysis needed for every program and policy issue before a decision is made. Therefore, analysts make choices daily about what will be examined and how deeply the issue will be analyzed. White compares this to a triage process: certain choices are obvious, both for inclusion and exclusion. In the middle ground exist a group of items where time pressures dictate less analysis and certain risks are taken so that the analyst can focus on the important, high-payoff policy sensitive issues (White, 1999, p. 481). The avalanche of work forces all administrators to be selective about what they challenge or they reevaluate. Senior analysts believe that to some extent the test of a good analyst is the items that he or she chooses to challenge. While they accept that a good analyst may adopt various role behaviors, they also suggested that some inexperienced analysts adopted role behaviors that were counterproductive. Two approaches cited as mistakes, but frequently taken by novice analysts were summed up as "watchdogs" and "isolationists." In the watchdog role the analyst challenges almost everything. One analyst said:

> The watchdog role might be appropriate when there is some history of manipulation or wrongdoing within an agency. But generally the watchdog role is a letter of the law approach, permits little exercise of good management practice and it is frustrating and annoying to both the analyst and the agency, and works against the full and free exchange of ideas and information. But more than that the analyst who chooses to play the role of watchdog had better know the program and the policy of the agency, as well as, if not better than, the agency personnel. And it is a rare analyst who can claim that —and even rarer, have it be true.[3]

An analyst who plays watchdog in challenging everything will review superficially and soon wear out his welcome. It is not good enough to challenge everything; not only is it extremely destructive of interpersonal relationships, but challenging everything means analyzing nothing. Time alone prevents it. Needless to say, agencies do not like analysts to take a watchdog posture. But, every once in a while, letting an agency know that you are looking at a request is a very handy posture for an analyst to adopt. For example, it is not a good idea to choose a strategy that says, "I won't look at any requests below $500.00 or I won't look at any non-personnel requests." An analyst always has to give the impression that he is looking. Once in a while when there is a questionable request that could be let go through because the analyst knows the people and the agency, it helps make his reputation as a detail person to send that request back and ask questions about it: "I once received a travel voucher claim back because when entering the beginning and ending mileage from my odometer, I switched the numbers and put the ending mileage in place of the starting mileage. The travel claims office sent it back and had me fix it. I had mixed emotions. First, I thought any fool could see it was a clerical error on my part and it would have been better for me if they had sent me the money. After all, I had paid for the expense out of my pocket and I was due the reimbursement. On the other had, the voucher was clearly wrongly made out. As much as I wanted my money back, I had a sneaking admiration for whomever caught the error and sent it back. I never made that mistake again." Everyone who works in a bureaucracy has tales like this. From an analyst's perspective, even if the main concern is policy and program achievement, a reputation for being a good detail person does not hurt a bit.

The isolationist approach is usually adopted by the analyst when overloaded by assignments. In budget bureaus the overload tends to be the rule rather than the exception. Therefore, the budget analyst simply becomes a paper processor. "Unquestioning and unknowing, he simply processes everything. To the self-sufficient agency he seems like a godsend. He doesn't ask questions, he doesn't slow up the paperwork during the non-budget season, for he lets the agency be about its business, but he also causes that agency much concern during the budget session." It is here in the budget session that the isolationist must be able to interpret to the decision maker the thrust and the aim of the agency's plans. He can be easily led astray or become confused by any question that deviates from the substance of the agency's budget presentation. "Being ill-informed, his recommendations are often ill-advised." He doesn't know the agency. By challenging requests, by interacting with the people the budget analyst gets to know the agency.

No set pattern exists for the characteristics and personality traits that make a good budget analyst. Zody suggests that the good budget analyst has character, meaning personal integrity, is an excellent listener, is inherently questioning (Who, What, Where, Why, When), is cautious, avoids the emotional aspects of a disagreement (relies on reasonable assumptions, sound logic and verifiable information in argument), is neither miserly nor extravagant and focuses on the three Es: Economy, Efficiency, and Effectiveness, is parsimonious with public resources and knows that simply adding more resources will not solve problems, even if resources were inexhaustible.

The good "budgeteer" according to Zody has prudent judgment and seeks reasonable certainty, seeks to do the honest thing ("looks in the mirror and knows the honest thing has been done"), and has a passion for excellence, accuracy, precision, and timeliness (Zody, 1998a, pp. 251–252). One budget supervisor suggested that some key words describing the ideal analyst would include: effort, patience, flexibility, service, respect, communication, and selectivity. Patience is difficult, but it is important. Line agencies are sometimes filled with relatively inflexible people and dealing with them demands patience. They have a task to do and they tend to have "tunnel vision" about that task. Or they may be people who are not as adept at thinking up new ideas as the budget analyst herself. Or they may be people who have seen many new ideas come and go and are a little bit rigid in picking up another new idea. Flexibility meant, for one analyst the "...ability to say you are wrong when you are wrong. The better you get, the more difficult it becomes to say you are wrong."

We have included a competence test for a budget analyst as a checklist used by a supervisor of budget analysts to see how his analysts were doing.[4] The first question tests the analyst's knowledge of the leadership in the analyst's agency. The second assesses the extent of the analyst's program knowledge. The third seeks to ascertain how well the analyst understands current efforts. Only the fourth question is a pure budget question; it asks about the size of the budget and the potential increment of change. The assumption is that the analyst who cannot answer these questions is so out of touch as to be almost useless. This supervisor believed that, "An analyst should need no more than 30 seconds to answer these questions." Budget supervisors feel that the continuous interaction with the agency over critical matters in budget execution and preparation makes it easy for the budget analyst to learn the people and the programs in his agencies. Budget analysts deal with time and money; since both are in usually in short supply; conversations between the analyst and his agencies quickly penetrate the superficial. As one analyst said: "You just get to know people really well, really quickly. Who can be trusted, who can't. What words mean to them. It's always good to know when 'yes' means 'yes, but...' or a nod means 'I heard what you said', and not 'I agree with you.'"

Another budget analyst supervisor commented that, "The ideal relationship requires continual effort on the part of the agency and the analyst, and must be developed over time ... I also believe that analysts often unwisely choose to use a watchdog or isolationist approach in budget analysis." It is easy however to slip into these roles. New analysts especially fall prey to these approaches, until they have developed the experience to recognize what the real issues are and whose word can be trusted.

There is no doubt that good budget analysts have the ability to influence policy. To do this takes experience and sensitivity to political issues. There is no preferred prototype for the budget analyst, other than that he be a good communicator, analytic, and a quick study. While no discipline is significantly more valuable than another, the increasingly analytic thrust of public administration and affairs programs has certainly increased the attractiveness of that discipline as a training ground for potential budget analysts in recent years, but economics, business administration and even liberal arts majors also work out.

To conclude this discussion, we offer Zody's (1998a) thoughts on budget ethics (p. 251). We have argued that budget analysts have great power to influence political decisions. Power must always be accompanied by ethical behavior. Because budget analysts hold power rather anonymously and cannot be held accountable through the electoral process, ethical behavior is particularly important for them. Hard work is not enough. Thus Zody quotes from *Hamlet*, Act I, Scene III:

> Neither a borrower nor a lender be;
> For loan oft loses both itself and friend,
> And borrowing dulls the edge of husbandry.
> This above all, to thine ownself be true;
> And it must follow, as the night the day;
> Thou canst not then be false to any man.

This is as good place as any to start when looking for injunctions for ethical behavior for budget analysts.

CONCLUSIONS

Budget analysis is part science and part intuition. Budgets are complex as are the tasks faced by analysts. In this chapter we have attempted to provide a perspective on budget analysis from the analyst's level. In addition, we have reviewed many of the tasks and dilemmas faced while playing the role of controller or gatekeeper in the budget process. As with any profession there are a number of tricks of the trade that may be learned only from experience. In budget analysis, experience with the budget cycle improves the insight and quality of analysis. Sustaining a career as a budget analyst requires an "iron stomach" some have observed. However, in this chapter we have shown that many of the tasks of budget analysis are relatively routine. Also, it is important that while budget analysts wield considerable power and influence, their role in essence is to provide the best information possible for the real decision makers in the Executive and legislative branches of government to make the decisions for which they are responsible and should be held accountable to the public.

However, this is not to say that budget analysis is not political; just the opposite is true. Virtually every major option posed in the budget is laden with political implications. Thus, the budget analyst must be fair and attempt to present all sides of issues so that decisions may be well informed. In the end, we quote Zody on ethics because the budget analyst and analysis pose constant ethical dilemmas. Budgeting, like politics, is the art of compromise. Budget analysts, at their best, facilitate the process of political negotiation and compromise that allows political resolution to difficult policy and resource problems.

EXHIBIT 1
A Hypothetical Competence Test for Budget Analysts

1. Who are the major division and section heads of the agency? Tell us something about each of them. The analyst should have at least five phone numbers of agency personnel that he has used so often that he has them memorized.

2. Describe the major efforts of the department in the past year and in the past month. When a major proposal emanates from an agency head the analyst should be able to find out who originated the proposal before it was adopted as the policy of the agency. This implies the existence of some informal contacts within the agency and a posture of trust of the analyst on the part of some agency subordinates.

3. What major problems—administrative and/or policy—face the agency at this time? What is the agency doing about them? The analyst should need no more than 30 seconds to answer these questions:

    A. If only a single piece of legislation affecting the agency could be passed in the coming year, what bill would it be?

    B. What single function of the agency is least worthwhile?

    C. What single function would be most desirable to expand if additional funds were made available to the agency?

    D. Assuming that reorganization by Executive fiat were possible, what functions of the agency ought to be transferred to other agencies and what functions of other agencies ought to be transferred to that agency?

    E. What outside organizations would be most upset if the agency's budget were halved overnight?

4. If the agency were to submit an annual budget today, what would the analyst estimate to be the dollar amount requested? What changes from the present budget would he or she see? In other words, what is his or her focus and what is his or her level of understanding of budget content and cost?

NOTES

1. Much of the material in this chapter is drawn from the experience of the authors as operating budget analysts in state government, from conversations with students who later worked as budget analysts, and from ongoing research with budget analysts about budget analysis at federal, state and local governments. The perspectives shared by budget analysts and their supervisors are drawn from all levels

of government and both central budget office and line agency settings. Insights are drawn from current data and from historical sources. While nothing is true everywhere, the authors suspect that most who function as budget analysts will be able to relate to most of the concepts in this chapter. J. McCaffery would especially like to thank David Head who initiated him into the world of budget analysis long ago and whose comments helped shape this chapter. There is now a significant body of literature on what budget bureaus and budget analysts do. Some dates from early description of the Bureau of the Budget and OMB, such as those by Paul Appleby (1957) and Percival Brundage (1970) to the more recent work of Bruce Johnson (1984) and Al Killeen (1990). There is also a significant and recent body of literature concerning state and local budgeteers, including work by James Gosling (1985), Kurt Thurmaier (1995) and Katherine Willoughby (1993). The reader interested in this area will find the work of these authors a rich place to begin. For an excellent discussion of the functions of a budget bureau and budget analyst, which is still valid generically, see Davis and Ripley (1967), and Wildavsky (1979).

   2.   Derthick (1975, p. 85). Also, please note that because many of the quotes in this chapter come from personal interviews with budget analysts, under assurance of anonymity, in many instances no citation references are supplied.

   3.   This quote and the discussion of the watchdog and isolationist roles is taken from a memorandum to J. McCaffery from David Head.

   4.   This is from a state budget office memorandum reportedly authored by Paul Dommel.

CHAPTER VII

BUDGET STRATEGY

INTRODUCTION

One of the myriad challenges that confront the manager in the complex world of government is the responsibility for devising strategies for constructing and presenting budgets successfully in a highly charged political context. Without budget strategy, programs will not be created or funded to the extent that funding is required. Budgeting is a process of matching needs to money. However, it also requires considerable strategic thinking about what issues and policies are more or less likely to be funded in any given political context. Managers are responsible for the formal calculation of what needs to be done to execute programs and for controlling costs to match resources available. A key lesson in budgeting is to try to get the exact amount of funding appropriated and allocated that can be executed to the 100% level. This demonstrates efficiency, need, the ability to calculate and execute effectively, and enhances confidence in the reliability of the agency. The task of this chapter is to examine how managers cope with the task of building budgets, to examine budget presentation practices, and to suggest how managers may profit in future budget decisions. The perspective of this chapter is that of the practicing manager who must daily confront program realities and budgetary boundaries, developing strategies that will work given the incentives of the systems within which they work.

In devising budget strategy, managers may be responding to demands rising in the greater society; they may be directed by forms, time guidelines and fiscal constraints from the central budget office. Their budget requests may be reviewed, changed, and legitimized by other participants in the executive branch and in the legislature, and the courts (Straussman, 1986). However, theirs is the basic task of weaving together in a formal structure the numbers of workload, clients, and dollars, the intention to do more or less, the desire to provide more or less government to society within the context of a winning strategy. They are guided, reviewed, and controlled by law and by other parts of the political system. Their task is complicated by growing entitlements, top down budget routines, and fiscal shortfalls. Still, they have the basic data producing function, i.e., of building the budget—what Charles Levine termed "specification of the technical alternatives of programs." (Levine, 1985, p. 256.) Where fiscal stress reduces the resources available and constrains potential programs, the task of devising the winning budget strategy for presentation, negotiation, compromise and execution becomes even more critical.

This chapter does not attempt to detail all aspects of budget strategy. For a comprehensive analysis of strategic budgeting, see the work of Roy Meyers (Meyers, 1994). The chapter begins by focusing on one aspect of budget strategy: the counterpart to representation, i.e., *misrepresentation*. Budget winning strategy requires both effective representation and some degree of competitive behavior that stretches the limits of rules to outwit opponents competing for the largest share of the budget they can obtain. Thus, misrepresentation is considered here in the context in which it occurs as a legitimate part of the budget game in virtually all contexts of government. Does strategic misrepresentation in budgeting, which ranges from the mundane and routine to outright "gimmerickery," as Wildavsky and Caiden refer to it (Wildavsky & Caiden, 2001), bring ethical issues to the forefront of our consideration? The answer is that it does so to the extent that it warrants the special attention at the beginning of this chapter. After considering aspects and examples of strategic misrepresentation the chapter then moves on to a more comprehensive analysis of budgetary strategy.

STRATEGIC MISREPRESENTATION IN THE PHASES OF THE BUDGET PROCESS

Published research on the practices of strategic representation in budget formulation and negotiation is so abundant and this topic has been viewed from so many angles that we believe we have little to add to what has already been written and rewritten over the past fifty years. It is necessary to cite only a few works to provide an introduction to budget representation and strategies for winning resources in competition with other agents (see, e.g., Wildavsky, 1964; Wildavsky & Caiden, 2001). However, research work on misrepresentation is far less numerous (Anthony, 1985; Jones & Euske, 1991; Meyers, 1990, 1994).

Initially, how do we define strategic misrepresentation? To do so we draw on the work of Howard Raifa who investigated and taught the use of misrepresentation in game theory, until he was hounded out of this area by critics who alleged he was teaching students and readers how to cheat and win, which was not what he intended to do in his teaching and research. Practitioners and academics alike know where budgets may be padded and how to do it. Practitioners are rewarded for this knowledge, but academics may be punished if they are not careful how they teach this material, lest they be accused of "teaching how to cheat." Academics who avoid the subject altogether may feel more comfortable, but their students enter the real world at a competitive disadvantage to those already there and to those teachers who understand that strategic misrepresentation must be a topic for discussion.

In essence, we define strategic misrepresentation as intentionally planned lying and cheating justified by the view that in a competitive environment the opposition will engage to some extent in the same types of behavior. The classic example is in labor negotiations where a union initially asks for a higher wage increase than it expects to receive and the employer offers a rate lower than what he expects eventually to have to pay. Both sides plan and execute to the best of their abilities strategies, supported by data and arguments, that misrepresent in anticipation of similar behavior by the opposing agent. In budgeting, the use of strategic misrepresentation ranges from simple to highly complex initiatives. This chapter reports only a small number of the many ruses used to compete for resources in budgeting at all levels of government and in all nations in the world (Jones et al., 2001). The key issue in consideration of strategic misrepresentation is that the rules of the budget game provide incentives for the behaviors that result. Without these incentives, the use of strategic misrepresentation would vanish. In essence, strategic misrepresentation is employed because it is permitted and often it succeeds. And when it does not succeed, there is almost always the ploy of plausible deniability in politics (and accounting and budgeting) to cover up the tracks of risky practice. After all, what good is a strategy that does not provide an out for failure? At its core, strategic misrepresentation is simply an intentional approach to strategic planning and execution that involves acceptance of higher risk to obtain greater results.

Examples of misrepresentation, such as inflating proposals to ask for more than is really justifiable so that an agency eventually gets something closer to what it actually needs, or generalizing the justification of cuts to cover virtually any budget reduction action, a typical ploy in Executive branch budgeting, are only tips of the misrepresentation iceberg. The approach we adopt in this chapter is to classify examples of strategic misrepresentation temporally, that is, according to when they occur in the budget cycle, e.g., in budget preparation instructions when executive analysts specify inflation adjustments below levels that are likely to be present in future budget years. On the one hand, this conditions program advocates to inflate their budget requests. On the other hand, budget proposals often attempt to hide new programs and costs within the base to avoid the exceptional scrutiny given such proposals in budget review.

Perhaps one of the most effective forms of strategic misrepresentation in the budget formulation phase occurs when the executive, through his or her budget office, specifies new rules for the entire budget game. Thus, the installation of zero-based budgeting may be justified on the grounds that it will cause real program priorities to surface and allow the base to be examined with the same care as the increment. With this high-minded objective, a new set of rules is to give advantage to the rule makers at the expense of the rule learners. Program advocates are at a disadvantage in competition with budget examiners in that they do not fully comprehend how the game is to be played. Budget examiners take advantage of the predictable uncertainty wherever it occurs with the resulting effect of allowing the executive to target budget reductions at their discretion, for example, at programs that are ideologically or politically unacceptable but for which there are not sufficient grounds to reduce or eliminate on the basis of efficiency or ineffectiveness (Jones & McCaffery, 1989).

Another predictable ploy in budget formulation is for the executive or legislative branch to intentionally overestimate or underestimate revenues or expenditures. This is done to provide the excuse for budget cutting or to support the case that the proposed budget will be more in balance than is likely to obtain when actual revenues are received and expenses are incurred. In the federal government, the U.S. Congress has repeatedly accused the executive branch of overestimating revenues to minimize the annual budget deficit. The estimates of the Congressional Budget Office (CBO) have been regarded by Congress as much more reliable than those provided by the President's Office of Management and Budget (OMB). This is a result not only of Congress having more confidence in its own staff; ex post evaluation has in many, but not all, instances shown CBO to be more accurate since creation of the Office in the 1974 Congressional Budget Impoundment and Control Act.

An example of misrepresentation in the politics of revenue estimation is available from California prior to enactment in 1978 of Proposition 13, the act that stimulated a wave of property tax reform and reduction across the nation (Levy, 1979). The Governor of California misinformed the public on the level of the state budget surplus in the apparent belief that if the actual size of the surplus were known, voters would choose property tax reform to retrieve the surplus. The governor's fears proved well founded as property tax reform was approved by voters despite misrepresentation of the level of the surplus.

Analysis of the budgetary politics of negotiation and enactment permits the segregation of decision contexts and issues into macro- and micro-categories. The macro-politics of the budgetary process typify the debate over high profile issues that command great public attention. Reform of the Social Security Tax or provision of aid to Contra forces in Central America are examples of macro-level policy issues debated between and within the executive and Congress. The micro-level issues are just as political as the macro level issues, but they are negotiated between agency budget officers and executive and legislative budget analysts. The allowable inflation adjustment is one such issue, as is the attempt to conceal new programs in the base. Other similar ploys at the micro-level include intentional agency miscalculation of the budget or a failure to adjust downward on items as directed to put the onus of budget compilation and the rationalization of components to the whole on the backs of budget examiners. Computers have assisted budget examiners with the task of defining the base and incremental adjustments relative to a set of budget instruction parameters, but computers do not always catch cleverly disguised "efforts" of this type.

Typical ploys in budget negotiation include inflating constituent group size and consequent demand for the program and use of organized lobby organizations to magnify the case for spending by applying pressure to the reelection calculus of elected officials. The age-old use of campaign funds and other types of benefits to trade for legislative votes providing employment in an elected official's state or district supports misrepresentation of client demand. Clientele groups with the best lobby typically are rewarded in the budget process when their effort is carefully coordinated with the program justification of the agency sponsor of the program. What is lamented by political scientists as the evil of pork-barrel politics is democracy in action from the viewpoint of many client groups.

Budget execution to some degree has a life of its own in most government organizations. The manner in which spending takes place and the services or assets acquired often do not relate directly to the proposals approved and promises made in budget formulation and negotiation. Agency and department program managers and budget officials typically reveal a strong preference for maximizing discretion in the application of resources to programs. They prefer to be as free as possible from the constraints applied by elected officials and controllers in the executive and legislative branches unless control provides necessary protection. Strong preference for discretion over the program for which managers are responsible is exactly what the precepts of management control recommend, that is, that managers be held accountable for the successes and failures of their programs relative to outputs achieved rather than to "political" variables (Anthony & Young, 1984; Euske, 1984).

A reward structure that emphasizes outcomes motivates managers to take ownership of their programs and to become more results-oriented. Budgetary discretion permits managers to apply resources where they are deemed to produce the desired mix of output. Output is contingent upon a technical core designed to solve problems that inhibit generation of output or block achievement of organizational goals. Program managers try to insulate and protect the critical technical cores of their organizations from interference, or political "noise," intruding from the resource decision environment (Thompson, 1967). Noise is reduced through the application of various ploys to gain budget execution freedom and to insulate against external interference.

Where a tight system of oversight, control, and audit is applied to budget execution and where program managers are strong protectors and supporters of their "technological cores" of problem solvers, pressure is placed on managers to misrepresent both factors of production and details of budget execution from oversight, audit, and program evaluation (Jones & Thompson, 1986). Motivation to behave in this manner typically is related legitimately to the desire to solve real problems (Euske & Euske, 1993). Implicit in the argument made here is the assumption that the incentives for strategic representation and misrepresentation are not produced exclusively by the executive or the legislative branches of government or that they are the product of one or the other side of the political spectrum. And it should not be inferred that only budget and program advocates or budget controllers engage in strategic misrepresentation. Rather, strategic misrepresentation is a type of behavior in evidence across the board in the game of budgeting as a result of incentives established and reinforced by the dynamics of the public budgetary process.

Furthermore, it must be reiterated that all budgetary advocacy or control does not involve or require strategic misrepresentation and that all strategy in budgeting does not involve misrepresentation. Rather, misrepresentation is a contingent strategy employed in response to a set of incentives present under specific circumstances. Implied in this analysis is that reform of the rules of budgeting is necessary to reduce or eliminate it.

PATTERNS OF STRATEGY

Budgets are fixed, periodic events for managers. They have organizational cycles and legal roots. Managers must respond to budget calendars. Not all managers respond the same way, nor are they all similarly motivated. Economic analysis of bureaucracy has produced a picture of the manager as a budget maximizer who gauges self-interest in terms of budget expansion. On the one hand, he expands his budget because his tenure in office is determined by his sponsors and clientele who expect to maximize the budget. On the other hand, he maximizes the budget because of the rewards it brings him and co-workers in terms of salary, power, reputation, and the other rewards a "wealthy" organization can provide its workers. As a result of these two themes, public-sector budgets are larger than they ought to be. In response, administrative theorists argue that when bureaucrats attempt to maximize utility, they do it not for personal gain and survival, but because they are motivated by duty, a picture of the good society, and the satisfaction of having contributed to helping attain that society. Sigelman (1986) summarizes and tests this argument, concluding that the maximization of personal utility does not necessarily lead to maximized agency budgets, finding that those who did call for expansion did so because they believed that all state functions ought to be increased. Those who scored high on professional commitment were more likely to advocate more growth and those who spent more time with the agency's clientele also were more supportive of larger increases, as opposed to those who were less committed professionally and those who were more limited in their range of client contact. Place in the organization counts, as does professional commitment, as does the concept of the role of the state. Certainly the picture of managers asking for more money because they identify more closely with their clientele, or because they are more professionally committed is more appealing than that of the manager budgeting for a new carpet or salary increase.

Historical research in budget patterns discloses that aggressive agencies tend to get more in the budget struggle than do less aggressive agencies (Sharkansky, 1968), and that the outcome of the budget struggle tends to be incremental (Wildavsky, 1964), although precise measurement of just what incremental means has been a source of extensive debate (Bailey & O'Connor, 1975; Tucker, 1982) Wildavsky's study found more than half of the increases within 10% of the previous year's base (1972, p. 14). However, this is analysis of aggregate budget totals. Research into outcomes of agency patterns has shown great fluctuation within individual agency budgets (LeLoup & Moreland, 1978; Natchez & Bupp, 1973) as well as an investigation of the base by reviewers (Gist, 1977; Kamlet & Mowery, 1980; Lauth, 1987). Thus although budget patterns tend to show incremental growth in the aggregate, the prudent manager can expect questions to probe the base as he or she presents justification for budget needs. LeLoup and Moreland's study of budget trends in the U.S. Department of Agriculture is especially interesting since it clearly demonstrates the range of intra-agency behavior.

The aggregate pattern is for agency budgets to grow at an incremental rate and the jurisdiction's budget office to cut because resource requests exceed available resources. The legislature tends to cut more from the proposed budget while mainly taking its cues from the executive budget. While Wildavsky (1964) emphasized the relationship of the agencies to Congressional committees, more recent research indicated that BOB/OMB was more powerful than the agencies or Congress in determining the size of the agencies annual increments (Kamlet & Mowery, 1980; Tomkin, 1983). This trend was intensified by David Stockman and his emphasis on an ideological budget driven by top-down decision procedures (Heclo, 1984; Wildavsky, 1988). This is the outline of the budgetary ritual. Within this framework *agencies rely on code words and behavioral repertoires to get what they think they need.*

Wildavsky (1984b, p. 64) sees that technical data supporting budget requests is not enough: what matters is how good a politician you are. The elements of being a good politician include cultivating a clientele to support your requests, developing other people's confidence in your work, and sharpening skills in following strategies designed to present your requirements in the most convincing fashion. Confidence involves trust. The complexity of the budget process dictates that some people must trust others, because they can only check up on them a small part of the time and because no one can be an expert in everything. In a fascinating study of state budget outcomes Duncombe and Kinney (1987) found that for agency officials in five western states budget success was not measured by getting the largest amount or percentage appropriated, but rather by getting enough to meet current needs with a few improvements and in maintaining good relationships with the legislature and its budget staff, and with the Governor and the executive budget staff. This is a reaffirmation of the need for confidence, trust, and competence in the budget process. Duncombe and Kinney suggest that their findings may have been distorted by the recent climate of fiscal scarcity in the states surveyed; however, if this is true, that only makes their conclusions more important, for in bad times is when the system has to work. In good times, enough organizational slack exists to overcome mistakes, misunderstandings, and misfits.

CONTINGENT STRATEGIES

Wildavsky (1964) also identified another group of behaviors that were designed to react to the conditions of the moment—time, place, and circumstance. These he called contingent strategies. On a fundamental level, contingent strategies are ways of combining the perennial concerns of an organization with the language and perception of current events. Public organizations administer laws; they are not free to choose what they will do from an unlimited list of possibilities. Their needs often outrun their resources, so they must choose. When they choose, they couch that choice in words reviewers are used to hearing. This simplifies information transfer. Janet Weiss (1982) submits that efficient decision makers sort through numerous alternatives to give serious attention to only one or two and that new information is pre-filtered by what has occurred before; decision makers simplify by "seeing" a problem as another case of something seen before and already understood. Weiss also concludes that decision-makers master a repertoire of skills and use these skills in combinations appropriate to the decision at hand. In budgeting, this repertoire of skills includes contingent strategies.

Contingent strategies are the shorthand ways managers tell reviewers what is happening in their programs relative to what reviewers want to hear. Contingent strategies are detailed explanations of causation. They are responses to organizational and environmental demands, comparable to private sector marketing strategies and tactics. The ubiquitous strategies of clientele, confidence and competence establish the environment for belief and the contingent strategies attempt to establish causation. They explain why the budget should be changed from one year to the next in terms that the reviewer is used to hearing and comprehending.

Casual observation suggests that these contingent strategies are agency specific—not all agencies can make a profit—and change over time. Wildavsky (1975) examined types of justifications in the outdoor recreation budget from 1949 to 1969. Twelve different justification categories were discovered in 1949. The most frequently used justifications were facilities and personnel inadequacy, and increased user pressure. These two themes accounted for over half of the justifications. In 1958, the largest single category was increased user pressure. In 1969, the total number of strategies tripled. User pressure was third, with two new strategies taking first and second place. These were enhancement of social, spiritual and educational values and alleviation of city problems. Wildavsky argues that these new justifications were a reflection of current social thought in 1969, but user pressure persisted for two decades as an explanatory budget strategy. This illustrates the persistence of agency budget themes.

Gloria Grizzle (1986) found an integrating theme in budget decisions. Examining how budget format influenced budget review, Grizzle found that irrespective of format, questions about management dominated discussion, even under a program budget format which is designed to produce questions of a planning orientation. Straussman's examination of the courts' role in the budget process displays the courts basically making workload oriented management decisions, for example in rulings on prison staffing (1986). The point here is that although the repertoire of contingent strategies might seem unlimited, most cluster centrally around the basic elements of management specific to an agency. For a tax department this may be processing tax returns, for a fire department putting out fires and fire prevention, for a social work department, caseload and clientele counseling. Each function has different imperatives, but budget people learn to connect them by speaking a universal language. Contingent strategies are part of that language.

EXAMPLES OF CONTINGENT STRATEGY ELEMENTS

This section explores some of the powerful contingent strategies and potential responses to them. Some of the most prominent are as follows:

- *Workload:*   Workload justifications often are linked to historical statistics, demographic trends, and forecasts. Their logic is simple: workload growth must be handled. "Eight auditors did 80,000 audits; our forecasts indicate we will have to do 90,000 audits, therefore, we need one more auditor. Each auditor keeps one clerical position busy with typing, filing or billing..." The logic is seemingly inescapable; to do what was done last year to this year's clientele requires another person. Reviewers may argue that the manager can find ways to absorb this growth or they may argue that funds are too scarce and irrespective of consequences, no new personnel will be authorized. Another variation of this theme is to tell the agency to decrease its workload by decreasing program intensity.
- *It makes a profit:*   A manager may argue that auditors generate revenues far in excess their salary. Reviewers may reject this appeal by arguing simpler forms would increase voluntary compliance, thus allowing the auditors to concentrate on the real criminals. Making a profit is a good justification but most government agencies do not make a profit and hence cannot use the strategy.
- *Spend to save:*   At this point the manager may argue that spending on the audit function now will encourage people to pay promptly now—thus getting the money in on time—and discourage people from not paying in the future, thus guaranteeing future streams of revenues and avoiding costly crash audit programs to catch up for the lack of auditing. This strategy is often employed in the natural resource area in the areas of flood, fire, and reforestation where a dollar spent now will avoid spending many dollars in the future. Reviewers tend to like the logic of this kind of argument, but not to buy it unless some clear documentation exists. Hardheaded reviewers often try to talk the manager into estimates of how soon the "saving" will begin, with the tighter the resource situation the sooner the saving being the criteria. Some jurisdictions ban "spend to save" justifications, unless the

agency is willing to put dollars saved into the current budget or specify a definite and near time frame.

- *Equity*:   In this instance, the manager might argue that the law
requires all the clientele be audited and hence another auditor is
needed to keep in compliance with the law and provide equity
among taxpayers. This can be turned back by asking if differences do
not exist among the returns and if the "no problem" returns or the
simple documents cannot be sorted and processed quickly enough
so that no additional people are needed but the dictates of the law
are fulfilled. Another way is to simply change the interpretation of
the law. When Defense proponents argue that treaties obligate us to
a certain level of spending, one response is to agree that the treaties
bind us to commitments, but not to a precise level of spending and
that the commitment can be fulfilled with a cheaper mix.

- *Backlog*:   Backlogs are generally bad business, particularly if they are
composed of critically ill people. In many government functions the
need to meet a backlog is less clear. For example someone is certain
to ask what difference it will make if a backlog occurs in an audit
function. The rejoinder ought to talk about equity—the legal responsibility to subject all of a class of citizens to audit—or and making a
profit and putting money in the state's coffers. Then again, someone
may ask if the workload could not be sorted so that the backlog is
composed of relatively harmless returns. Backlog and workload justifications tend to look alike in their written form, but the distinction
between the two is very important for the analyst. A true workload
increase will probably have to be met with either increased personnel
or changed policy, barring a stunning managerial improvement. A
backlog may be solved with temporary personnel who cost less and
who can go on to other jobs and do not constitute a permanent
increase in the personnel budget. If a backlog will continue to
increase, then it must be solved with a more fundamental measure,
including by hiring permanent personnel or a change in policy;
nonetheless it is very important for the analyst to be able to distinguish between a backlog and a workload change. The possibility
exists that a backlog once taken care of will stay taken care of; thus, it
would be inappropriate to use permanent resources on it. The practicing incrementalist is likely to use temporary measures such as overtime or temporary help before resorting to a less flexible solution.
The reviewer does not want to give away something for nothing.

- *The crisis*:   The crisis is a good justification when a crisis exists. Polio
was a crisis in public health in the early 1950s and AIDS is in the
1980s. Most agencies do not have crisis themes to present. When they
do, they present reviewers with difficult choices. Unable to make a

crisis vanish, reviewers can argue about the level of spending being too high to be usefully spent out or put to work in the fiscal period under consideration. Thus, another theme recurs: if the item is unbeatable, try to decrease the level of support. Crises however do exist: Kemp(1984) found that accidents and scandals had an important effect on regulatory policy and budgetary outcomes in three regulatory agencies—the SEC, FAA, and FCC.

- *The increase is small.*   Allusions to size may seem effective when the increase is small compared to the total size of the budget, but professionals do not take this line of argument seriously. Increases are either justified or they are not. In one hearing, one reviewer said "let's split the difference and give her 5%" and the other jumped in saying "what for? He hasn't made a case for anything yet." Moreover, he who argues the increase is small may be urged to absorb it.

- *Strategies.*   Strategies built around cutting the most popular program or threatening all or nothing are high-risk strategies. In the late 1950s and early 1960s cutting sports programs or kindergarten was an effective threat for a school superintendent to make; in 1987, San Francisco's school district used a "cut the athletic program" approach to its benefit. Fiscal necessity has seen such programs cut with seemingly little effect, but in the right circumstances, this remains a powerful strategy. The Washington Monument ploy—turning off the lights or even closing it—is the standard against which all "cut the popular program" tactics are measured. All or nothing is a powerful but limited strategy. The manager who takes an all or nothing approach has to be prepared to live with the consequences of a "nothing" decision. If the manager states he cannot do function B if function A is cut, he may find he has just offered budget reviewers another item to cut: function B.

- *Mandates and commitments.*   Superior levels of government have been fond the last two decades of levying requirements upon subordinate levels of government, not always with the necessary funding to accompany the workload. A manager who is in the possession of a mandate has a strong case, but reviewers can always argue the fiscal level of concurrence, again complying with the letter of the mandate, if not the spirit. Managers who were persuasive in convincing their reviewers to buy into federal grants sometimes were surprised when the continuing costs for maintenance bills came due. Now reviewers must fully examine the total and continuing costs of the grant.

This list of strategies is not meant to be exclusive. The point to remember is that while many strategies are generic and cross subject matter boundaries (e.g., workload) others are subject matter specific: health and human services agencies strategies are oriented around saving lives, not making a profit; a tax department can claim to make a profit, but not to save lives. The challenge to a manager in developing and presenting budgets lies in bringing forth the most compelling themes in the administrative area and being able to deal with the dialogue that surrounds those themes in the political environment. While the retrenchment literature is rich in crisis management insights (Behn, 1980; Levine, 1978a). Lewis (1984) found that cutback budgetary strategies did not appear significantly different from expansionary strategies. A further indication of the staying power of the contingent strategies can be found in a close reading of Wildavsky's *New Politics of the Budgetary Process* (1988; 1992). Familiar ploys appear: the wedge (p. 232), what they do affects what we do (p. 184), spend to save, all or nothing (p. 182), it's so small (p. 183). However, many things have changed and the federal process of the 1980s has been replete with rather transparent gimmicks, e.g., moving payroll dates and funding for less than a full year in order to come to totals either selected through the top-down budget process or as a result of deficit reduction targets, as well as choosing the base number most useful for one's policy position.

ADVANCING STRATEGIES

Managers must also be able to present their positions effectively, be it in clear concise prose or in a budget hearing. Since the latter is a crucial stage, rehearsing the budget presentation makes sense. Hearings take place both within administrative settings and in the legislature. Contact with the budget bureau will usually warn the agency what the budget bureau's concerns are. Scouting budget hearings also makes sense in order to see what items interest the budget committee; if they are asking everyone else about fee revenue and outsourcing, it stands to reason they will ask your budget presenter also—be prepared to answer those questions. Contact with the committee or its staff is also useful to prepare for the hearing. Veteran observers usually advise that the agency play it straight, not spring any surprises, give the committee some warning in advance of the key issues, and make sure the department's position unrolls the way the documents sent to the committee predict so they are both working from the same script. They urge that the presenter be organized, that only a few people testify for the agency and that testimony be choreographed so that the agency not look confused and that the right things get said at the right time. They recommend that budget people answer only the questions they are asked. Glittering generalities, ambiguous phrases, and pious references to the general welfare are seen as inappropriate. Clear, direct presentation of program, supported by accomplishments, and solid justification of changes from the base are what is necessary. Mastering the budget means mastering detail; detail then allows for consideration of the policy that guides the budget. What if all agencies follow the prescriptions recommended above? Does that mean that budgets automatically increase? Should spending increase simply because managers have become effective budget advocates? The answer is not necessarily affirmative, for equally effective analysts can sit on the other side of the table. Not only can they know and respond to arguments the agency makes, but they may have developed a budget system that helps them in their battle to satisfy needs and hold down spending.

SOME PRESCRIPTIVE CONSIDERATIONS

Manager perceptions of how to approach the budget decision vary. In one study, managers explained how they decided how much to ask for. Most took a textbook approach (McCaffery, 1987a): they determined what needed to be done, decided on production objectives, estimated how it would be accomplished—staff, supporting expenses—found the cost factors and then wrote budget justification. Their budgets were driven by many of the conditions analyzed earlier: workload, mandates, and local fiscal conditions.

Others took a different approach, one suited to the context and to relational factors in the budget decision rather than linear thinking about what needs to be done. One said that she knew her project was a pet project, and she would get most of what she could justify. Then she tried to find out how much her reviewers had to distribute. Then she built a budget based on program needs, but padded it a little bit because she knew the person who reviewed it believed that everyone asks for more than they need: "I know I'll be cut so I pad a little." She concluded that budget supplements were not too hard to get and if she did not get what she wanted in the main budget battle she could get it as a supplemental. She added that since training was a "buzzword" that year, she wrote as much of her justification as she could around training.

What was remarkable here is the step-by-step isolation of the key variables in the process. These included the identification of the project as a pet project, an estimate of how much there was to get, the necessity to pad a little and the knowledge that supplementals always were available. This manager seemed relatively comfortable with the budget process. This may be because of the pet project syndrome, or it may be because she had confidence in the insight to operate the budget mechanism to advantage.

Another participant in the study said that his most effective budgetary strategy was to project himself into the role of his superior. He said that he examined their environment, and their philosophy, both personal and institutional. By that time he had already decided what he needed. He then went through a process of building a case for all or part of what he needed such that it made sense to his superiors from their point of view and was "approveable" within their environment.

The test of approveable was how they would feel defending the request: "I try to make sure that I give them reasons they will feel comfortable using if someone asks them why they approved my request" (McCaffery, 1987a, p. 119).

He then enumerated a list of principles he followed. These included being honest in determining need and avoiding the temptation to define what he needed by what it was "safe" to ask for; being honest with the request and not scheming by asking for two in order to get one; by recognizing their authority and responsibility and the right to say no; but by not settling for a plain no. If a request were denied, he asked for alternatives or a better way of accomplishing the task, or acceptance of the consequences of saying no.

This is valuable advice for the student of budgeting and a wise caution to the veteran convinced of the compelling power of numerical arguments such as workload growth. The managers quoted above approached the budget decision as an ongoing situation. People who imitate them are likely to be less frustrated and more successful in the budget struggle than if they approach budgeting as a simple technical calculation where clear answers produce victories based on workload measures or sophisticated benefit/cost analysis.

However, where the line is drawn between giving "them" what "they" can approve and recommending what is technically necessary is critical. If the budget-maker does not tell the political decision maker what the model program should be, then all that is left to compromise over is what cost the public will accept, not what needs to be done. Certainly one proper role for the civil servant is to ask for what is necessary and let elected officials decide what to do, based on their appreciation of what the public will pay for and needs. Nonetheless, putting oneself in the place of one's superior is a useful technique for the budget craftsman as the budget is prepared.

CONCLUSIONS

Managers cannot magically close deficits, invent new revenue sources, or make workloads vanish. However, they do have a fiduciary responsibility to do well with what they control. Irene Rubin describes the impact on a group of federal agencies of budget cutbacks. She found that rather than fighting the cutbacks with end runs to Congress, they followed the President's directives even to the point of cutting their own agencies (Rubin, 1985). Joseph White (1988) calls this reality "agencies as victims" and suggests that agencies do not dominate budgeting but that those few federal agencies who were successful in the early 1980s had strong clientele support. For the person responsible for the agency budget, conclusions about his weight in the total picture are almost irrelevant; he, as White concludes, exists to budget. His values are likely to be conservative values, e.g., efficiency, effectiveness, performance, regulation of inputs, because he has many demands to satisfy. Moreover, his values are comprehensible and important to all other players in the system.

Managers choose their budget strategy and level of risk; some will be aggressive, some will not—what Jones (1986) termed the difference between proactive and reactive strategies. Some will be content to say to funding sources: "if this is what you want me to do, here is what I need." The more aggressive will attempt to specify what more needs to be done. Both types need basic budget skills. Technically, the budgeter must write good justification, make accurate calculations and maintain interpersonal communications within the system as a part of viewing the budget decision as an ongoing situation rather than a unique event. With the realization that the concept of budget base is more ambiguous than had been previously realized, doing the numbers alone is no longer so easy (Albritton & Dran, 1987; Wildavsky 1988, p. 201), but then none of it is easy. Duncombe and Kinney have more advice for budgeters especially vis-à-vis the legislature—to be absolutely honest and not predict dire consequences if they are not likely to happen, and to maintain good relationships and the perception of being a team player. They also urge that the budgeter try to get greater flexibility in the use of funds: "keep agency expenditures within appropriations if at all possible, carry out legislative intent, and manage budgets wisely" (Duncombe & Kinney, 1987, p. 36). While this may not seem as persuasive as buying low and selling high, it is the public sector moral equivalent. Indeed, it is more than that, for following these injunctions will tend to increase the gain for everyone.

CHAPTER VIII

RESTRUCTURING AND BUDGETING UNDER FISCAL STRESS

INTRODUCTION

This chapter defines restructuring and its application and explains why restructuring is the primary method by which public organizations in the United States and elsewhere have managed fiscal stress and budget restraint over the past three decades. To restructure an organization initially entails defining all of the skill areas and work processes where an organization has special or unique skills and knowledge, i.e., its core competence relative to the capability of other organizations. Secondly, restructuring requires an assessment of those core competence areas that fit within its overall mission and objectives. Thirdly, under restructuring the organization contracts out non-core competence work that needs to be done to fulfill its mission to other organizations, including those in the private sector, that have core competence comparative advantage. The comparative advantage of contractors may lie in the superior quality of their products or services, or may be the result of ability to produce products or services at lower cost with no loss of quality. Finally, restructuring meets its goals only where the organization then eliminates everything else that does not contribute value to the services and products delivered to the citizens and stakeholders served by the organization, i.e., non-core competence work processes and that work not contracted out.

At the beginning, restructuring requires a careful assessment (typically a reassessment) of the mission and objectives of the organization, an evaluation of the organization's strategy relative to its target markets for products or services, definition of criteria for determining core competence, and value engineering to define what work materially contributes to mission and goal achievement, and the extent of the contribution. Restructuring demands a comparison between the costs and performance of work performed by the organization and that of potential alternative service suppliers. This step is essential to decide where to contract out, or where a service or product should not be supplied by the organization at all. And, because restructuring requires cost and performance comparison, activity based-cost analysis, or what is termed "responsibility accounting" in the public sector, must be employed to permit such comparisons to be made. Responsibility accounting, budgeting, and management control are techniques or methods that enable the organization to define its core competence and costs of product and service production.

According to the principles of mission or responsibility accounting, budgeting, and management control, the components of the organization should be classified according to their primary mission or responsibility, e.g., mission centers, revenue centers, expense or cost centers, internal service centers, investment centers. Each is evaluated in terms of its contribution to the delivery of services that meet citizen demand. Restructuring may result in significant "delayering" or flattening of organizational structure, considerable delegation of authority, responsibility, and decision making on day-to-day operations to levels of the organization closer to its constituency. Restructuring usually means shedding jobs. Indeed, large-scale productivity improvement in government may depend upon the elimination of hundreds of thousands of jobs. However, restructuring also should include increased employee education and training, especially in the use of new technology and work processes.

WHY RESTRUCTURE?

Why should public organizations restructure? Part of the answer lies in the significance and relative performance of the U.S. services sector. Services now constitute 75% of GDP. This means that the United States must increase service productivity to grow wealthier and in recent decades increases have been glacial. Government productivity poses an especially severe problem. The 20% of the American workforce employed by government generates less than 15% of GDP. Value-added per worker is only 5% lower in private services than in manufacturing, but government productivity lags manufacturing productivity by a third. In contrast, in 1958, value-added per government worker was 40% higher than in the goods sector.

A second part of the answer goes to the organization of service delivery. Arguably, bureaucracies were once relatively effective. Bureaucratic organizational arrangements successfully provided security, jobs and economic stability, ensured fairness and equity, and delivered the "one size fits all" services needed during the era of government infrastructure development that lasted from the turn of the last century to the mid-1960s (Osborne & Gaebler, 1992, p. 14). During crises such as the Great Depression and two world wars, bureaucracy saved us. In the meantime, however, the hierarchical, centralized, rule-driven organizational arrangements invented during the industrial era have become increasingly anachronistic.

Global economic competition, international capital mobility, and breathtaking improvements in telecommunications and information storage, processing, and retrieval are producing a knowledge-based economy—one where workers demand autonomy and citizens/customers demand high quality products, superior service, and extensive choice. Old-fashioned business bureaucracies cannot meet these demands; neither can old-fashioned government bureaucracies. Meeting these demands requires flexible, adaptable, innovative, and customer-focused organizations that offer an array of high quality goods, tailored to individual wants and needs. However, few public officials or managers have had much experience restructuring. Consequently, better methods for management are needed. Additionally, better evaluative frameworks against which reduction options and actions may be assessed also are required.

In the United States, starting in the mid-1970s and continuing through the 1990s there was considerable public discussion of the need to reduce the size of government and scope of government activity. The causes of government financial stress and retrenchment during this period appear to be essentially economic in origin. However, politics always plays an important role in influencing and then reflecting public opinion. Criticism of the pervasive social and economic role of government in general, and the adequacy of public service performance specifically is born from political ideology.

Under certain conditions, politicians are able to orchestrate the public frustration that results from reduced economic opportunity and uncertainty into a crescendo of voter support for government budgetary control, but whether control is subsequently exerted is another matter. Over the period in question government expenditures were limited in a number of ways: by economic recession that reduced tax revenues; by tax limitation measures approved through popular vote in the wake of such mandates as Proposition 13 enacted in California in 1978; by reductions in federal government transfer payments to provincial, state and local governments; and by changes in government funding priorities for domestic service and social assistance programs. For example, expenditure cuts made by the provincial government in the early 1980s in British Columbia resulted from reductions in tax and non-tax revenues as well as the application of a different philosophy regarding the value of some social programs and services.

The political motivation to curb or redistribute government expenditures, or to actually reduce spending levels nominally or in constant dollars, may be viewed to emanate from a variety of factors and not just as the result of public dissatisfaction with government and the public administration performance. The dilemma in facing financial stress in the public sector results in large part from the fact that over the past thirty years or so in North America our society and economy have become accustomed to and dependent upon growth in government. Growth fits well with both the motives of political decision makers seeking support on the basis of providing jobs, public works projects and welfare assistance, and of citizens desiring the benefits of political expenditure decisions. The retrenchment game is not particularly attractive to politicians no longer able to reward constituents, public managers desiring to preserve their programs and jobs, or to citizens benefitting from the provision of transfer payments and services by government. It is little wonder that we avoid thinking about retrenchment, given that its outcomes are likely to displease great numbers of citizens and political actors.

Among the issues that must be addressed when governments have fewer revenues to spend are the following: Should the scope of public policies, programs and organizations be reduced? Why do government policies become immune to review, modification and termination? How can we tell which policies and programs should survive and which should be modified, reduced or terminated? How should decision-makers attempt to reduce or terminate public policy programs or organizations where this appears desirable? Public managers and policy analysts are beginning to face the necessity for reducing policies and programs. However, few public managers have much experience in cutback management. This chapter provides information to public managers, policy analysts and others on methods for improving the management of financial stress, and forms a framework against which actions may be evaluated.

A FRAMEWORK FOR ANALYZING FINANCIAL STRESS

Analysis of public financial and program restraint may be divided into (a) the causes of financial crisis; (b) methods for managing financial crises; (c) issues and dilemmas faced by public administrators in attempting to manage restraint; and (d) methods to both achieve and avoid policy, program and organizational reduction termination. The second of these subjects, methods for managing financial crisis, is of most immediate concern to public managers and analysts.

The range of non-mutually exclusive financial stress management alternatives includes (1) doing nothing, which is likely to work only for a short time if the financial crisis persists; (2) increasing revenues; (3) reducing expenditures; (4) increasing employee and organizational productivity; and (5) employing a set of more innovative responses that are productivity-related. The fifth category of productivity-related responses includes the co-optation of other organizations, programs and constituents; cooperation; volunteerism; program or mission reorganization and merger; joint purchase and service agreements with other governments, contracting; and privatization.

Before developing plans to manage financial stress, prudent managers will attempt to define the seriousness of the financial crisis. A general framework has been suggested by Schick. A modification of this framework produces the following categories of financial crisis: (a) relaxed scarcity where revenues in constant dollars just equal expenditures for a period of one to five years; (b) chronic scarcity where revenues fall short of proposed expenditures by less than 5% for a period of one to five years; (c) short-term acute scarcity where revenues fall short of proposed expenditures by greater than 5% for one or two years; and (d) prolonged acute scarcity where revenues fall short of proposed expenditures by greater than 5% for more than two years. Two additional categories may be added where they occur: (e) long-term austerity, and (f) financial recovery and continued austerity. However, definitions of these states are less precise than those for categories (a) through (d). Long-term austerity may be defined as a condition where revenues and expenditures are constrained in constant dollars relative to previous patterns of growth for a period of five years or longer. It is a condition that many governments are likely to face over the next decade and perhaps beyond. Financial recovery and continued austerity is the condition in which governments have adjusted to reduced revenues through reduced expenditure, program modification and improved financial management.

In this context it may be useful to note that the terms "financial stress" and "crisis" may be differentiated to indicate the former as a state in which difficulty is experienced in balancing revenues and expenditures over a long period of time, while the latter indicates a sudden event in a short period, such as the inability to meet debt service payments resulting in default on bonds and the concomitant loss of credit rating and borrowing capacity. In this chapter the term financial crisis is used to characterize both stress and crisis conditions as defined above unless otherwise stated.

FISCAL STRESS MANAGEMENT APPROACHES

The two most prominent financial stress management options are to increase revenues and to reduce expenditures. Included in the revenue option is the examination of existing revenue sources, with more attention to potential political support for alternative ways of increasing revenue, to new pricing policies reflecting the elasticity of demand of consumers of public services, and the equity implications of price increases. Recognition that pricing policy is of strategic importance may be a revelation to some public managers accustomed to the idea that pricing ought to concern only private sector managers. In addition, the revenue option includes the search for new revenue sources, including new fees and services charges, and definition of what may be termed the "revenue rights" between public organizations and different layers of government. This latter task creates a new set of challenges in intergovernmental relations. General expenditure reduction options include across-the-board reduction, specific program reduction, and program-policy merger and termination. Expenditure reduction typically includes careful examination of legal, regulatory and other intergovernmental mandates to differentiate those that may be ignored without incurring lawsuits and loss of revenue. The additional management options listed above (increasing productivity and various others included under the rubric of innovative responses) are discussed subsequently in presentation of a general model of phases of recognition and management of financial crisis in public organizations.

For those interested in studying other management options in depth, a body of work too extensive to summarize here has emerged in the past few years. This literature draws heavily upon applied social science research conducted over more than thirty years in political science, economics, political economy, public administration, sociology, organizational theory and behavior, anthropology, psychology and other disciplines. While studies of financial stress in public organizations by researchers in the field of public policy and management have a distinct professional and applied focus, this work has its origins in and owes a considerable debt of gratitude to traditional social science theory.

A MANAGEMENT RESPONSES MODEL

A general sequence of events appears to characterize the recognition and management of financial crisis in public organizations. The following portion of this chapter provides a summary of phases of recognition and management characteristic of public organizational response to financial crisis and prolonged stress. This is a scenario-based model of financial stress-coping methods in time sequence. As a general model it is subject to all of the errors of generalization, omission and potential inapplicability to specific cases and circumstances that pertain to models of this type. Despite these weaknesses, the model is useful for identifying and ordering many of the events that appear to characterize financial crisis management in public organizations. Discussion of phases of recognition and management in this chapter elaborates the model. It emphasizes the most significant components of the model in an integrative way, similar to the manner in which financial crisis is encountered and accommodated by public managers.

How has the public sector tended to approach restructuring in the past? A reasonably similar pattern or sequence of events appears to characterize the restructuring initiatives of many public organizations. The first response to restructuring typically involves denial. This is usually followed by short-term measures to reduce spending, accompanied by efforts to assign blame. Organizations at this point must choose between reducing services and cutting positions. Many public officials balk at this choice, arguing that budget cuts should be made gradually, that organizations are better off relying on employee attrition, withdrawal of vacant positions, cuts in support budgets, and even deferral of maintenance than on across-the-board personnel reductions or cuts targeted at specific programs or services. When push comes to shove, they cut "soft" services first. Then they cut things that are invisible to the public, e.g., in support operations and maintenance, employee training, and capital asset replacement. These cuts eat up an organization's accumulated capital and often demoralize its employees who understand that ignoring maintenance and investment will lead to higher costs later. Nevertheless, massive layoffs are also costly. When severance pay, outplacement costs, loss of morale and valuable skills, not to mention the dislocation experienced by the employees who lose their jobs, are considered, staff reductions through attrition may actually be more cost-effective than termination—especially poorly targeted terminations.

The next phase of restructuring usually involves deeper, across-the-board budget cuts, often accompanied by hiring and salary freezes, increased use of part-time and nonpermanent employees, and other initiatives to reduce total salary costs. However, the across-the-board strategy tends to weaken organizations throughout. It is especially damaging in that high-demand programs and high quality personnel are cut the same amount as programs with lower demand and quality (Jones, 1984; Jones & Bixler, 1992; Jones & McCaffery, 1989). Unfortunately, many public organizations and their employees appear to prefer the across-the-board and attrition approach, with nonessential services cut first and the last-hired employees the first to lose their jobs. Application of length of service rather than merit criteria often eliminate less experienced and younger staff. Unfortunately, these employees may be more adaptable to change than those with longer records of service. Employees cut in this phase may include a higher proportion of new entrant women and minorities than is represented in the total organizational workforce. There also may be an accompanying loss of highly skilled employees who find better employment opportunities elsewhere in a less stressful working environment.

HOW SHOULD RESTRUCTURING BE MANAGED?

A number of variables in addition to those mentioned at the beginning of this chapter must be addressed in restructuring management. Once the organization has reviewed and assessed its strategic and market plans, determined its core competence areas, performed value chain analyses, decided on what work processes will be retained, contracted out or eliminated, then it must begin to address a number of issues related to managing reduction. Typically, the first issue is how to deal with personnel reduction. As noted previously, personnel may be reduced by attrition or by layoff and termination. It is essential for the organization to develop a deliberate strategy on personnel reduction and then stick to it. Public organizations often attempt to reduce through attrition, a slow yet effective method given that the costs of this approach can be afforded. Attrition takes longer and is more costly in the long-term; termination appears to be more cost-effective in the long-term but costs more up-front because of the necessity for paying employees for accrued benefits, and, in some instances, bonuses. Legal constraints, union contracts and other strictures make termination more difficult in the public versus the private sector. Numerous political and other constraints seem to force public organizations toward the attrition approach. However, it should be kept in mind that termination is used more often in the private sector because of its apparent long-term cost advantage and for other reasons, including sustaining employee morale for those not terminated and the advantages gained from shifting the organization rapidly toward the achievement of new goals and market opportunities. With respect to strategy, we advocate use of both attrition and termination, in short depending on the circumstance and degree of political and market pressure to change.

To manage employee reduction, the criteria for cuts and rules on how cuts will be made must be developed and communicated clearly to employees. Some public organizations have developed procedures to mix length of service and merit criteria in determining layoff or employment termination schedules. Employee performance evaluation systems may be designed so that employees generate service credits for high performance ratings. These credits are then added to other credits earned through length of service and total service credits are then used to define employee layoff order and rights to move into the positions held by less senior employees in the same or similar job classification elsewhere in the organization.

The service credit system also may be used to set priorities for employee reassignment to new positions within the organization, either at the point where personnel cuts are made or after a period of layoff. While reduction-in-force rules often include the provision of replacement or "bumping" rights across organizational units, unlimited bumping is stressful, disruptive and may cause serious losses in employee morale and productivity. A "single bump within class" system that restricts movement rights to a single choice and compares the qualifications of those seeking to replace other employees with requirements for the contested positions appears to be a preferable option. Union contracts may constrain the close application of qualification and requirement definitions, as may civil service rules.

One of the most important dimensions of personnel management under restructuring is the extent to which the organization invests in education, training and placement of employees whose jobs have been cut. Education and retraining may be necessary to enable reassignment of employees to new positions within the organization. Investment in education, training, and placement services, and job search assistance is costly but desirable in most instances. Responsible management of job loss can build rather than reduce morale, and may help sustain or even promote the productivity of employees whose jobs are not cut, particularly for those who continue to face the threat of elimination.

We have stressed that strategic planning and the establishment of both program and personnel priorities should guide restructuring. Maintenance of service quality and the retention of valuable employees must continue to be of paramount importance to the restructuring organization. Under conditions of program reduction and termination, enforcing priorities requires strong political support, effective strategic planning, a sophisticated information base for decision making, and considerable attention to negotiation with employees, citizens receiving services and stakeholders. All of this can be assisted through definition of critical mass program and core resource operation levels, i.e., resource levels below which programs cannot operate and still achieve their mission and objectives satisfactorily (Jones, 1985).

Evaluation of value-added to the services delivered to citizens and employee and stakeholder participants is critical to effective restructuring. The capable manager will recognize that cuts ought not to be based on organizational prestige, program longevity and employee seniority, budget size or other convenient but non-value added criteria. Regrettably, the program information needed to do otherwise is often lacking. At this point, the implementation of a strategic planning process that generates accurate and reliable information about market and citizen demand patterns and

shifts in demand and enables comparisons between programs, service production costs and productivity is critical. The planning process and strategic plans also ought to fit with longer-term financial, debt management
and capital planning. In attempting to plan and execute restructuring
effectively, managers are likely to be frustrated as they recognize the extent
to which they have under invested in or simply squandered valuable
accounting, planning, program and policy evaluation, information technology and other analytical resources in the past.

The issue of participation in restructuring decision making is sensitive
and may be dominated by management-labor contracts to a considerable
extent. Arguments for broader participation of employees are often made
on the grounds of fairness, contribution to employee morale and adherence to democratic management values. A much stronger argument for
participation is that employees and program constituents have information
that needs to be assessed by program managers in deciding whether and
how to restructure. Many of the best suggestions on how to save money and
increase efficiency are likely to come from program managers, their staffs,
and citizen consumers if they are asked.

Centralization of planning and the reassessment of priorities are typical
in public sector restructuring. Prolonged dependence on one or a few individuals to make restructuring decisions can result in reintroduction of
many of the bureaucratic weaknesses that contributed to the need to
restructure in the first place. A "Chinese mandarin" system of management
by personal influence is inimical to effective restructuring because of its
effect on workplace morale and on the openness of the organization to
restructuring, reengineering, reinvention, redesign and rethinking. However, the degree of centralization of authority in restructuring may be less
important than other variables in explaining successful restructuring.
Smoothing the impact of cuts, continuity of leadership, the extent to which
restructuring is politicized, ability to define and communicate organizational mission and goals, the extent to which service priorities are established and budgeted, form of government, and degree of cooperation
between executive and legislative arms all appear to be more important
variables than centralization per se.

The dilemma of centralization of decision authority versus broader participation in restructuring comes down to a fundamental tradeoff—either
centralize and limit representation for purposes of decision and execution
efficiency, or allow decision participation to be more open and, consequently, open to greater fragmentation and delay. Open access and participation in restructuring more fully utilizes the knowledge extant in the
minds of employees, those served by the organization and stakeholders.
However, broad participation often limits the ability of public organizations
to establish new priorities quickly and to target cuts. Broad participation

may make significant restructuring impossible as all parties have the opportunity to articulate reasons why the organization should remain as it is rather than adapting to new market, social and political conditions. Either way, something of value is sacrificed, which reinforces our view that the best approach may be a combination of the two wherein politicians and managers cooperate but employ a procedural mechanism to limit choice and constrain the time in which choices can be made and appealed. In the closure of military facilities in the United States, the Congress and Executive branches of government used such a constraining procedural mechanism to close hundreds of military bases, the specifics of which had been debated in some cases for decades (Thompson & Jones, 1994).

RESTRUCTURING UNDER FISCAL STRESS CONDITIONS

Where the organization faces fiscal stress or financial crisis, prolonged, acute mismatches between jurisdictional means and policy commitments may severely inhibit the ability to continue in the status quo. Budget deficits may accrue and interest payments increase as a percentage of total revenues and spending. Credit ratings may suffer, and the ability of public organizations to finance capital construction and to borrow to meet short-term cash shortages may be impaired. In many instances, the need for restructuring may not be recognized until the government as a whole or specific public organizations face a financial crisis and cannot continue to earn revenues either through the political/budget process or from the market, then the need for restructuring becomes readily apparent. Where public organizations, including those in state and municipal governments, rely in part on deficit financing and borrowing, the ability to get credit from external lenders may become impaired or lost.

Where the confidence of elected officials is lost in ways that affect budget decisions and willingness to fund programs, and where loss of external market user revenues and credit worthiness has occurred, longer-term financial planning and action is needed to evaluate the effects of program and service demand shifts and, from a financial perspective, to improve cash flow, cash management and investment practices. Under conditions of fiscal crisis, special attention must be given to insure entitlement and pension fund solvency, to limit debt load to fit tax base and debt service capacities, to assess property and equipment leasing or liquidation options, to develop accurate capital asset depreciation and replacement costs and schedules, to improve inventory management and, in some cases, to establish sufficient fund reserves to support the budget in the event of future revenue shortfalls.

Long-range program and financial planning may require the counsel of financial management consultants and may involve the participation of other public entities, bankers, municipal bond market advisors and others to rebuild confidence in the accountability and credit worthiness of the enterprise. Public organizations often discover, as have many private organizations, that long-term productivity improvement requires risk capital for investment in new equipment, employee training, additional program analysis and market research. Because restructuring requires analysis of service value, additional costs for accounting system modification, data collection, analysis and decision making is inevitable. Of course, some organizations are penny wise and dollar foolish—they avoid these costs by cutting deeply across-the-board without regard to the capacity to deliver quality services in the future. This approach is not a model for successful restructuring despite the obvious advantages of expedience and ease of compromise it gives to elected and appointed officials. Indeed, it is possible only where governments practice cash rather than accrual accounting, which means that organizations can convey a false impression of fiscal health by playing games (often in violation of the law) with the timing of income and expenditures, e.g., in New York City in the fiscal crisis of the mid-1970s. Fiscal smoke and mirrors sometimes will suffice to persuade the news media and the public that a crisis has been averted, apparently without serious long-term loss. Unfortunately, the costs of mismanaging the financial component of restructuring are high and are borne for a long time, e.g., as in Orange County, California.

OPPORTUNITIES FROM RESTRUCTURING

The most important contribution restructuring can make to increased productivity may come from the replacement of out-of-date technology. In many public organizations shortsighted, across-the-board budget cuts made over a multi-year period create substantial technology and employee education and training gaps.

Under restructuring, some of the ideas proposed to resolve organizational and citizen problems may initially appear to be too radical but may later prove to be workable. For example, under the pressure of fiscal necessity, the City of Oakland, California sold the public building that housed its museum to private investors. However, the City continued to provide museum services under lease agreement with the new owners. Similar sale and lease-back agreements have been successful for other cities. These arrangements enable local governments to reduce their maintenance and operation costs while private investment incentives help to insure proper maintenance and care for facilities. Users of facilities may be required to bear a larger proportion of costs through user fees. Better cost accounting can help in setting prices and appropriate fee levels relative to measures of ability to pay.

Justifications for provision of services by government must be thoroughly reevaluated by public officials in making decisions about user fees, program reductions, or whether to continue provide the service at all. The trend toward privatization has been driven by recognition that many of the services provided traditionally by government can and ought to be provided by the private or not-for-profit sectors of the economy. Restructuring, contracting out and privatization are compatible in many instances as a means of reducing the scale and scope of government.

In general, restructuring has to be managed taking into account the rigidities and constraints built into hierarchical public bureaucracies. Typical manifestations of such constraints include overspecialization of function, devotion of inordinate amounts of time to self-defense rather than to problem solving, problem avoidance through obfuscation, resistance to the implications of new information, and a fear of adaptation to new social and economic conditions. Inability to adapt reduces the probability of survival. Recognition that these rigidities and constraints exist should cause us to devote more resources to the study of restructuring and to the education and training of public decision-makers, managers and service providers in methods for diagnosing the need for and managing public organizational change.

THE CONTEXT FOR RESTRUCTURING THE PUBLIC SECTOR

Beginning in the United States in the mid-1970s and continuing through the 1990s, considerable public discussion of the need to reduce the size, scope and role of government in the economy was undertaken. To a considerable extent the debate in the United States paralleled that occurring elsewhere in the world. Examples of this may be found in the debate in this era that took place in the United Kingdom, Sweden and selected other European nations, Canada, Australia, New Zealand and elsewhere. The stimulus for dialogue about the size, scope and role of government and the need for government restructuring during this period appears to be essentially economic in origin, as we have noted. However, politics always plays an important role in influencing and reflecting both economic crises and public opinion. Views on the pervasiveness and relative disadvantage resulting from the broad social and economic role played by government in general, and perceptions of inadequacy of public service performance specifically are subject to interpretation based on different political and ideological perspectives. Further, the condition of the economy may be, in some cases, somewhat independent of views on the need for restructuring government. In the United States, political demand for restructuring continued during a period of unprecedented economic growth that produced a balance a federal government budget in the late 1990s.

Where public dissatisfaction increases, typically some politicians are able to orchestrate public frustration resulting from reduced economic opportunity, or uncertainty in the case of the U.S. economy in the 1990s, into a voter support for greater government programmatic and fiscal control and restructuring. Over the period in question in the United States and globally, public sector revenues and expenditures were constrained or redirected for number of reasons including (a) economic competition and recession that reduced economic growth, employment and tax revenues; (b) major political change (e.g., the end of the Cold War and corresponding economic and social reformulation in Germany, Central Europe and the nations of the former Soviet Union), (c) tax limitation measures approved through popular vote (e.g., Proposition 13 in California); (d) reductions in federal government transfer payments to subordinate governments; (e) changes in government funding priorities for domestic services, social assistance, health care, defense and other programs. Expenditure cuts and shifts in policy priorities made by governments in this period resulted in part from reductions in tax and non-tax revenues as well as from the application of different social philosophies regarding the costs and value of many services provided by government. Political motivation to curb or redistribute government expenditures, or to actually reduce spending levels nominally or in constant dollars, may be viewed to emanate from a variety of factors independent of public dissatisfaction with government and the public sector performance.

The dilemma in facing the need for restructuring the public sector results in large part from the fact that for more than fifty years Western societies and economies have become accustomed to, and to some extent dependent upon, continued growth of government. Growth has fitted well with both the motives of political decision makers seeking electoral and financial support on the basis of providing jobs, public works projects and welfare assistance, and of citizens desiring the benefits of political representation for their causes, needs and preferences. Restructuring is not particularly attractive to politicians who, because of it, are no longer able to reward constituents. Neither is it attractive to public managers desiring to preserve their programs and jobs, or to citizens benefitting from the provision of transfer payments and services by government. It is little wonder that, collectively, we tend to want to avoid thinking about public sector restructuring given that its outcomes are likely to displease great numbers of citizens and politicians.

CONCLUSIONS

Among the issues that must be addressed when public sector officials and managers face restructuring in response to economic challenges and changes in patterns of political and social demand that threaten or actually reduce or shift revenues are the following: Should the scope of public policies, programs and organizations be reduced? Why do government policies become immune to review, modification and termination? How can we tell which policies and programs should survive and which should be modified, reduced or terminated? How should decision-makers attempt to reduce or terminate public programs or organizations where this appears desirable? Elected officials, public managers, policy analysts and the public have had to respond to the necessity for changing policies, cutting or shifting spending and restructuring organizations since the 1970s. However, before this era, few public officials or managers had much experience in restructuring. And we may wonder to what extent the lessons from success and failure produced as a result of having to cope with the challenge of restructuring during this period have been learned and internalized so that we may do better in the future.

This chapter has provided information that elected officials, public managers and others need to understand to better assess alternative methods for improving the management of economic and fiscal stress through restructuring. Evaluation of restructuring may be segmented into the determination of: (a) the causes of economic and fiscal stress, (b) methods for improved management of restructuring, (c) the issues and dilemmas faced by public officials and managers attempting to manage restructuring, and (d) methods for either achieving or avoiding restructuring. The range of non-mutually exclusive approaches to management of restructuring includes:

- Doing nothing, likely to work only for a short time if economic and fiscal stress persists,
- Increasing revenues and/or reducing expenditures,
- Increasing employee and organizational productivity and employing a set of more innovative responses that are productivity-related of the type presented in this chapter.

The third category of productivity-related responses includes a number of approaches not discussed to any extent in this chapter but important in restructuring the role of government as a whole. These include increased cooperation between and networking with other organizations, programs and their constituents, strategic co-optation of other organizations, increasing citizen volunteerism in provision of services to the public, mission and program reorganization and merger, joint service and purchase agreements within and between governments, contracting out, and privatization.

Finally, before developing plans to manage restructuring, prudent elected officials and public managers will attempt to define the components of demand for restructuring. In doing so, they may respond to this demand in a holistic manner rather than in the piecemeal fashion that has characterized many unsuccessful attempts to restructure the public sector and public sector organizations in the past.

CHAPTER IX

BUDGET PROCESS REFORM

INTRODUCTION

Once the budget is enacted, the categories that money will be spent on are clear and unambiguous. The number of personnel and their salary are set. What will be bought to service them is also clear, by item in capital outlay, and by dollar amount of goods and services in the other supporting categories. The budget is built by relying on documentary evidence from previous year budget execution patterns and by estimating future needs. Even though all these documents do not accompany the budget display, it is assumed that the budget will be executed as it was built, save for those explicit contrary instructions the budget accrues as it passes various levels of review. It is easy to see how even for small jurisdictions, line item budgets quickly become large and forbidding. As the size of the jurisdiction and its budget increases, the line item display is forced to more and more levels of summarization, until it becomes unintelligible.[1] The data are there, and if not readily apparent, can be resurrected, but the question now becomes "what does all this mean?"

In the last fifty years, various budget formats have been developed to answer this question. In the 1950s and again in the 1990s an emphasis on costs, activities and outcomes led to "performance" budget experiments. Sandwiched between these two performance budget experiments were such systems as Program Budgeting; Planning, Programming, and Budgeting (PPB); Management by Objectives; Target-Based Budgeting; and Zero-Based Budgeting. None of these were persuasive enough to gain universal adoption, although remnants of some systems exist in later systems, and some, e.g., zero-based budgeting, are re-adopted under the appropriate conditions. For example, the ranking system of zero-based budgeting with its levels of effort below the current level finds its way in many systems that would not think of doing a comprehensive, zero based review each year. However, when fiscal conditions are difficult, ZBB has its uses, particularly at state and local levels.

Performance Budgeting, Program Budgeting, and PPBs all were systems that were originally oriented toward defense. Performance Budgeting focuses on activities accomplished, outputs and unit costs. In the 1950s performance budgeting did not get a lengthy trial in defense, but it did see some success in local government. Its Achilles heel seemed to be the masses of calculations it took to derive unit cost data; in this it made budgets less rather than more comprehensible. More importantly, not all government programs had measurable outputs, or even items that could stand as surrogates. The Department of Defense went on to focus on programs with program budgeting which presented budgets in terms of programs, rather than activities or objects of expenditure, but it too frustrated analysis at the aggregate level and gave way to PPBs. This is an extremely complex resource allocation system used within the Department of Defense where it combines threat assessment, planning for the appropriate force structure and buying the goods and services and providing appropriate training to the people who will be able to avert or overcome the threat.

Civilian sectors of the federal government had a short flirtation with PPBs, as with management by objectives as a budget system, and Zero-Based Budgeting (see Rose, 1976; Schick, 1973, pp. 148–149; 1978, pp. 177–180). PPBs was abandoned at about the time when more and more of the federal budget was directed toward mandatory expenditures and the systems which followed it were even less well equipped to answer the important questions about budget policy. Remnants of PPBs survive in attempts to estimate benefit and costs and to do long range planning, but few non-defense functions have a threat-based world with which to contend and threat assessment and modifying force structure must be seen as the heart of the PPBs apparatus.

Under the Government Performance and Results Act of 1993, the federal government embarked on a performance measurement experiment that may lead to performance budgeting. In this iteration, strategic planning and customer/clientele involvement have been added to activity groupings, the search for appropriate outcomes and the effort to cost outcomes and evaluate changes in outcomes that might come from adding additional dollars. The strategic planning and customer involvement facets of this iteration are important changes. In the 1950s, performance budgeting tended to focus on costs of activities, implicitly assuming that cost per unit numbers would eventually lead to more centralization of the budget process and allow a few people to make good judgments about all activities by following the changes in a few key numbers. Under GPRA, this iteration of performance measurement and strategic planning in the 1990s seems more open to decentralization of goals throughout the organization and to forcing customer/client desires to percolate up into consideration at higher levels. The promise of a more useful and effective system seems tantalizingly close. This promise has attracted subordinate levels of government in the United States (Florida, Texas, Arizona) and elsewhere (New Zealand). However, the record of budget innovation suggests that one ought not be too optimistic about reform. Ultimately, object of expenditure data still remain linked to the accounting system, hence, when worst comes to worst, the data for line item analyses can still be found. Particularly for legislators, line-item analysis seems to have an enduring appeal.

THE CRISIS IN BUDGETING

Naomi Caiden has suggested that public budget systems are "excellent barometers" indicating the current condition of the prevailing political environment. Caiden notes that where resources are available to accommodate most goals, where participants agree on most issues, and where it is possible to predict the future with some confidence, budget processes tend to be stable and routine and budget reform manifests itself as technicians attempting to make marginal adjustments to a generally satisfactory situation. When the converse of these conditions occurs, Caiden suggests that budget reform may be highly controversial, challenging the appropriateness and viability of the budget process itself (Caiden, 1991, 1982, 1983). Aaron Wildavsky has said that the budgetary norms of balance, annularity, and comprehensiveness have been shattered beyond recognition and that the assumptions behind these norms—accepted limits on taxes and spending, predictability for a year, and departmental control of spending no longer hold (Wildavsky, 1992, p. 397). For the U.S. federal budget the 1995 budget process seems a worst case scenario; the norm of annularity was fundamentally shattered, major segments of the government were temporarily shut down and the Secretary of Treasury was forced to extraordinary actions (he borrowed from pension funds) to avoid a default on U.S. government bonds. The good news was that the political system adjusted to these disruptions, the people did not riot, credit markets did not collapse and eventually there seemed to be agreement that some of the philosophic decisions forced in the budget process were so fundamental that they would be better addressed in 1996 by the Presidential and Congressional candidates.

BACKGROUND ON REFORM

In the early 1980s, Naomi Caiden observed that budget reformers were concerned with uncontrollability of certain federal expenditures, budget numbers that "seemed to move of their own volition" and items that were not on-budget. Moreover, the budget process exhibited each year undue complexity, confrontations, delays, and threats of process breakdown. Caiden concluded that the major problems with the federal budget process were associated with the large percentage of the federal budget deemed uncontrollable, instability of budget numbers given their linkage to a volatile economy and the multitude of places in the budget process where one can begin calculating, and the impossibility of doing adequate scrutiny of every program due to the size and fragmentation of the budget. Other problems included the fact that many federal activities are carried out by other levels of government or carried out through loan and credit activities that are not on budget and the repetitiveness of the process in Congress. Caiden observed that the goals of budget reform stressed, "Cohesive policy making, long-term decision making, clear information and analysis and deliberate choices between competing claims" (Caiden, 1983, p.16). Caiden warned that some of these goals are in conflict with characteristics of the U.S. political system, which some contend emphasizes ambiguity, preservation of options, blurring of issues and avoidance of conflict in order to reach resolution. Thus, appropriate budget reforms could be undermined by contravening political norms. Even in the area of budget reform, Caiden observed that there were tradeoffs and "such key reform concepts as flexibility, planning, control and responsiveness cannot be accommodated simultaneously" (p. 5).

Caiden's Reform Agenda

Notwithstanding the slippery nature of the path to budget reform, Caiden suggests that ways need to be found to cope with long-term commitments, instability of budget numbers, fragmentation of the budget process and repetitiveness of the process in Congress. After examining a number of reform proposals, Caiden distills a set of recommendations that would probably satisfy most reformers. These include:

1. A **foresighted** budget—budget horizons that extend beyond the annual budget.
2. A **responsive** budget—a budget that has the flexibility to respond to changing economic conditions.

3. A **credible** budget—a budget with numbers that are clear and consistent, accurate, and where variances are analyzed; effective scorekeeping and no manipulation for political purposes.
4. An **influential** budget—control is emphasized and expenditures are made as intended by the budget; programs are assessed for their goal attainment; efficiency and effectiveness come from relating resources and programs.
5. A **consistent** budget—consistent choices should be made in an orderly way on tax and spending policies.
6. An **integrated** budget—logic means that aggregates control details, overall priorities guide detail choices, and early choices control choices later in the process;
7. An **optimal** budget—long- and short-term choices sometimes conflict, hence budget reform is not a stable end-state, but should be expected to be a series of "unstable dynamic tradeoffs, shifting according to the requirements of the time" (Caiden, 1983, p.16).
8. A **neutral** budget—budget reform is political and may involve changes of political power; hence reforms tend to add on to present structure in order not to take power away from present power holders (or because they cannot).
9. Accomplishment of reform within the **traditional** framework—the annual, unified budget. Caiden warns that this latter point may not be sustainable if conditions change dramatically.

In the years that have passed since the publication of Caiden's article, it is hard to see which of these suggestions was more seriously compromised. Budget horizons were lengthened, but annual appropriations remained the norm, with most fiscal years beginning with continuing resolutions and appropriations bills being passed one or two months into the fiscal year. Hardly anyone would assert that the last decade of federal budgeting was credible or that choices on taxing and spending policies were made in an orderly way. If the process of the last decade with its deficits, missed deadlines, and executive-legislative deadlocks represent a series of unstable, dynamic tradeoffs, few would be attracted by the nature of such a model for the long term. On the positive side, it is hard to specify how much long-term damage has been done by this fractured budget process. Mandatories remain about the same percentage of the federal budget as they did in 1983, while the national debt has quintupled from 1980 to 1998; as a result, interest on the national debt became one of the larger budget categories. However, the deficit declined as a percentage of GDP from 1983 on and by 1998 the federal budget was in a surplus position, resulting in substantial amounts of the debt being paid down. Moreover the projected ten year surplus totals to 2011 gave rise to tax cut competition in the Presidential election of 2000, which resulted in the one of the largest tax cuts in U.S. history in 2001, with some assurance that more of the debt would be paid down.

While reforms that directly addressed limiting deficits, such as Gramm-Rudman-Hollings, the Budget Enforcement Act of 1990, and the Deficit Reduction Act of 1993 did not seem to be successes at the time, they probably served to hold down annual spending and deficits, while at the same time complicating the budget process. Both the reforms of 1990 and 1993 contained significant deficit reduction measures, but the growth of health care costs and other demographic trends meant that there was still significant work to do before a balanced budget could realistically be foreseen. In fact, few observers predicted the booming internet economy which came to the rescue of the budget in the late 1990s. Conventional wisdom now gives government action (particularly that in 1990 and 1993) about half the credit for the surplus of 2000, with the unexpected power of the economy given credit for the other half. Meanwhile two rather significant fundamental reforms were being put in place. The first of these was the passage of the Chief Financial Officer's Act of 1990 that addressed internal issues of financial management and control and the second was the Government Performance and Results Act of 1993. These are long term efforts to add rationality to federal financial management and budgeting. The outcome of the CFO act will eventually provide an auditable statement of what is bought for what is spent. The GPRA will eventually provide agency strategic planning linking mission statements to performance measurements and dollars.

The Government Performance and Results Act of 1993 (see, Wolfgang, 1994; see also McCaffery & Wolfgang, 1995) seemed to be a direct return to performance budgeting and the linking of inputs to outputs. On August 3, 1993, Congress passed Public Law 103-62, the Government Performance and Results Act (GPRA). The purpose of the act was to shift the focus of federal government management from inputs to outputs and outcomes, from process to results, from compliance to performance, and from management control to managerial initiative. In 1994, OMB Circular A-11 warned that budget requests for increases without performance data would be difficult to justify. OMB encouraged agencies to use output and outcome-based performance measures in the budget decision-making process and budget justification statements. In 1995, OMB held a performance review of many key programs and in a memorandum to the heads of Executive Departments in September, Director Alice Rivlin said that FY97 budget requests needed to contain significantly greater amounts of useful performance information to help define both funding levels and projected program results. Still more performance information was to be included in the FY1998 budget. This would set the stage for a decision about government-wide implementation of performance budgeting or simply the use of performance measures to clarify and support budget requests for FY99.

Initially this appeared to be a return to the concepts of performance budgeting on a federal government wide basis. In one sense, this is true; in another, it is not. While GPRA emphasized the development of performance information as crucial to the budget process, it links performance measurement to the strategic planning and managing process. In September of 1995, a strategic planning guidance was added to A-11 as a new part two of the budget preparation circular. OMB Director Rivlin's cover memo stated that there was "no more important element in performance-based management than strategic plans." According to the memo, agencies were expected to use strategic plans as a means for unifying various performance initiatives into an integrated effort. Initiatives mentioned included performance agreements, customer service standards, and performance partnerships. This brand of performance budgeting is built upon linking measurement to the governmental objectives developed in the strategic planning process and carried out as a part of the strategic management process. Additionally, pilot programs examined in 1994 and 1995 manifested a heavy reliance on issues of customer service and satisfaction. Consequently, the analyst who expects the old brand of performance budgeting as a cost per unit of work performed will be surprised by a much more comprehensive apparatus linking strategic planning, strategic management, performance measures and measures of customer satisfaction.

Some advantages mentioned by participants in pilot projects included improved planning, more effective administrative control, decentralized decision making, improved public relations from clearer program information, better focus on the activities of the organization, and provision of more precise quantitative measures. Some disadvantages were also noted. Performance budgeting was not equally applicable to all agencies. For example, an agency involved in basic research did not have workload data that was easily quantifiable.

Secondly, efficiency was not guaranteed by using unit cost data. Administrators could use a performance budget to identify problem areas or wasteful agencies, but this by itself did not increase efficiency. Third, some units found it very difficult to agree on an appropriate set of performance measurements. Many indicators proved to be inappropriate and some agencies had to go through several iterations of defining measures before they could agree on a good set of measures. Fourth, measures of effectiveness and outcome or impact are extremely difficult to develop and get agreement about. Fifthly, agencies did not find this a cheap system to operate; staffing time and costs associated with developing and monitoring several indicators was burdensome for the smaller agencies.

This reincarnation of performance measurement has focused from the start on external relations. Every person interviewed in one pilot program identified customer satisfaction measures as a major strength of the new performance measurement system. Many also mentioned the value of having a shared sense of vision from the top to the bottom of the organization. These two points alone are significantly different from the performance measurement and budgeting efforts of the 1950s. Even if GPRA does not lead to a complete performance budgeting system, it appears it will add more performance information to the budget process, a linkage to strategic planning and management, and measures of clientele satisfaction.

This is an attractive starting point for budget reform and some states have also been active on the performance budgeting front, including Texas, Arizona, and Florida. Arizona, in legislation in 1993 and 1995, instituted a system that required formal identification of all programs and compels agencies to develop strategic plans and performance measures to support their budget requests (see Franklin, 1995). This information provided a basis for evaluating program efficiency and effectiveness. In 1993 more than 1200 programs were identified. As agencies began to develop their strategic plans in 1994, many made changes to their original program structure, de-emphasizing some and emphasizing others. Performance measures were directly related to a program's mission, goals and objectives. While measures of inputs and outputs remain important, greater emphasis was placed on efficiency, quality and outcome measures. A key provision of this process was to make information on agency strategic plans and performance results more readily available to the Governor and Legislature. A master list of all state programs was presented to the legislature each budget session along with the budget. In budget development, there was a schedule that linked budget requests to agency strategic goals. Agencies also provided a schedule of performance measures with the most important designated as caseload/budget drivers. The Legislature identified a process for systematic review of program authorizations very much like a zero base budget review of program necessity. The outcomes of these reviews were recommendations to retain, eliminate or modify funding and related statutory references for the programs. In 1995, Arizona had a budget of about $11 billion, with $6 billion from federal sources.

However, like the CFO Act, this new brand of performance budgeting is an internal professional reform that is removed from the legislative-executive spotlight where so much of the budget process has come to grief. While it may produce better numbers and measures indicating how satisfied clients are, it may have little impact on the big issues which the budget process must confront—adjusting to economic variations and coping with growing entitlements or rising health care costs and the level of support that citizens have come to expect from their entitlement programs. The new performance budgeting may be a good reform, but it is unlikely to be a sufficient reform.

Another model for improving the budget process by improving information may be found in the annual award program administered by the Government Finance Officers Association. Each year GFOA tests budgets against a set of standards and gives awards for the outstanding budgets (Rickards, 1990, pp. 75–77). These standards include criteria that evaluate budgets as:

1. A Policy Document
   - General government and specific unit statements of policy (goals, objectives, mission statements, strategies)
     a. Changes in policy since last budget
     b. Budget process itself explained
2. An Operations Guide
   - Link of budget programs to line items by organizational unit
   - Organizational chart and work force
   - Capital spending impact on daily operations and operational budgets
   - Specific objectives given to department heads of line managers
   - Means to measure performance accomplishment
3. A Financial Plan
   - Major revenue sources
   - Bases for forecasting, including factors that will influence forecasts
   - The organization of funds used by the government
   - End of year projection of financial condition
   - A capital financing element … separate capital budget
   - Consolidated picture of operations and financial activity
   - Debt management issues
   - Accountability basis used by the government
4. A Communication device
   - Availability of a draft of the budget prior to its adoption
   - Clear summary information on the budget
5. Aids to understanding the budget: a budget message, a table of contents, a glossary of terms, an identification of the basic units of the budget, charts and graphs with narrative explanations, key assumptions used in preparing the budget, a cross index and supplemental information, including statistical tables.

GFOA gives out awards each year to state and local jurisdictions that score high on these criteria. Ricards took this template and examined cities and counties in Texas. His examination of 69 city budgets in Texas using these criteria concluded that Texas cities had, on average, acceptable budget presentations, but counties had weak ones. The biggest shortcoming appeared to be the readability of the budget presentations (Rickards, 1990, pp. 72–87). The problem with this program is that it assumes that better information presented in a better format will lead to better budgeting. Given the dynamics of policy formation, this may not be so. Some may argue that more clarity in information simply increases the difficulty of compromise when fundamentally different philosophies are in conflict. It is difficult, however, to argue that less clarity usually is a benefit to the budget process.

WHY BUDGETING IS CONTRARY

The quest for budget reform has to encompass both information production and process. In 1995, Roy Meyers (1995) was able to suggest a series of difficulties with the federal budget process not too much different from those that Caiden had suggested in 1983. Meyers suggests that a good budget process must be comprehensive in scope, honest in its numbers and projections, perceptive by including both near and far term events, cooperative with other policy making processes (should not dominate them), accountable in reserving important decisions to legally appropriate authorities, responsive in adopting policies that match public preferences, constrained in the amount of money needed each budget period, judgmental in getting the most effects for least cost, timely in completing tasks when expected and accessible in being understandable without excessive effort. Meyers suggests that the federal budget is high in comprehensiveness and low in constraint, judgment, timeliness, and accessibility; Meyers ranks the other characteristics as medium. At this point it is appropriate to pause and consider why analysis of budget process reform is so confusing.

Nowhere is the budget process totally satisfactory. Something about it unsettles both practitioners and policy analysts. For some, it is the sheer untidiness of the process; for others it is the perception that outcomes do not accurately reflect the desires of the community that the budget process serves. Some may fear the budget process gives unfair advantage to certain skilled players; others may be frustrated by the suspicion of unfair advantage gained through a presumptively open and accessible process. In any case, the quest for a good budget process continues, notwithstanding that budget reform has been aggressively pursued since the late 1800s in the United States.

Budgeting is not a science. Certain factors complicate the search for a good budget process. First, what students learn about it does not seem to be sequentially collectable and usable as is research in most sciences. For example, the search for a balanced budget has roots that go back to the founding of the republic. Aaron Wildavsky suggests that a balanced budget norm was born out of the deliberations of the founding fathers and governed much of subsequent American budgetary practice, notwithstanding that the federal government budget was rarely balanced and states often achieved balance by separating operating from investment accounts. The cyclical nature of this budget debate can be seen in the movements for a balanced budget in the 1980s and 1990s. Since it is not a science, progress toward a good budget process does not seem to be linear.

Budgeting in modern democratic states is not very old.   It is still evolving. Aaron Wildavsky (1975a, p. 272) suggests that the appearance of a formal budgeting power may be dated from the reforms of William Pitt the Younger. As Chancellor of the Exchequer from 1783 to 1801, Pitt was faced with a heavy debt load as a result of the American Revolution and continuing struggles with France. Pitt consolidated a maze of customs and excise duties into one general fund from which all the government's creditors would be paid. He reduced fraud in revenue collection by introducing new auditing measures and he instituted double-entry bookkeeping procedures to track both debits and credits in one system. Pitt established a sinking fund schedule for debt repayment and altered the basic schedule of taxes and customs to reduce the allure of smuggling.

Until the Revolution, the American colonies generally followed English practices (McCaffery, 1987b). Colonial legislatures set the salaries of royal governors and other officers, but neither expenditures nor taxes were heavy. England could and did impose duties and customs intended to regulate trade and navigation. After the revolutionary war, the Colonies vested power in various legal arrangements in the legislative branch, to the initial exclusion of the executive branch. Under the Articles of Confederation, the central government was weak and the legislative branch of government carried out both the legislative and executive functions of government. The colonists had just waged a war to escape rule by a monarch and they were not interested in substituting another strong executive in place of the King. Under the Articles of Confederation, Congress basically prepared all revenue and appropriation estimates, enacted them into law, and then attempted to execute what had been enacted. This system did not work very well. The revolutionary period was marked by a scarcity of hard coinage, various paper money schemes, a dependence on debt and letters of credit, an aversion to national taxes, and some degree of negligence, wastefulness, disorder and corruption. While some may find some of these same characteristics in current day processes, the main point is that the budget process is a power shared between the executive and the legislature; neither can go it alone and either can make the process very difficult.

Budgeting is a negative power.   This is a very old characteristic of the budget power and may be traced to the Magna Carta that constrained the revenue raising power of the King of England. Subsequent to the Magna Carta, the development of the budget power in England as a check on the power of the King was evolutionary. By the middle of the fourteenth century, the House of Commons had been established and was passing broadly phrased revenue acts; once the money was raised, the King's ministers could spend the money as they wished. The next step was for Parliament to insert appropriations language in Supply Acts stating the particular purposes for which the money could be used. Rules were made for the proper disbursement of money and penalties imposed for noncompliance. Progress in setting up a budget process was not linear and a full-fledged system would have to wait hundreds of years. The historical development of the budget power in England and the United States was very different; in England the process involved a gradual diminution of the power of the King; in American the process involved a gradual diminution of the power of the legislature in favor of the executive. The fact that budgeting is a negative power leads to an emphasis on the status quo, or even the status quo ante, and much debate, deliberation and delay before new projects are attempted. This frustrates those who see emergent needs and would use the power of government to meet them. While program advocates build, budgeteers cut. For them the essence of a good budget is built on frugality, thrift, efficiency, and a budget like last year's in dollar amounts. For most budget technicians, the triumph in budgeting is to discover and abort or contain a program that starts small, but would have growing or even open-ended out year expenditures. Because all demands cannot be met, budgeting has a negative culture. When this culture is confronted with a strong demand, it is forced to react positively to it. Thus, budgeting also has a reactive component to it that further disturbs the orderliness of its cycles.

Conflict is inherent in the budget process. Conflict leads to both a messy process and ambiguous outcomes. No one gets 100% of what he started after. Conflict within a benign environment had beneficial outcomes, as is depicted so well by Wildavsky and others in the United States from the 1950s to the early 1970s where stable routines were developed in a stable and moderately growing economic climate and there was consensus on basic policy ends. The benefit of conflict in this setting was that it drove a stable set of behaviors between claimants and controllers in the budget process. Allen Schick (1990a) has argued that claiming and rationing are at the center of the budget process. Individuals and groups articulate demands on government for services. If the government can satisfy all demands, no budgeting process is necessary. Conversely, if government is so poor it can satisfy no demands, then no budget process is possible, necessary, or feasible. History offers few examples of societies so rich that all demands can be accommodated, and perhaps even fewer where the power holders of that society wished to accommodate all such demands.

Aaron Wildavsky's (1964/1984b, 1988/1992) classic portrayal of the budgetary process suggested that the overwhelming complexity of the budget drove an incremental approach, where programs were reviewed a piece at a time, with different parts being reviewed in different places, and reviewers relying on participant feedback to tell them if they had cut too much from one program or another. The complexity of the budget process dictated that some people must trust others in this process because they can only check up on them a small part of the time and because no one can be an expert in everything. Wildavsky saw man's inherent intellectual limits making an incremental approach a necessity. This view assumed constant making and remaking of the budget, with a heavy concentration of review on what is changed in the current year from the previous year. The picture of an incremental process with specific roles for budget participants dominated how observers interpreted the budget process in the United States in the last third of the 20th century and to some extent misled them, for the United States from the early 1970s on had to cope with external economic shocks, internal demographics that made some of the promises made early more difficult to keep and a gradual fraying at the boundaries of commonality in policy ends.

The budget process is a planning process.   At its heart, budgeting is about the future and what should happen in the future. For agencies, this planning process might involve estimates of how many audits or accounts will be done in the next year; for welfare advocates it might involve estimates of what it will take to provide a decent standard of living to the poor; for defense agencies it might involve appreciations of foreign policy and defense resource planning about threat capacity and potential responses involving everything from aircraft carriers to tanks. While numbers give the budget document the aura of precision, it is still a plan and the outcomes of this plan are often substantially different from what the plan predicted. While this is a natural phenomenon, it has not done the reputation of the budget process much good. In the United States, participants can intervene at various stages in the budget process to modify original budget plans. The struggle to keep these plans on track is also seen in budget execution when agencies attempt to execute the budgets they have prepared in an environment which is usually changed slightly from the one in which the budget was developed. Budget systems usually provide some capacity to modify the enacted budget during budget execution; these range from fund transfers and reprogramming, to emergency bills and supplementals, to emergency legislative sessions.

No magic formula for a good budget process has been discovered despite strenuous efforts.   Reformers have made major efforts at reform of process and outcome of the process for more than 100 years. At the federal level, the development of an executive budget system would have to wait until the passage of the Budget and Accounting Act of 1921, which established the Bureau of the Budget and gave the President the power to submit a budget to Congress that would represent all the needs of the federal government for the coming year. The stimuli for passage of this act may be found in the deficits incurred in W.W.I and the various reform movements rising out of local governments and the Progressive movement. It also had a national background. Irene Rubin (1993) suggests that some part of federal reform came from efforts to oversee the railroads at the end of the nineteenth century. Railroads were big and important to the public for carrying goods and passengers. With the quick expansion of railroads and the consolidation of one railroad by another, it was not always easy to tell if a railroad was making a profit, or, indeed, if the railroad was solvent. This meant it was also difficult to tell if the rates that were set for freight and passengers were fair. Thus in the 1880s the Interstate Commerce Commission was put in the position of regulating rates, but to do this it had to develop better accounting tools in consultation with the railroads. Once these procedures had been implemented for railroads—considered the largest, most complex and most sophisticated of private corporations, government was then urged to make similar improvements for its own operations (Rubin, 1993, p. 440).

Frederick Cleveland at the New York Bureau of Municipal Research continued these reform efforts in the first decade of the twentieth century as did President Taft's Commission on Economy and Efficiency in 1912. Long before the federal government had passed the Budget and Accounting Act of 1921, many American cities had passed local budget reform acts that prevented city councils from appropriating money outside the confines of a budget. As early as 1899, the National Municipal League drafted a model municipal charter that incorporated a budget system under the direct supervision of the mayor (Burkhead, 1956, p.13). In the United States, twentieth-century budget reform spread from the local level to state and national levels.

Reforms have involved both process and outcome. Much of the history of budget reform involved finding ways to present budget information to decision makers in a more meaningful way so that better decisions can be made about how to allocate scarce resources. These reforms have included performance budgeting, program budgeting, zero-based budgeting, Planning-Programming-Budgeting and various systems focused on target or mission-based budgeting. Some reforms have focused on the budget process itself, in the belief that better staff or a more timely process would provide a better budget process. Paramount among these sorts of reforms would be the Budget and Accounting Act of 1921 and the Congressional Budget Reform and Impoundment Act of 1974.

Dissatisfaction with budget outcomes, usually in respect to growing deficits, has resulted in a different type of budget reform basically attempting to mandate a balanced budget, one where spending equals revenues. Examples of this kind of budget reform include the Gramm-Rudman-Hollings Acts of 1985 and 1987 and the Budget Enforcement Acts of 1990 and 1993 and several attempts at a Constitutional Balanced Budget Amendment at the federal level. These efforts were not without some adverse consequences. Attempts to meet the GRH targets often involved optimistic estimates of spending and revenues and certain gimmicks like shifted paydays which probably did more to damage the budget process than reform it, especially since few if any of the GRH targets were met.

Only nine times from 1930 to 1998 had the U.S. federal budget been in a situation where revenues exceeded spending (see *A Citizen's Guide*, 1995). The great depression of the 1930s and the intense effort of World War II appear to mark a turning point in American society; from that period on policymakers appear to have become committed to a larger role for government. In practice this has meant that claims on the budget have exceeded available resources and the federal government has usually been willing to go into debt to meet those claims. In 1995, the national debt stood at $4.8 trillion, after quintupling from 1980, and annual payments for interest on the national debt was the fourth largest category in the federal budget. Rhetoric about the national debt and deficit reduction has provided a constant subtext to budget discussions from the mid-1980s to 1998. The turn of the century surpluses are haunted by the specter of approaching unmet needs in social security and medical care.

In the American context, many of the issues in budgeting have been issues for a long time; these include the type and extent of taxation; how large the national debt should be; what the relationship should be between the executive and legislative branches and how budgets should be presented—in lump sums, itemized detail, or in some other format that might lead to better decision making. These questions endure because they are important and not easily solved.

Budget environments differ and this makes a difference. Budgeting in an environment of high inflation (5% a month) is so different from budgeting in an environment of relative stability (3% inflation a year) that tests of goodness for the budget process are bound to be very different (see Caiden & Wildavsky, 1974). Tests for goodness of process may be impossible to state for such varying environments.

A common understanding of what budget means is elusive. At the federal level, the budget sometimes means the Budget Resolution, sometimes a Reconciliation Bill, sometimes the Authorization Bill, sometimes the Appropriation Bill; changes in entitlement criteria in substantive law outside of the foregoing measures can also affect the size and scope of the budget. Deciding how these elements should fit together into a good budget process is elusive. At subnational levels, there are operating and capital budgets as well as budgets supported by various funds or belonging to different special districts. A common test for goodness for all of these is difficult to envision.

Goodness of outcome is a value judgment. This can only be made as an artifact of the value structure of the judge. Goodness of process may be discoverable from information processing, engineering, and biological systems, but no ready parallels are obvious that will produce a useful test for goodness of outcome.

SOME PRESCRIPTIONS FOR THE BUDGETARY PROCESS

The fact that Caiden and Meyer's evaluations are not too dissimilar although twelve years apart in time is enough to give anyone pause who might wish to prescribe for the budget process. Having said this there would seem to be some appropriate indicators to look for in a good budget process. These are highly conditioned by the biases of the authors and even at that some of them are a very close call. Nonetheless for purposes of stimulating discussion, consider the following propositions:

1. Spending should equal revenue in the long run and the long run should not be too long. The idea here is that marginal deficits from year to year are all right, especially given the unpredictable nature of the economy, tax revenues, and emergency spending patterns. Small frictional deficits are all right. If they become a problem, then a rainy day fund might be considered. At the national level, it is easier simply to use a debt instrument, but the value being operationalized here involves not going in debt, unless intergenerational transfer issues make it a wise policy. Emergencies could be met with a special fund or with reserves generated by budgeting to 99% of the revenue sum. On a budget of $2 trillion, 1% would provide more than enough to cover the usual weather or defense-related emergency supplemental appropriation.

2. A small deficit is all right when it is oriented to investment accounts. The stretch to define investment must not be too great. In general, investing in bridge repair to help move goods to market is different from repairing covered bridges so that tourists might enjoy them, unless the multiplier effect for tourism is awfully high. Somewhere a line has to be drawn between the essential and the nice to have.

3. Time is important. The budget cycle should be a cycle. The public expects a budget cycle, as do bureaucrats. When politicians prolong the cycle past its natural end, public expectations are violated and this affects the fundamental legitimacy of the political system. Tim-

ing is really a trivial problem, given that the next budget will crowd right in on top of the last so why jeopardize the fundamental perceptual connection of the people to government over "late" budgets and politicians who "can't get anything done." Timing is important as an indicator to the public of the health of the political system, and the operators of the political system ought to respect that. A budget process needs closure. After all, how can the next budget process start, if the current one is not over? When the 1995 budget process finally ended in April of 1996, the public interest in it had long since moved on.

4. Simplicity is important, simplicity in format and numbers, because the actions of the players are complex. If the format, numbers (baselines and forecasts) and the process are too complex, then behavior begins to be seen as magical and unpredictable and unworthy. There is probably little realistic hope for this prescription; even "as simple as practicable" results in a very complex process.

5. The budget must be auditable and audited and a respected entity must say periodically "this is good or this is bad." All stakeholders need to know that someone is watching; this has to do with responsibility and legitimacy. In general, U.S. systems have done well on auditing for propriety.

6. There must be consensus on where the important numbers come from and on roughly what they are. This is not a simple task, but it is important. Schick's (1990a, p. 5) compelling description of baseline alchemy makes it easy to understand how an increase gets portrayed as a cut and why this is done. However, when major players come up with different numbers to measure the same phenomena, the public becomes disenchanted and disgruntled and legitimacy of the system suffers. Last year's actuals, this year's budget, the budget request, the baseline, and estimates of GDP growth, inflation and unemployment ought to be discoverable.

7. Access is important. Stakeholders ought to have access to the places where decisions are made that affect them. This is very difficult at the national level, less so at local levels. Publicity, notification, and open meetings are important. The media has a responsibility to learn about the budget process and report it accurately; they too serve the purposes of the republic.

8. Ownership is important. The budgetary entity should own as much of its revenue stream as possible. When state and local governments are given a high percentage of pass-through revenues or money from other levels of government, that money may be targeted for special purposes and thus not reviewed thoroughly. Even when it is not earmarked money, it is free money from another level and the

intensity of budget review will be diminished. In this example, a unit with a higher level of revenues from its own sources would get a higher grade on its budget process. Its taxpayers would certainly prefer more money from other levels of government, but all money belongs to someone, and taxpayers should not expect to pay their expenses with other people's taxes.

9. Competition is important. Special district budget processes intrinsically are not as good as general purpose budget processes because competition over resources is diminished. It is easy to see why special districts are created—they favor accomplishment of a special task—however, the competition for resources is among those who want more and those who want a lot more for that function. A low tax rate for a flood control district, local library district, pollution abatement district, fire control district, water district or what have you risks hiding inefficient and ineffective decision making. Just because the rate is low does not mean the right questions were asked or answered correctly. A good budget process is one where resource seekers compete with other resource seekers. While special districts may be seen as a sub-national phenomenon, there are moral equivalents to special districts in the federal budget too, only they are called social security, Medicare, Medicaid, the highway trust fund, and interest on the national debt. To the extent these are must fund categories, they diminish the amount of decision space available for meeting new needs or enhancing old programs and the level of competition is diminished.

10. Political systems ought to be frugal with the promises they make which endure beyond the time period of the budget process. Entitlements and special districts are created as a response by the political system to demands so great that the annual budget system is not deemed a safe enough vehicle to honor them. These are set asides that the political system deems so important that they have converted them into promises they intend to keep. Interest on the national debt has the same status; it results from a need deemed so special it was met with deficit funding with the promise to pay in the future, which is one reason why until recently federal deficits have usually resulted only from times of serious national crisis. A system that had many special districts and high deficit financing might score high on responsiveness, but low on responsibility.

11. The executive should propose a balanced budget. Proposing a balanced budget disciplines the executive branch to think in terms of balance and this thinking will filter down the administrative hierarchy so that lower level administrators who usually do not make the connection between revenue and expenditures will understand that

a budget process is a constrained process. Being a careful steward of funds is helped by understanding that funds are limited; this is an insight often lost in the bowels of bureaucracy where managers are busy planning and building without a sense of constraint. Without that sense, the glass is always at least half full, and the ethic is to ask for more; after all you may well get it. It is likely that this guidance will come in the form of top line constraint (no increases greater than 3% or new programs only if paid for out of old programs, or both). It can be argued that asking for more is an administrator's job, thus it is probably wise to make sure someone at the top of the hierarchy strikes a final balance. State and local governments generally propose balanced budgets and take actions during budget execution to keep them balanced, although each year a number of them end up in a deficit position, usually depending on the strength of the local economy and its affect on tax revenues and counter-cyclical payments. This is not a great change from existing practice for state and local governments. Perhaps it is enough to ask the federal government to limit its spending to changes in its income, i.e., GDP-linked growth limits.

12. When the executive proposes a balanced budget, the legislature should honor this commitment except in times of national emergency. When it decides on an emergency (or to pass an unbalanced budget) it should have to enact a separate clearance defining what constituted an emergency this year, prior to enactment of the bills that compose the budget. Perhaps this could be done as a legislative resolution which does not need executive level assent; from this point on, the executive can work to get the legislature to modify its intent, agree with it, or veto the implementing funding bills.

13. A good budget process probably includes an item veto (preferably one where the chief executive can veto all or some of the item) for the executive, as well as the impoundment power as it existed prior to the Congressional Budget Reform Act of 1974. The purpose here is to manage funds in the appropriation process (with an item veto) and during the execution stage with impoundment. Undoubtedly these strengthen the hand of the executive branch. Most Governors have an item veto power; in addition to frugality, governors do use it to change legislative policy, especially the reducing veto. At the national level, Congress persists in putting earmarks or funds marked for specific targets in appropriation bills; often these are very cleverly designed to appear to be somewhat general when in fact only one state or research institution or site fills all the requirements. Whether an item veto could reach all these is debatable, or whether if reachable the President would reduce it but leave some

money in there to show he was in favor of the idea too but just could not fully fund it is a possibility. In budget execution, current federal interpretation is that the executive must spend all the money appropriated, unless Congress agrees to rescind budget authority. Given time lags in budgeting, a wiser course would seem to be to return to the pre-1974 statute and allow the President to impound funds deemed not necessary by his managers, but perhaps to put percentage limits on the power. There is no doubt this increases executive power, especially the executive powers to meddle around the margins and to reward or punish individuals or individual constituencies, but it also allows for sensible budgetary management.

14. On the legislative side, legislative procedures should allow for focus on the budget. This means that the number of committees that handle the budget should be as few as necessary. At the federal level, this probably means there should be a set of budget committees to set overall targets and a set of appropriation committees to fund those targets. The authorizing committees fulfill an important function essentially giving shape to a program and taking a big picture look at a sector; the authorizing bill is seen by the authorizers as giving guidance to the appropriators, but it would seem that one of these two sets of committees is enough, and the comprehensive view of the appropriators is more important than the sectoral view of the authorizing committees. This sectoral view is often replicated by the budget committees in order to get to their functional totals in the budget resolution. Effectively what this might mean is a full set of important subcommittees for the budget committees, which in the Congressional process might endanger the timely passage of a Budget Resolution. In the name of comprehensiveness and unity, it might also be useful to take the social security program from the tax committees and give it to the budget and appropriators. If the appropriators are going to get 100% of the blame, they might as well have closer to 100% of the budget under their control.

For many years, Wisconsin had a joint budget committee consisting of a few members (13 total) drawn from both legislative chambers. It held hearings on the budget of each agency or program and passed on its recommendations to both houses, where its members were expected to be important players in the budget debate. It was a relatively small, powerful and very important committee, both on the budget and tax side. The tax committees tended to write technical corrections and major tax legislation to implement the budget only after approval by the Joint Budget Committee. Undoubtedly this was the legacy of a part time legislature based on a local government model, but it seemed to work. At the national level, this would be like reducing the size of the budget committees and authorizing them to hold joint hearings and produce recommendations on the President's budget. It could still produce a budget resolution, followed up by the appropriation bills. Perhaps considering the size and substantive domain of the federal budget (capital and operating budgets, defense, stabilization policy), this would not be a wise idea, but committee roles have changed over the nation's history and other arrangements are discussible (although the trend from the Civil War onward seems to have been toward creating more committees to decentralize power whenever one set of committees gained too much power).

15. Equity linkages should be made. Two kinds of linkages could be considered. On the macro-level, a rule could be used which would prevent the budget from growing faster than gross domestic product. This would connect spending to the growth in wealth of the polity. On the micro-level, entitlements should not grow faster than the wealth of those who have to pay for them; if the incomes of current taxpayers rise more slowly than what is paid out to those on entitlements, the possibility for great dissatisfaction exists on the part of the taxpayers. When fewer workers support more recipients, this condition is exacerbated. The budget process has changed since the 1950s at the federal level due to entitlements and the strain put on the budget process by them; people expect to get not only their "entitlement" but also a dividend that will hold them harmless from inflation. In describing this policy area, Wildavsky calls it the "collapse of consensus" (Wildavsky, 1988, Ch. 4). In the medical care area, another level of players, new technologies, often dramatic in their impact, and increased costs complicate notions of equity. This will not be an easy issue to solve in the budget process; it may be argued that it was skirmishing over these issues that brought the 1995 federal budget process to its knees.

16. The role of the legislature should be to represent the needs of the people, even when the people do not understand what those needs are. Administrators are good at picking up the little needs, e.g., more caseload, new rain gutters, a new fire truck, but they are not good at defining the macro-needs that face society; this is more properly the legislature's role. Legislators have to lead, identify emergent needs and seek ways to fund them. The reason people tend to be for a balanced budget in the abstract and against it in practice occurs when they learn approximately what price they themselves will have to pay and cannot be guaranteed that all others similarly situated will suffer equally. Legislators have to bridge these gaps; legislators have to educate people and lead them. In this

sense, the President is of course a legislator. No reforms will be effective if the system is going to be operated by people who intend never to compromise.

Budget systems demand compromise and accommodation, and a sense that what is not won this year may be won next year, even when that win is a reduction in spending. That is why timeliness and closure are virtues; without them people have difficulty standing back and measuring the outcome of the budget process in order to prepare for the next cycle. This is not so important to those in the bureaucracy; after all, they know which programs are carrying through at roughly the same level and what new things did or did not get funded and which new programs are still waiting legislative approval. However, it is much more difficult on the legislative and the greater public's side. Probably the balance of innovation in a political system comes out of the legislative process. The budget process should be operated by persons of good will and common sense who are willing to listen to new ideas and can articulate what must be done for the people who elect them.

CONCLUSIONS

In the budget process, there is an intersection where the tools of professional articulation meet the needs of political representation. Here participants describe desires with numbers. These numbers represent estimates of available resources, describe what was funded last year, and indicate what should be funded in the budget year. Forecasts, projections, and various financial calculations lend weight to these numbers. These are professional representations of how much is enough. No matter how accurately computed, these numbers may be deemed inadequate to answer demands that are expressed by participants in the political review of the budget. The fundamental problem of the budget process seems to be that there is always more to do: claimants always want more. Some claimants may subscribe to wanting less in general, but few want less for their own programs and the collection of individual programs adds up to more.

If the test of a good budget process is outcomes, then the good process will always be meritorious to the extent that it gives more to goals pursued by those who judge the process; however, so complicated are budget routines that programs can actually give clienteles more than last year, but less than an inflation adjusted baseline so that the clientele perceives more as less and is frustrated. If the provision of more (dollars, goods, services) is not enough to indicate the health of the budget process, are there simple process guidelines that indicate what makes a good budget process? What if a "good" process leads to bad outcomes as judged by a significant portion of the population? These are difficult questions to answer. Budget process reforms have been industriously sought for over a century at different levels of government in the United States, but the difficulty of making a smooth intersection of political representation and professional articulation indicates that the budget reform process is unlikely to be finished soon. It is to be hoped that this is a cyclical process, where the cycle leads to improvements in the budget process rather than simply adding redundancy and complexity. With a homogeneous population and a stable economy and no exogenous shocks, elected officials may still differ over the budget, but the scope of argument would be contained, there would be a definite majority at the center and the need for budget reform might be reduced. Casual observation would seem to indicate that not only is America very diverse, but it is growing more diverse. Iowa and California are very different places, as are Florida and Alaska. It takes great optimism to expect that one budget system will fit well over this diversity without many frictional adjustments. The realist might suggest that it is a wonder the federal budget system works at all.

NOTE

1.   For example, an observer calls the line item appropriation bill that finances Congress "...a monument to obfuscation" and compares understanding its various line items to trailing a cat through the "labyrinthine passageways of the capitol itself" (see Meyers, 1994, p. 61).

CHAPTER X

BUDGETING FOR RESULTS

INTRODUCTION

Management control is the process by which public managers and employees generally are motivated to advance the purposes and policies of the organizations for which they work. It is also a process for detecting and correcting unintentional performance errors and intentional irregularities, such as theft or misuse of resources. In many organizations the primary instrument of management control is responsibility budgeting, which embraces both the formulation of budgets and their execution.

Information and transaction costs make it necessary and desirable to decentralize some decisions in organizations. Decentralization in turn requires organizations to solve the control problems that result when self-interested persons do not behave as perfect agents, in accordance with the goals and rules of the organization and preferences of executives and other sponsoring parties. Capitalist economies solve these control problems through the institution of alienable decision rights. But because organizations suppress the alienability of decision rights, they must devise substitute mechanisms that perform its functions. Three functions are critical: (1) allocating decision rights among agents in the organization, (2) measuring and evaluating performance, and (3) rewarding and punishing individuals for their performance. Responsibility budgeting and accounting systems are the most widespread mechanisms for performing these functions.

In this following section we explain the nature of responsibility budgeting, its intellectual justification, its antecedents, and its present and future use in the public sector. This is not a straightforward task. We cannot simply explain how responsibility budgeting is used and how it works. Responsibility budgeting makes sense only as a part of a framework of structural, procedural, and monitoring/reporting relationships. We must, therefore, also explain the framework that gives it utility and power. At the same time, responsibility budgeting and accounting, or their functional equivalents, make an essential contribution to the efficacy of this broader framework of relationships. One cannot arbitrarily mix and match administrative relationships and expect that the outcome will be productive. The efficacy of administrative relationships depends upon their congruity with each other as well as with the purposes and products of the entity in question and the productive and information processing technologies available to it.

GOVERNANCE ARRANGEMENTS, ADMINISTRATIVE PROCESSES AND CONTRACTUAL RELATIONSHIPS

All governance arrangements and administrative processes are primarily mechanisms for motivating and inspiring people, especially subordinate managers, to serve the policies and purposes of the organizations to which they belong. This means that all governance arrangements and all administrative processes can be treated as contractual relationships and that administrative design and implementation can be thought of as negotiating and enforcing contracts.

One way of describing contractual relationships involves the language of principal and agent. This language implies a hierarchical relationship, in which a nominal subordinate (agent) serves the purposes of a superior (principal). On the presumption that behavior is largely self-interested, principal-agent relationships are problematic (give rise to agency costs) only where (a) the efforts of the agent cannot be perfectly observed; (b) the interests of agent and principal diverge; and (c) agents pursue their own interests, i.e., behave opportunistically.

One of the key goals of governance arrangements and administrative processes is the minimization of agency costs. Of course, agency costs also include all resources used to reduce divergences of interest, i.e., identifying collectively beneficial relationships, negotiating contributions, and devising procedures for monitoring performance and sanctioning defectors. Included here are a whole panoply of activities extending from the employment of security guards to the design and implementation of new or reconfigured accounting and reporting systems. Hence, minimizing agency costs means minimizing the sum of costs that result from opportunistic behavior plus the costs of avoiding or controlling that behavior (Zimmerman, 1977).

Traditional or Weberian bureaucracies rely on rules to govern or prevent opportunistic behavior. In other words, principals specify in detail what agents must do (or must not do), carefully monitor their actions, and sanction all deviations accordingly. The problem with this approach is that agents often have better information about some things than do principals. Principals hire agents because of their superior expertise and to spare themselves the burden of being perfectly informed about every aspect of an organization's operations. In neither case will principals have the knowledge needed to specify in detail what the agent should do without thereby sacrificing performance. This means that rules are not always a wholly satisfactory solution to the principal-agent problem. It is this fact that makes the application of agency theory to the public sector especially important, for it is in the public sector that the opportunity costs arising from detailed rules often seem highest.

Organizational economists do not generally advocate more rules as a way to control opportunistic behavior. Rather, they stress two alternative approaches. One is to improve principals' abilities to monitor agents. This is often referred to as improving "transparency." For example, full accrual accounting gives a truer picture of resource use than does standard government accounting and thus helps make government operations more transparent. The second is to seek ways to align the incentives of agents with principals' interests. This is the preferred approach of organizational economists and managerial accountants. As the New Zealand Treasury (1987) observed, "Incentives matter. … Well-designed policies will align the interests and actions of individuals with those of the nation."

AN HISTORICAL DIGRESSION: FROM TRADITIONAL BUREAUCRACY TO THE M-FORM ORGANIZATION

Most large-scale organizations in the American public sector are organized like turn-of-the-century railroads. Operating responsibility is delegated on a geographic or site basis, rather than a line of business basis. Regional chiefs report to an agency head. Small armies of administrative staff specialists also report to agency heads. Their job is to gather and process quantities of data for agency heads to use to coordinate activities, allocate resources, and set strategy. These structures can be traced directly to the administrative system developed by the Prussian bureaucracy under Heinrich von Stein, Gerhard von Scharnhorst, August von Gneisenau, and Helmuth von Moltke. The Prussian system included administrative innovations such as detailed centralized resource requirements planning (discretionary expense budgets), control by rules and standard operating procedures, functional organizational design, vertical integration, decomposition of tasks to their simplest components, sequential processing, and administrative centralization and specialization of administrative staff functions such as reporting, accounting, personnel, and purchasing.

The Prussian administrative system was once widely emulated by forward-looking businesses and governments all over the world. In the United States, among the first large-scale organizations to adopt this system were the railroads and the military departments. In industry early adopters of the elements of the Prussian administrative system consistently grew large as hierarchy and bureaucracy created massive economies of scale and scope. Economies of scale are produced by spreading fixed expenses over higher volumes of output, thereby reducing unit costs. Economies of scope are produced by exploiting the division of labor—sequentially combining highly specialized functional units in multifarious ways to produce a variety of products (Chandler, 1962; Rosenberg & Birdsall, 1986). In some cases the expansion of the early adopters occurred through the destruction of business rivals, in others by merger with them.

Not only did the Prussian administrative system make large, complex organizations relatively efficient; it seemingly made them inevitable. Only very large organizations could fully exploit the Prussian administrative system. Only they could capitalize on extreme task specialization or afford the throngs of staff experts needed to gather and process quantities of data for top management. Hence, for a long time it seemed that bigger organizations were necessarily better. And there seemed to be no natural limits to this conclusion. The planning and control system the General military bureaucracy under General Erich Ludendorff used to mobilize Germany's resources during World War I (the Kriegwirtschaftsplan) was merely an amplification of its peacetime arrangements. The centralized planning system, Gosplan, used in the Soviet Union to implement its long-term policies and strategic plans was an adaptation of the Kriegwirtschaftsplan.

Improvements in information processing, especially in the realms of accounting and finance, eventually limited organizational expansion, however. These innovations had the effect of increasing the relative efficiency of coordinating organizational activities and the flow of materials through arm's length relationships (as opposed to direct supervision), making it possible to avoid some of the opportunity costs inherent to rule-based governance systems.

The administrative system developed by Alfred Sloan and Donaldson Brown at General Motors in the 1920s demonstrated the maturity of these innovations. Sloan is best known for the multi-product or M-form organizational structure, in which each major operating division serves a distinct product market. Short-run integration under Sloan's system was achieved via buyer-seller relationships between GM's five automotive divisions and the divisions making automotive components (e.g., Fisher Body or Delco-Remy). Longer-run integration was achieved via the capital budgeting system devised in 1923 by Donaldson Brown, GM's chief financial officer.

GM's operating divisions were managed entirely by the numbers from a tiny corporate headquarters, using the DuPont system of financial control, also devised by Brown. Under this system, each division kept its own books, and managers were evaluated in terms of a return-on-assets target. The operating division managers continued to rely on control by rules and standard operating procedures and detailed resource-requirements plans. Sloan, however, believed that it was inappropriate, as well as unnecessary, for top managers at the headquarters level to know much about the details of division operations. If the numbers showed that performance was poor, it was time to change the division manager. Division managers with consistently good numbers got promoted, ultimately to headquarters. The divisional form of organization is not only a device to resolve a span of control problem; it also allows each division or business to be remotely controlled by the numbers from a strategic apex.

The general device that allows for remote control is a control system that aligns the incentives of operating unit managers with the purposes and priorities of the organization as a whole. For a remote control system to operate effectively, financial and cost information needs to be relevant. Establishing reporting entities corresponding to segmented business activities is the fundamental rule of thumb to be followed in the construction of such a system. A division is both a reporting entity and a segmented business activity. An ideal type—and even typical—division is one headed by a general manager who reports to the strategic apex and enjoys full line authority over the middle line and operating core.

THE ROLE OF RESPONSIBILITY BUDGETING AND ACCOUNTING

Responsibility budgeting and accounting is the most common remote control system used by large-scale organizations in the private sector. It is a form of internal contracting in which: (a) units and managers are evaluated relative to the targets they accept, (b) only financial measures are used to measure and reward accomplishment or punish failure, and (c) financial success or failure is attributed entirely to managerial decisions and/or employee performance. While private businesses were quick to learn bureaucratic control from government, governmental organizations have been slow to adopt remote control systems.

The digression is relevant here because responsibility budgeting is as much organizational engineering as it is financial management and accounting. Organizational engineering is concerned with the following three elements:

- *Administrative structure*—the structure depicted in an organization chart showing the organization's administrative units and their relationships to each other. Under responsibility budgeting, work can be arranged into administrative units according to mission, function, and/or region.
- *Responsibility structure*—the allocation of authority and responsibility to individuals within the organization. Under responsibility budgeting authority and responsibility must be unambiguously assigned.
- *The account or control structure*—the system of measuring and evaluating performance. Under responsibility budgeting, information on inputs, costs, activities, and outputs is critically important.

Under a fully developed responsibility budgeting and accounting system, administrative units and responsibility centers are coterminous and fully aligned with the organization's account structure, since the information it provides can be used to coordinate unit activities as well as to influence the decisions of responsibility center managers.

Under responsibility budgeting, two basic rules govern organizational design. First, organizational strategy should determine structure. Strategy means the pattern of purposes and policies that defines the organization and its missions and that positions it relative to its environment. Single mission organizations should therefore be organized along functional lines; multi-mission organizations should be organized along mission lines; multi-mission, multifunction organizations should be organized along matrix lines. Where a matrix organization is large enough to justify an extensive division of labor, responsibility centers should be designated as either mission or support centers, with the latter linked to the former by a system of internal markets and prices (transfer pricing).

The second basic rule is that the organization should be as decentralized as possible. Most students of management believe that the effectiveness of large, complex organizations improves when authority and responsibility are delegated down into the organization. Of course, authority should not be delegated arbitrarily or capriciously. Decentralization requires prior clarification of the purpose or function of each administrative unit and responsibility center, procedures for setting objectives and for monitoring and rewarding performance, and an account structure that links each responsibility center to the goals of the organization as a whole.

The biggest difference between government budgets and responsibility budgets is that government budgets tend to be highly detailed spending or resource acquisition plans, which must be scrupulously executed just as they were approved (Thompson & Jones, 1986). In contrast, operating budgets in the private sector are usually sparing of detail, often consisting of no more than a handful of financial targets. As we noted earlier, Sloan of

General Motors, one of the fathers of responsibility budgeting, believed it was inappropriate for corporate managers to know the details of responsibility center operations. The notion that responsibility centers should be managed at arm's length, by the numbers, from a small corporate headquarters, reflects the effort to delegate authority and responsibility down into the organization. As the OECD report, Budgeting for Results: Perspectives on Public Expenditure Management (1995), explains, delegation of authority means giving agency managers the maximum feasible authority needed to make their units productive—or, in the alternative, subjecting them to a minimum of constraints. Hence, delegation of authority requires operating budgets to be stripped to the minimum needed to motivate and inspire subordinates. Under responsibility budgeting the ideal operating budget would contain a single number or performance target (e.g., a production quota, a unit cost standard, or a profit or return on investment target) for each administrative unit/responsibility center.

In responsibility budget formulation, an organization's policies, the results of all past policy (capital budgeting, see Thompson, 1997) decisions, are converted into financial targets that correspond to the domains of administrative units and their managers (Anthony & Young, 1984, p. 19). In responsibility budget execution, operating performance is monitored and subordinate managers are evaluated and rewarded. Operating performance targets must be expressed in financial terms. This makes it possible to make comparisons across unlike responsibility centers, thereby permitting the relative performance of managers to be evaluated and increasing the motivational efficacy of internal competition. It also has the effect of keeping higher levels of administration ignorant of operating details, thereby discouraging them from meddling in the affairs of their responsibility center managers.

TYPES OF RESPONSIBILITY CENTERS

Responsibility centers are usually classified according to two dimensions:

1. *The integration dimension*—i.e., the relationship between the responsibility center's objectives and the overall purposes and policies of the organization; and
2. *The decentralization dimension*—i.e., the amount of authority delegated to responsibility managers, measured in terms of their discretion to acquire and use assets.

On the first dimension, a responsibility center can be either a mission center or a support center. The output of a mission center contributes directly to an organization's objectives or purpose. The output of a support center is an input to another responsibility center in the organization, either another support center or a mission center.

On the decentralization dimension, accountants distinguish among four types of responsibility centers based on the authority delegated to responsibility managers to acquire and use assets. Discretionary expense centers, the governmental norm, are found at one extreme; profit and investment centers are at the other. A support center may be either an expense center or a profit center. If the latter, its profit is the difference between its costs and its "revenue" from "selling" its services to other responsibility centers. Sells is in quotation marks here because the organization as a whole has not sold anything to an outside party. Rather, the responsibility center providing the service records revenue in its accounts and the center receiving the service records an expense. Revenue and expense cancel out when the organization consolidates its books. Money rarely changes hands in interdivisional transfer pricing. Responsibility centers don't get to keep "their" profits. Only the organization as a whole earns a profit. Selling to and buying from outsiders are the only activities that can generate real profits or losses for an organization.[1] Both profit and investment centers are usually free to borrow, and investment centers are also free to make decisions about plant and equipment, new products, and other issues that are significant to the long-run performance of the organization.

Discretionary expense centers incur costs. The difference between them and other kinds of responsibility centers is that their managers have no independent authority to acquire assets. Instead, the manager's superiors must authorize each acquisition. In the US system, under detailed line item budgets, acquisitions must be authorized by Congress and signed into law by the President. But all discretionary expense center managers are accountable for compliance with an asset acquisition/resource requirements plan (expense budget), whether written into law or not. Once acquisitions have been authorized, discretionary expense center managers are usually given considerable latitude in their deployment and use. Managerial accountants generally believe that administrative units should be discretionary expense centers only where there is no satisfactory way to match their expenses to final cost objects.

In some cases, expense center managers are evaluated in terms of the number and type of activities performed by their center. Where each of the activities performed by the center earns revenue or is assigned notational revenue (transfer price) by the organization's controller, these centers are referred to as revenue centers.

In a cost center, the manager is held responsible for producing a stated quantity and/or quality of output at the lowest feasible cost. Someone else within the organization determines the output of a cost center—usually including various quality attributes, especially delivery schedules. Cost center managers are usually free to acquire short-term assets (those that are wholly consumed within a performance measurement cycle), to hire temporary or contract personnel, and to manage inventories.

In a standard cost center, output levels are determined by requests from other responsibility centers and the manager's budget for each performance measurement cycle is determined by multiplying actual output by standard cost per unit (see Thompson, 1997). Performance is measured against this figure—the difference between actual costs and standard costs.

In a quasi-profit (or pseudo-profit) center, performance is measured by the difference between the notational revenue earned (transfer price) by the center and its costs (Kaplan, 1991). For example, let's say a Veteran's Administration hospital department of radiology performed 500 chest X-rays and 200 skull X-rays for the department of geriatrics. The notational revenue earned was $25 per chest X-ray (500) = $12,500 and $50 per skull X-ray (200) = $10,000, or $22,500 total. If the radiology department's costs were $18,000, it would earn a quasi-profit of $4,500 ($22,500 – $18,000).

In profit centers, managers are responsible for both revenues and costs. Profit is the difference between revenue and cost (or expense). Thus, profit center managers are evaluated in terms of both the revenues their centers earn and the costs they incur. In addition to the authority to acquire short-term assets, to hire temporary or contract personnel, and to manage inventories, profit center managers are usually given the authority to make long-term hires, set salary and promotion schedules (subject to organization wide standards), organize their units, and acquire long-lived assets costing less than some specified amount.

In investment centers, managers are responsible for both profit and the assets used in generating the profit. Thus, an investment center adds more to a manager's scope of responsibility than does a profit center, just as a profit center involves more than a cost center. Investment center managers are typically evaluated in terms of return on assets (ROA), which is the ratio of profit to assets employed, where the former is expressed as a percentage of the latter. In recent years many have turned to economic value added (EVA), net operating "profit" less an appropriate capital charge, which is a dollar amount rather than a ratio and is more generally consistent with the value-creating purposes of organizations (Kaplan, 1991).

Formerly, in most large complex organizations in the private sector, individual production units were typically standard cost centers; staff units were typically discretionary expense centers. Indeed, only mission centers were allowed to be investment centers. The reasons for this are complex, but they go to difficulties associated with expensing intermediate and joint products. Mission centers in private sector organizations produce final products that are easily priced and that are expensed following generally accepted accounting practice. In contrast, support centers produce intermediate products and these were, until recently, hard to cost, let alone price, with accuracy. Attempts to do so were often either excessively arbitrary or prohibitively costly. Now, however, advances in information technology, managerial accounting, and organizational design have made it possible and, in some cases, beneficial to treat every responsibility center in an organization as an investment center (Thompson, 1997).

Paradoxically, public sector organizations are a mirror image of large complex organizations in the private sector. We know now how to treat support centers in most organization as quasi-profit or even investment centers (Lapsley, 1994; for additional public sector examples, see Anthony & Young, 1984, pp. 371–374; Kaplan, 1991). But, because the final products of government's core mission centers are public goods that are passively enjoyed, pricing final outputs remains for the time being and for the foreseeable future either excessively arbitrary or prohibitively costly. This means, for example, that, while it might make sense to treat military depot maintenance, spare parts management, or facilities support centers as investment centers,[2] it will continue to be necessary to treat the armed forces' combatant commands as discretionary expense centers. Fortunately, as far as exhaustive expenditures are concerned, about 75% of the activities performed by the U.S. federal government fall into the support category and, for the most part, state and local governments are not in the business of supplying pure public goods.

Transfer Pricing

Under responsibility budgeting, support centers provide services or intermediate goods to other responsibility centers in return for a notational transfer price, organizations are structured to take advantage of specialized knowledge and local conditions, center managers make decisions and are held responsible for the overall financial performance of their centers. Sound transfer pricing is, therefore, the key to aligning the incentives of responsibility center managers with organizational interests.

Transfer pricing is also important to transparency within organizations. It helps to determine the costs of services provided by one unit to another, which is central to measuring performance relative to a financial target, and therefore plays a major role in establishing, as well as manipulating, the incentives facing responsibility center managers. Transfer pricing also reveals the internal costs of service decentralization where costs are incurred in transferring decision rights to others within an organization. When one subunit transfers tangible assets, knowledge, skills, etc., to another, both units calculate the cost as a means of revealing their liquid and tangible asset use internally and in external provision of service.

There are two common approaches to transfer pricing:

1. Laissez-faire transfer pricing: buying and selling responsibility centers are completely free to negotiate prices, to deal, or not to deal; and
2. Marginal or incremental cost pricing: the responsibility center selling the service is required to charge the buying responsibility center whichever is less of market or incremental cost.
3. (A third method is based upon fully distributed average cost of the service or product.)

However, the circumstances that justify large complex organizations—economies of scale and scope—render these simple transfer-pricing mechanisms problematic. Scale economies are usually the result of large, lumpy investments in specialized resources—technological knowledge, product specific research and development, or equipment. These investments tend to give rise to bilateral monopoly, a circumstance that provides an ideal environment for opportunistic behavior on the part of suppliers and customers.[3] For example, once an intermediate product producer has acquired a specialized asset, customers may be able to extract discounts by threatening to switch suppliers. In that case, the supplier may find it necessary to write off a large part of the specialized investment. Or, if demand for the final good increases greatly, the intermediate product supplier may be able to extort exorbitant prices from customers. Hence, where the relationship between intermediate product supplier and customer is at arm's length, opportunistic behavior may eliminate the payoff to what would otherwise be cost-effective investments. For example, the 1994 Report of the Commission on Roles and Missions of the Armed Forces (Thompson & Jones, 1994) suggested that budget authority should flow through the combatant commands to the military departments. Were that the case, lacking a long-term credible commitment on the part of the Joint Chiefs and the combatant commanders, the Navy's investment in specialized assets like aircraft carriers would permit it to be exploited in peacetime. In wartime, of course, the tables would be turned.

The new economics of organizations tells us that vertical integration occurs because it can mitigate this problem, in part through the substitution of direct supervision for remote control. Studies of military procurement demonstrate that specialized investments are critical to vertical integration. Where intermediate products were both complex and highly specialized (used only by the buyer), there was a 92% probability that they would be produced internally; even 31% of all simple, specialized components were produced internally. The probability dropped to less than 2% if the component was unspecialized, regardless of its complexity.

Unfortunately, the problems that arise in arm's length transactions where there are few alternative suppliers/customers also arise where one attempts to replicate free market forces within the organization, allowing buying and selling responsibility centers complete freedom to negotiate prices (laissez-faire transfer pricing). Traditionally, economists have argued that services should be transferred at marginal or incremental cost to the buying responsibility center. But this can seriously distort the evaluation of support center performance and tend to eliminate incentives to improvement.

As a result, organizations face a serious dilemma. They can maximize short-run performance by using marginal cost in internal transactions, thereby seriously distorting performance measurement and incentives, which will cause shortfalls in long-run performance. Or they can sacrifice short-term performance by relying on laissez-faire transfer pricing, thereby obtaining superior measures of the support center's contributions to organizational performance, and improve the chances of maximizing performance in the long term. Organizations can, promote short-run performance by using incremental cost pricing or they can promote long-term performance by using laissez-faire pricing, but they cannot do both simultaneously using either of these simple transfer pricing mechanisms.

In theory, bilateral monopoly can be governed quite satisfactorily by unbalanced transfer prices, multi-part transfer prices, or quasi-vertical integration. Under unbalanced transfer prices, the selling responsibility center is credited with the full cost of the transacted item (often standard cost), plus an agreed upon markup, the buying center is charged its marginal cost, and the organization's accounts are adjusted to reflect the difference between the two. Unbalanced transfer prices are rarely used, however, where market prices are available. Under, multi-part transfer prices, the service delivered is decomposed to reflect underlying cost drivers and priced accordingly (your home phone bill is an excellent example of a multi-part tariff). Under quasi-vertical integration, the buyer invests in specialized resources and loans, leases, or rents them to their suppliers. Quasi-vertical integration is common in both the automobile and the aerospace industries, and, of course, it is standard procedure for the Department of Defense to provide and own the equipment, dies, and designs that defense firms use to supply it with weapons systems. Other organizations that rely on a small number of suppliers or a small number of distributors write contracts that constrain the opportunistic behavior of those with whom they deal.

In still other cases, desired outcomes can be realized through alliances based on the exchange of hostages (e.g., surety bonds, exchange of debt or equity positions) or just plain old-fashioned trust based on long-term mutual dependence. Toyota, for example, relies on a few suppliers that it nurtures and supports (Womack, Jones, & Roos, 1990). They have substantial cross-holdings in each other and Toyota often acts as its suppliers' banker. Toyota maintains tight working links between its manufacturing and engineering departments and its suppliers, intimately involving them in all aspects of product design and manufacture. Indeed, it often lends them personnel to deal with production surges and its suppliers accept Toyota people into their personnel systems.

Toyota's suppliers are not completely independent companies with only a marketplace relationship to each other. In a very real sense, they all share a common purpose and destiny. Yet Toyota has not integrated its suppliers into a single, large bureaucracy. It wanted its suppliers to remain independent companies with completely separate books—real profit/investment centers, rather than merely notional ones—selling to others whenever possible. Toyota's solution to the bilateral monopoly problem appears to work just fine (Womack, Jones, & Roos, 1990). In fact, with the exception of unbalanced transfer prices, none of the solutions to the bilateral monopoly problem noted here presumes vertical integration. All that is required is full access to cost and production information (Milgrom & Roberts, 1992). Of course, all of these solutions to the transfer pricing/organizational design are potentially available to government organizations. Indeed, many of them were pioneered by federal acquisitions personnel or imposed by public utility commissions. They are not, however, widely understood or appreciated by public administrators and financial managers.

RESPONSIBILITY BUDGETING IN GOVERNMENT

The origins of responsibility budgeting and accounting in government can be traced to the Planning, Programming, and Budgeting System (PPBS) era in the U.S. Department of Defense (1961–1967). Responsibility budgeting and accounting was the centerpiece of Project Prime, perhaps the most promising of the organizational design and development efforts initiated under Secretary of Defense Robert McNamara. Project Prime was the brainchild of Robert N. Anthony, who succeeded Charles Hitch as defense controller in September 1965. Anthony saw the need for clarification of the purpose of each of the administrative units that comprised the Department of Defense, their boundaries, and their relationships to each other, and for an account structure that would tie the entire organization together. DOD Comptroller Robert Anthony proposed that the Department of Defense:

1. Classify all administrative units as either mission or support centers;
2. Charge all costs accrued by support centers—including charges for the use of capital assets and inventory depletion—to the mission centers they serve;
3. Fund mission centers to cover their expected expenses—including support center charges;
4. Establish working capital funds to provide short-term financing for support units; and
5. Establish a capital asset fund to provide long-term financing of capital assets and to encourage efficient management of their acquisition, use, and disposition (Thompson and Jones, 1994, p. 128).

The principal formal device by which a measure of intraorganizational decentralization was and is accomplished within the Department of Defense is the revolving fund. These funds involve buyer-seller arrangements internal to the Department of Defense. They have actually been in use for some time. The Navy had a revolving fund as early as 1878. Modern-day revolving funds date to the 1947 National Security Act, which authorized the defense secretary to use them to manage support activities within the Department of Defense. Two kinds of funds were established under this authority: stock and industrial funds (since replaced by Working Capital Funds). Stock funds were used to purchase supplies in bulk from commercial sources and hold them in inventory until they are supplied to the customer—usually a military unit or facility. Industrial funds were used to purchase industrial or commercial services (e.g., depot maintenance, transportation, etc.) from production units within the Department of Defense. Both kinds of funds were supposed to be financed by reimbursements from customers' appropriations.

Anthony's proposal would have expanded the scope of this device and enhanced its effectiveness by establishing rules for setting transfer prices prospectively rather than retrospectively and by making support center managers responsible for meeting explicit financial targets. Internal buyer-seller arrangements encourage efficient choice on the part of support centers, as well as the units that use their services, only if prices are set ahead of time and support centers charge all of their costs against revenues earned delivering services. Furthermore, their managers must be fully authorized to incur expenses to deliver services, and held responsible for meeting the stated financial goals of their centers (Bailey, 1967, p. 343).

Project Prime was not implemented as Anthony designed it. One reason for its failure is that the U.S. federal government accounts for purchases, outlays, and obligations, but it still does not account for consumption.[4] Full value from the application of responsibility budgeting can be obtained only where government adopts a meaningful form of consumption or accrual accounting (measuring the cost of the assets actually consumed producing goods or services). Because the U.S. government does not account for resource consumption, its cost figures are necessarily statistical in nature (i.e., they are not tied to its basic debit and credit bookkeeping/accounting records). Without the discipline that debit and credit provides, these figures are likely to be satisfactory only for illustrative purposes or where a decision maker must make a specific decision and a cost model has been tailored to the decision maker's needs. Another reason for the failure of Project Prime is that U.S. appropriations process does not perform the capital budgeting function satisfactorily, a problem that PPBS did not really address and certainly did not fix. Besides which, the existing process procrusteanizes every operating cycle to fit the fiscal year.[5]

Responsibility budgeting next surfaced in the United Kingdom, as part of the Thatcher government's Financial Management Initiative, announced May 17, 1982 (Lapsley, 1994). The Financial Management Initiative called for a radical change in the internal structure and operations of government agencies. Objectives were to be assigned to responsibility centers. Costs were to be systematically identified. They were to be measured on an accrual basis (i.e., matching resources consumed to services delivered) and include not only the direct costs of service delivery but overheads as well. This identification enabled those responsible for meeting particular objectives to be held accountable for the cost of the resources they were consuming.

The scope of responsibility accounting and budgeting in the UK was further extended in 1988 by the Thatcher government's Next Steps Initiative. In the last eight years, much of the British civil service has been reorganized into a set of executive agencies that have been given considerable administrative and fiscal flexibility and expected to meet annual financial performance targets. The heads of these executive agencies are no longer career civil servants. They are recruited from either the private sector (about 25%) or public sector, hired on short term contracts, with pay and tenure contingent on their success in meeting annual performance targets. By April 1996, there were 125 executive agencies in the UK, with 37 more candidates under consideration, covering about 75% of the British civil service.

Following the launch of the Financial Management Initiative in Great Britain, other governments—Australia, Canada, Denmark, Finland, and Sweden—have adopted responsibility budgeting and accounting. None, however, has moved as far or as fast as New Zealand. Moreover, New Zealand's reformers explicitly recognized their debt to agency theory.

New Zealand

Most of the external attention given to New Zealand's public management reforms has focused on its efforts to improve transparency: the adoption of accrual accounting and reporting on performance. New Zealand was the first country to publish a full set of standard financial statements, including a balance sheet of assets and liabilities and an accrual based operating statement of income and expenses. However, the changes made in the structure of the government of New Zealand designed to promote effective resource use and investment are even more significant than are the changes in financial reporting. First of all, New Zealand's Parliament privatized everything that was not part of the core public sector. The residual core public sector now includes a mix of policy and regulatory and operational functions and the military services, policing and justice services, social services such as health, education, and the administration of benefit payments, research and development, property assessment, and some other financial services.

Second, Parliament redefined the relationship between it and the heads of government agencies. Agency heads lost their permanent tenure and are now known generically as "chief executives." They are appointed for fixed terms of up to five years, with the possibility of reappointment. Each works to a specific contract, the conditions of which are negotiated with the State Services Commission and approved by the Prime Minister. The State Services Commission also monitors and assesses executive performance. Remuneration levels are directly tied to performance assessment.

Third, Parliament changed the way it appropriates funds for use by the remaining government agencies to link appropriations to performance, allowing Parliament fiscal control, but, at the same time, providing greater fiscal flexibility for agency heads. The basis of appropriation depends on the agency's ability to supply adequate information about its performance. Three modes of appropriation are possible, recognizing that some agencies provide goods and services that are more commercial or contestable than do others.

All agencies started out in Mode A, but most have progressed either to Mode B or C. Under Mode A, agencies were discretionary expense centers and Parliament appropriated funds for the purchase of resources. Indeed, the only change from the budget process in effect before 1989 (or, for that matter, the budgets used by most governments throughout the world) is that separate appropriations were provided for expenditures for plant and equipment. This mode remained in force until the agency developed a satisfactory accrual accounting system and identified its outputs, both of which are needed for performance assessment.

Under Mode B, most agencies are quasi-profit centers. This mode is designed for agencies that supply traditional, noncontestable, governmental services: the central control agencies, including the State Services Commission, most regulatory and police functions, and some justice services, i.e., policy agencies and activities that include an element of compulsion for the buyer. Under this mode, Parliament appropriates funds retrospectively to reimburse agencies for expenses incurred in producing outputs during the period covered by the contract, whether for the government or third parties. Costs are measured on an accrual basis; they include depreciation, but exclude taxes and the return on funds employed. Changes in an agency's net asset holdings are also explicitly appropriated.

Under Mode C, agencies are investment centers. Appropriations pay for the outputs produced by the agency and for any changes in the agency's net assets. Agencies in Mode C are required to pay interest, taxes, and dividends and must establish a capital structure. Mode C agencies are set up in a competitively neutral manner so that their EVAs can be assessed by comparison with firms in the private sector. The prices paid for the outputs supplied by Mode C agencies are supposed to approximate fair market prices. In general, this means that agencies must show that they are receiving no more than the next best alternative supplier would receive for providing the outputs. Mode C agencies are not permitted to borrow on their own behalf or to invest outside their own areas of operation. Each month, each agency reports on its financial position and cash flow and resource usage and revenue by output. Variances are calculated and explanations provided. Under Mode B, managers are free to make some decisions about investments in plant and equipment; they may make even more decisions under C. The fact that their financial performance is one of the main bases upon which managerial performance is assessed helps insure that those decisions will be sound.

Government's key decisions remain firmly in the hands of Parliament. The decisions that have the most significant future consequences for the government of New Zealand's stakeholders are clearly those that have to do with the kind, quantity, and quality of service provided by the citizenry. Under the existing system of appropriations and financial reporting, those issues must be explicitly confronted when cabinet enters into long term contracts with agencies, state owned enterprises, and firms to deliver service outputs and its consequent liabilities must be stated in present value terms.

The United States

Responsibility budgeting and accounting was adumbrated in the United States and influenced the now defunct Defense Management Report Initiatives of the Bush/Cheney era in the Department of Defense, and arguably the content of both the Chief Financial Officers Act and the National Performance Review's calls for mission-driven, results-oriented budgets and, more recently, performance based organizations (OECD, 1995, p. 230). Still, thus far it has had little practical effect in this country.

There are two explanations for this fact. The first is that many students of the expenditure process reject the notion that remote control can be reconciled with the American legislative budgetary process. Some people even assert that it can be practiced only by responsible unitary governments on the Westminster model, although that claim is belied by the Swiss and Swedish examples (Schedler, 1995) and various state (Barzelay, 1994) and local governments here in the United States (Kaplan, 1991). It would not be easy to reconcile responsibility budgeting with the U.S. legislative process, but we do not believe that they are necessarily incompatible. A second possible explanation for its failure to leave its mark on government accounting and budget practices in the United States is that, unlike most other countries, the United States has large, well-organized corps of government accountants, auditors, budgeters, program analysts, and teachers of government accounting and budgeting. All of these groups have vested interests in differentiating public from private practice, because that difference gives value to their expertise. A third reason seems to be that many people, in and outside of government, evidently believe that "public" necessarily implies Prussian-style bureaucracy. Where the purpose of the organization in question or the technology available to it make Prussian-style bureaucracy inappropriate, they will hear of no alternative short of full-scale privatization.

In the Clinton Administration's second-term, government reform efforts attempted to advance the concept of performance-based organizations (PBOs) modeled after Britain's Financial Management Initiative. The main theme of this reform effort is the use of contracts to hold PBOs accountable for financial performance. The progress of this effort was glacial. When legislation for the first PBO candidate, the Patent and Trademark Office, was sent to Congress, it aroused an intense debate between the administration and the chair of the House Judiciary subcommittee on courts and intellectual property regarding the relative merits of the PBO model versus a corporate model. This debate has been reproduced in various venues for successive PBO candidates.

FLEXIBILITY CHASING THE TAIL OF CONTROL

It is somewhat ironic that governments are beginning to embrace what may be termed "remote control" at the same time many well-managed businesses are abandoning it. These businesses have abandoned remote control because they are no longer compartmentalized the way they once were and it simply doesn't reflect the way they are now put together (Bruggeman, 1995; Otley, 1994; Bunce, Fraser, & Woodcock, 1995). Arguably, decompartmentalization is being driven by the information revolution, which is breaking down economies of scale and scope built upon functional specialization (Reschenthaler & Thompson, 1996). According to Michael Hammer, modern data bases, expert systems, and telecommunications networks provide many, if not all, of the benefits that once made internal specialization of administrative functions like personnel, finance, accounting, etc. attractive (Hammer, 1990, pp. 108–112). To the extent that the provision of these services requires specialized skills, they are increasingly contracted out to specialist firms. The people in the organization who actually do its real work perform the rest.

Hammer claims that jobs should be designed around an objective or outcome instead of a single function; that functional specialization and sequential execution are inherently inimical to expeditious processing; that those who use the output of activity should perform the activity and the people who produce information should process it, since they have the greatest need for information and the greatest interest in its accuracy; that information should be captured once and at the source; that parallel activities should be coordinated during their performance, not after they are completed; and last, that the people who do the work should be responsible for decision making and control built into job designs (Hammer, 1990).

Decompartmentalization has led to smaller, flatter organizations, organized around a set of generic value-creating processes and specific competencies. Some single-mission organizations are now organized as virtual networks, some multi-mission organizations as alliances of networks. Evans and Wurster refer to both of these kinds of organizational arrangements as hyperarchies, after the hyperlinks of the World Wide Web (Evans & Wurster, 1997, p. 75). Evans and Wurster assert that these kinds of organizations, like the Internet itself, the architectures of object-oriented software programming, and packet switching in telecommunications, have eliminated the need to channel information, thereby eliminating the tradeoff between information bandwidth (richness) and connectivity (reach). Evans and Wurster describe virtual networks (structures designed around fluid, team-based collaboration within the organization) as deconstructed value chains, and alliances of networks (the pattern of "amorphous and permeable corporate boundaries characteristic of companies in the Silicon Valley") as deconstructed supply chains, in which "everyone communicates richly with everyone else on the basis of shared standards."

The system used by IBM at its plant in Dallas, Texas, is an example of an existing virtual network. It has been designed to mimic a market-like, self-organizing system. Everyone in the organization plays the part of customer or provider, depending on the transaction, and the entire plant has been transformed into a network of dyads and exchanges. Each exchange is a closed loop involving four distinct steps: request from a customer and offer from a provider, negotiation of the task to be performed and the definition of success, performance, and customer acceptance. Until this last step is completed, the task remains unfinished. Each closed loop of workflow is further broken down into subloops. Under this system, even simple tasks give rise to dozens of loops and interconnecting lines; more complex tasks, such as modifying a major product, to hundreds; and managing the entire Austin plant to thousands. IBM uses powerful computers to keep track of all of these loops and lines, to chart all activities and operational flows within the plant, to keep track of progress being made at each stage of each transaction, and to prod tardy participants into action—this is control built into job design with a vengeance.

The effect of this system has been to break down departmental boundaries, eliminate bottlenecks, and to empower employees to take initiatives and coordinate themselves. As a by-product, the computer systems that keep track of all these loops and lines also identify the resources going into a particular job, almost entirely eliminating the need for cost allocation. Moreover, this information is available both prospectively and retrospectively to anyone in the organization.

Some well-managed multi-mission organizations such as Johnson & Johnson, 3M, and Rubbermaid have already organized themselves into loose alliances of networks, sharing only their top management, a set of core competencies, and a common culture (Quinn, 1992). The control systems used by these organizations are like those of centralized bureaucracies in that they collect a lot of real-time information on every aspect of operations, including nonfinancial information, but unlike the control systems of stove-piped centralized bureaucracies, which were erected on the premise that the exercise of judgment should be passed up the managerial ranks, this information is used to push the exercise of judgment down into the organization, to wherever it is needed, at the point of sale, at delivery, or in production (Simons, 1995). From top management's perspective, the primary purpose of this information is to provide them with insight into the integrity, competence, and morale of their network managers and employees so that they can allocate their best people to the most important jobs.

How far hyperarchy will go is an open question. Evans and Wuster (1997) claim that it will destroy all hierarchies, whether of logic or of power, "with the possibility (or the threat) of random access and information symmetry." If hyperarchy is where we are all heading, responsibility budgeting and accounting is at best an intermediate stage. It is now apparent, as it really was not before, that responsibility budgeting restricts the upward flow of operating information within organizations—making decentralization a necessity as well as an ideal. In contrast, networks and alliances are information rich environments. For the most part, access to information is symmetrical in fully networked organizations—equally available to all the people in the organization.

Why not skip the intermediate stages and go directly to networked organizations? It has been suggested that some governments might be moving in that direction, with the trend toward performance efforts and accomplishments reporting and the widespread acquisition of so-called enterprise resource planning (ERP) systems built around common data structures and centralized information warehouses, which permit data to be entered and accessed from anywhere in the organization (SAP, PeopleSoft, Oracle, etc.). Robert Kaplan (1991) argues, however, that organizations that try to move directly to a system where everyone communicates richly with everyone else on the basis of shared standards, without passing through a recommended period of experimentation with operational-feedback and cost-measurement systems, will almost surely fail.

We are less certain that this is the case. Nevertheless, we would point out that decentralization can work in an information-rich environment only where top management attends to top management functions—strategic planning, organizing, staffing, the intellectual and cultural development of the organization—and refrains from meddling in the conduct of operations. This takes self-restraint, and self-restraint must be learned. For that reason, it may make sense for governments to experiment with responsibility budgeting rather than going directly to new modes of organization and control. Few have had much experience with decentralization and almost none with self-restraint (Johansen, Jones, & Thompson, 1997).

CONCLUSIONS

In conclusion with respect to responsibility budgeting and accounting, it must be reiterated that the type of responsibility and control structures to be implemented in public organizations depends on what is appropriate given the operating environments and the customer-service strategy of each. The costs and benefits of alternative responsibility and control structures and budgeting and accounting methods must be thoroughly evaluated to make these choices. Where the organization's administrative and control structures are not aligned with its strategy, performance will be sacrificed.

A comprehensive understanding of the appropriate application of budgeting and management control techniques is necessary to implement realignment. In our view, the employment of responsibility budgeting and accounting is a significant step forward in this regard for most public sector organizations. However, as noted, there are alternatives to this approach, and risks associate with its implementation. Marginal applications will inevitably be preferred to more comprehensive efforts. As with any reform, public sector decision makers are challenged to embrace comprehensive rather than marginal reform if they want more responsive, transparent and results-oriented government.

NOTES

1.   This is a very important practical point. In the US federal government revolving fund agencies are prohibited from earning a "profit." Instead, they are generally directed to operate on a breakeven basis. The motivational effect of this maximand is to cause their actual costs to exceed standard cost in the majority of instances. In contrast, if they were directed to maximize "profit" and, assuming that they continued to base per-unit user charges on historical fully distributed average costs, the effect would be to encourage them to save budget authority for their internal customers and dollars for the U.S. Treasury. It might also have the effect of ratcheting their unit costs down, instead of permitting them to creep gradually up as is now typically the case. Clearly, the breakeven policy does not make sense and probably reflects the failure to understand the simple point that selling to and buying from outsiders are the only activities that can generate real profits or losses for the organization. Interestingly, many revolving fund agencies are permitted to earn a profit for their parent organization when they sell outside the organization.

2.   These are in fact currently revolving-fund operations; they tend to be treated like revenue centers, except when they "lose money," which is often the case.

3.   When factors enter into joint production, they typically develop a degree of specificity with respect to each other. Specificity gives rise to a Williamsonian "Fundamental Transformation" from an ex ante competitive relationship to an ex post bilateral monopoly (see Milgrom & Roberts, 1992; Williamson, 1985).

4.   OMB's Justine Rodriguez (1996) would fix this problem by creating a new set of accounts along the lines of the fund accounting systems used by nonprofit schools and hospitals. For example, each department could have one or more *capital asset acquisition accounts*. Outlays to acquire capital assets would be charged to these accounts, which would hold assets, but perform no operations. These accounts would also be permitted to borrow from Treasury to acquire assets. The assets they held would be rented/leased to programs, so each program account would show the cost of using assets, but this rent would net out of department totals because of offsetting collections to capital acquisition accounts. In cases where large inventories were acquired, they could be held by intragovernmental support revolving funds (e.g., franchise or working capital accounts) and "sold" just-in-time to programs. Employee pension funds already receive accrual payments from departments. Retiree health benefits could be treated the same way. Similarly, Rodriquez argues that we could require clean-up liabilities be paid to an account that would finance future environmental restoration. To connect resources with

results, program budget accounts would be aligned with programs providing goods, services, and transfers to the public. Support budget accounts (e.g., for personnel, legal, and computer services) would be financed by intragovernmental support revolving funds. Under this system, nearly all resources, except perhaps those to the agency head for policy coordination, would go to programs, which would buy their support competitively from their own department, from other departments, or from the private sector. Program outlays would then approximate program costs and could then be fairly related to program outputs.

5. GPRA and the CFO Act, when successfully implemented, would fix two of these problems (Jones and McCaffery, 1998). The third would require changes in budget law and executive orders (see Thompson, 1994).

CHAPTER XI

BUDGETING FOR PERFORMANCE

INTRODUCTION

Performance budgets emphasize activities performed and their costs and include various performance measures in the budget to document what is gained from what is spent. These measures usually include unit cost comparisons over time or between jurisdictions. Performance budgeting tends to emphasize measures of efficiency and effectiveness. Broader measures (outcomes) are often difficult to define and measure, particularly in human service functions. Nonetheless performance budget concepts have proven persistent.

General acceptance of the concepts of performance budgeting may be dated from the recommendations of the Commission on Organization of the Executive Branch of the Government (commonly called the Hoover Commission) in 1949. Among other recommendations, the Commission recommended that "...a budget based on functions, activities, and projects, called a 'performance budget,' be adopted..." (Hoover Commission, 1949, p. 8). The Commission observed that if the federal budget were prepared on a performance basis, focusing attention on the amount of work to be achieved, and the cost of this work, Congressional action and executive direction of the scope and magnitude of different federal activities could then be appropriately emphasized and compared in the resource allocation process. Additionally, the costs and achievements of the federal government would be furnished to the Congress and the people.

Performance budgeting was initially mandated by amendments to the National Security Act in 1949. These amendments required the Department of Defense to install performance budgeting in the three military departments (63 Stat 412, 1949). The federal government as a whole entered into performance budgeting as a consequence of the Budget and Accounting Procedures Act of 1950. This act required the heads of each agency to support "budget justifications by information on performance and program cost by organizational unit" (64 Stat 946, 1950).

While the federal government was developing performance measures and moving toward performance budgeting, some state and local governments quickly adopted the concept. Early attempts included Detroit, MI, Kissimmee, FL, San Diego, CA, and various states including Oklahoma, California, and Maryland (Seckler-Hudson, 1953, pp. 5–9). The City of Los Angeles has provided a noteworthy case study of this era from 1952 to 1958.

In 1951, Los Angeles created the position of City Administrative Officer (CAO) and filled it with Samuel Leask, Jr. Just one year after his appointment, Leask had instituted a performance budget system throughout the city. The heart of the Los Angeles system was a performance contract. This contract was based on goals and targets developed in the budget process. The parties to this contract were the mayor, city council and the CAO, on the one hand, and department administrators on the other. These performance contracts were monitored by the CAO during budget execution to ensure goals were being achieved (Eghtedari, 1959, p. 83).

The contracts were based upon work programs that became the starting point from which questions about timing, size and nature of expenditures could be framed. Departmental appropriations were based on work programs and a government wide reporting system was used to compare units of work performed to man-hours expended in the budget execution process. This was the final check on actual versus proposed performance (Eghetdari, 1959, p. 83).

A study of this system conducted primarily in the Building, Safety, and Library Departments found that the performance approach resulted in a strengthening of the executive budget, program planning and central control of decisions going into the executive budget. Measurement of work in a governmental jurisdiction was found to be practical and feasible, with positive benefits gained from such measurements (Eghtedari, 1959, pp. 82–88). In this case perhaps the major finding of the study was in the value of creating and staffing the Office of City Administrative Officer (CAO). The study found that the CAO had "...improved the quality of program planning, had brought about a higher degree of coordination among the essentially independent departments than ever before existed, and has made some contribution to the overall efficiency of municipal operations" (Eghtedari, 1959). Additionally, the new budget process assisted in increased control for the city administrator by creating the performance contracts. Perhaps the most important result of the Los Angeles experiment was the proof that a performance style budget in a governmental agency was feasible and beneficial.

During this period, the United States was not alone in its recognition of the potential of performance budgeting. As various state and local governments continued to experiment with versions of performance budgeting, nearly fifty countries implemented various aspects of performance budgets in the 1960s. Among the leaders in this endeavor were Sweden, Britain, Canada, and France. Most attempts in foreign nations merely supplemented the traditional budget and were usually issued as separate documents (Axelrod, 1988, pp. 272–273). Meanwhile the performance budget experiment in DOD was integrated first into Program Budgeting and then the Planning-Programming-Budgeting System (PPBS).

PERFORMANCE BUDGETING

Performance budgeting requires an administrator to separate programs into the basic activities in which the agency engages, decide what performance measures best fit each activity and develop budget costs for each measure. The typical performance budget has narrative describing what the unit does, performance measures which indicate activities and trends, and a breakdown by typical budget category. Exhibit 1 is a typical, if mythical performance budget. A "pure" performance budget would consist of activity classifications, workload data, other measures of performance, unit costing data, and program goals. Other data typically found in budgets that are modeled after performance budgets consist of narratives discussing the activity or program, several years of data for comparisons, mission statements, and desired outcomes. It should be noted most budgets which are called performance budgets are not of the pure format. Exhibit 1 illustrates how a typical performance budget might appear.

Once programs have been separated into activities, measurements for performance must be generated for program evaluation. There are five generic performance measures used with performance budgeting. These include input, workload, efficiency ("doing the thing right"), effectiveness ("doing the right thing"), and impact or outcome measures. Input measures describe the resources, time, and personnel used for a program. They typically appear in the budget as dollars for salary and supporting expenses. They also might be presented as staff training hours and number of person years expended on an activity.

Workload measures are volumetric measures of what an agency does. Such items as number of audits done, returns filed, checks issued, number of arrests made, or miles of highway constructed are typical workload measures. Workload measures are the lowest form of performance measure-

EXHIBIT 1
A Typical Performance Budget Display

Narrative
This unit is responsible for evaluating, inspecting, and licensing potential widget makers. As a result of dedicated analytic efforts all our unit cost indicators have shown a decrease from last year to this year.

Activity and Performance Measures

		UNIT COST		
ACTIVITY	ITEMS	BUDGET	This Year	Last Year
Evaluating	800	$15,000	$18.75	$19.00
Inspecting	18,500	$40,400	$ 2.18	$2.30
Licensing	2,600	$16,475	$ 6.34	$6.50
Total		$71,875		

Budget Accounts

Personal Services	$57,500
Supporting Expenses	$14,375
Capital Outlay	0
Total	**$71,875**

ment. The trouble with workload measures is that there are a lot of them and they do not tell anyone very much without further analysis. While workload measures do describe the activities of a program, they do not define how well the program is accomplishing its mission. To do this, workload measures must be converted into measures of efficiency, effectiveness and outcome.

Efficiency measures take workload data and merge it with cost data to develop unit cost measures. Then efficiency can be gauged on such items as the cost per arrest made, the cost of issuing a check, or the cost of flying an aircraft per hour. Efficiency is a much better indicator of performance than simple workload data since it gives outputs a direct cost relationship. These costs per unit can then be compared over time or against other similar activities to gauge competitiveness or improvement. This is important since it allows administrators a simple way to keep track of complex programs. At higher levels, the legislature can track efficiency measures to keep costs down, and the public can be assured its taxes are being spent efficiently. Efficiency, however, does not necessarily indicate effectiveness.

Effectiveness measures are used to mark output conformance to specified characteristics. Such items as quality, timeliness, and customer satisfaction fall into this category. These measures require the manager to determine goals for the particular program activity and to identify who the customers are and what type of characteristics customers would want within the products or services delivered to them. Then effectiveness measures indicate how well the agency is satisfying these needs. Effectiveness measures are better than efficiency measures in that the primary focus of effectiveness is on the customers, whereas the primary focus of efficiency is the organization. If efficiency focuses on cost per unit, effectiveness measures tend to focus on rates of accomplishment, e.g., percent of satisfied clients or ratio of clients helped as opposed to ratio of clients seen. Effectiveness is associated with the quality of service and includes such things as responsiveness, timeliness, accessibility, availability, participation, safety, and client satisfaction. If efficiency measures are largely internal, effectiveness measures connect the operator to his clientele, the citizen to his government.

Outcome measures are the most difficult level of measure used in a performance budget system. These are measures of outcome, impact, or result. They attempt to capture performance based on achieving what the program wanted to do as a whole. Simply put, they ask if the program achieved the mission it set out to do from the start. Has the city become cleaner, the streets safer, students more knowledgeable and customers more satisfied? In the 1970s several cities took photographs of their city streets and used a standardized photograph rating scale to judge if their streets were actually getting cleaner as a result of sanitation efforts. This information could then be compared against historical data or against a rating for a different neighborhood. After all, it is possible to collect many more tons of trash and to have the unit cost drop, but have the city streets getting dirtier. The photo scale technique was meant to provide an outcome measure. As a practical matter, outcome measures have proved to be very difficult to develop and maintain. They tend to be particularly difficult in human service areas, like education or public safety, where global statements are easy, but precise measurement difficult. Additionally, in the budget process, even where measurement is easy, sometimes it is difficult for policymakers to decide how many dollars it will take to move up an increment or two on a rating scale and if it is worth it. This further assumes more clarity in cause and effect relationships than may be possible in the real world. Constructing and evaluating measures adds technical difficulty to the budget process which many participants view as complicated enough in terms of determination of cost and political preference.

Early versions of performance budgeting focused simply on measures of workload and efficiency. In other words, the indicators focused primarily on the agency itself and were primarily internal measures of what the agency did and what it cost. These were input and workload measures, like salary cost and tons of trash collected, with efficiency ratios developed to measure the change in cost of collecting a ton of trash from one year to the next. Recent attempts at performance budgeting include measures of effectiveness and outcomes or results and have a focus on the clients and customers of the agency, with some measures constructed to evaluate client or customer satisfaction or response time to customer demand. Whatever measures are used, they are compared between similar agencies or over several years to measure competitiveness or improvement.

This type of budget aims to assist managers in wisely spending such that maximum output is achieved with as little input as possible, with the focus shifting from objects of expenditure to program activities as the basis for budgeting. Therefore, instead of budgeting for salaries, utilities, and travel expense; the manager would base the budget upon the activities his unit performs and policy makers would judge which activities should be increased or decreased.

GPRA AND PERFORMANCE MEASUREMENT

On August 3, 1993 Congress passed P.L. 103-62, the Government Performance and Results Act of 1993 (GPRA). The purpose of the act was to shift the focus of government management from inputs to outputs and outcomes, from process to results, from compliance to performance, and from management control to managerial initiative.[1]

The significance of this Act is evident in the Office of Management and Budget's (OMB) FY96 Circular No. A-11 (Preparation and Submission of Budget Estimates). Under these guidelines, justification of programs and program funding now require the use of performance indicators and goals as set forth by the GPRA. In issuing Circular A-11 in 1994 to control the preparation of the FY96 budget, OMB reported:

> Without performance indicators, performance goals, or some other type of performance data, agency requests for significant funding to continue or increase an ongoing program are difficult to justify. (OMB, 1994)

For the FY 1996 Budget submission, OMB encouraged agencies to use output and outcome-based performance measures in the budget decision-making process and budget justification statements. These guidelines agree with the general provisions of the GPRA.

The apparent long-term goal for GPRA is to implement performance budgeting as a means of resource allocation for all federal agencies. Performance budget pilot projects were conducted for FY 1998 and FY 1999 under the auspices of GPRA. In the following section, we evaluate some of the outcomes from one of the early pilot projects undertaken in DOD.

In the Department of Defense seven units were selected as pilot projects. The units had to volunteer, be selected by the Secretary of Defense and then be approved by the Director, Office of Management and Budget (OMB, 1995). The pilots nominated and selected were the Defense Logistics Agency (DLA), Defense Commissary Agency (DeCA), Air Combat Command (ACC), Army Research Laboratory (ARL), Commander in Chief, U.S. Atlantic Fleet (CINCLANTFLT) Carrier Battle Group and the Department of the Army, U.S. Army Corps of Engineers Civil Works Operation.

Of the commands selected, two are major combatant commands, one is a research facility and the others can be classified as service oriented agencies. This diversification in types of commands was thought to be useful in discovering how different types of agencies respond to performance measurement and what types would have problems. Conventional wisdom is that it is easier for the service agencies than the research or operational commands to develop performance plans/reports. The difficulty with performance measurement in the research and operational cases lies in outcome measurement.

A comparative analysis of the first set of plans submitted by each agency was conducted. Table 1 is a synopsis of the analysis results. The first column indicates the command or agency engaged in the pilot project. The second column indicates the primary orientation of the command (i.e., is the pilot unit service-oriented, or operational, etc.?). The third and fourth columns show the level of resources used by the agency in the form of budget and personnel. Column five shows the total number of measures included within the pilots' first performance plans.

The last five columns of Table 1 represent the five types of performance measures as described earlier. They are arranged on a spectrum from least difficult to capture (input) to the most difficult (outcome). Indicated for each pilot is the percentage this measure takes of the total number of measures in its plan. (Percentages may not add up to 100% since they were rounded to the nearest whole percent.) For example, ARL has included six output measures in its FY95 plan. This makes up approximately 32% of the total measures in the plan.

Some rather interesting results can be gleaned from Table 1. First, a comparison of the agency size with the number of measures used might be useful. By far, the largest pilot as measured by resources used is DLA. It is approximately three times the size of the nearest pilot in both budget and personnel. Twenty-two measures for an agency this size does not seem unreasonable. However, DLA does not have the largest plan with regard to number of measures. ACC tops the list with thirty-two measures in all. The budget authority covered by these thirty-two measures is less than one-

Table 1. Pilot Performance Measure Comparison

Command Agency	Type	Budget	Employees	Total Measures	Input	Output	Efficiency	Effectiveness	Outcome
DLA	Service	$14.6 Billion	~58,000	22	0%	36%	27%	36%	0%
DeCA	Service	$5.9 Billion	~20,000	11	27%	27%	18%	27%	0%
ARL	Research	$570 Million	~3,600	19	52%	32%	5%	11%	0%
AAA	Service	$44 Million	~700	7	14%	14%	29%	43%	0%
Corp of Engineers	Service	$1.7 Billion	~14,000	6	0%	17%	17%	67%	0%
ACC	Operations	$120* Million	13,500*	32	19%	6%	22%	50%	3%
TOTAL/ AVG %	N/A	N/A	N/A	97	21%	22%	20%	37%	1%

Notes:

* These resources represent only those being applied to the pilot project air wings, not the entire commands available resources.
** CINCLANTFLT had not yet submitted a performance plan at the time of this analysis and thus is not included in Table 1.

Source: Wolfgang (1994).

tenth that of DLA's. ARL also has a large measure/resource ratio (which is simply the number of measures divided by the resources employed) as compared to DLA. With nineteen measures, just short of DLA's twenty-two, ARL is measuring the performance of resources with a value of about 5% of DLA's. In fact, DLA has the lowest measure to resource ratio of all the plans. Overall, the trend appears to be toward more, rather than fewer, numbers of performance measures in this group.

Another interesting result taken from Table 1 is how different types of agencies chose measures in the spectrum of those available. The service type commands tended to choose measures more evenly distributed across the entire spectrum of measures. This contrasts with the research and operational commands. The research command, ARL, included 84% of its measures in the input/output categories. The operational command shifted to the opposite end of the spectrum in that 72% of its measures were effectiveness and efficiency indicators. However, one exception to this generality was the Army Corps of Engineers, which used four of six measures of effectiveness. As seen by the bottom row of Table 1, the plans as a whole spread across the spectrum evenly. Input, output and efficiency measures all have about 20% of the total. Effectiveness measures are used approximately twice as often as the others. The one glaring exception is the lack of outcome measures provided. Despite the shortage of outcome measures, the plans consisted of almost 60% higher order measures (i.e., efficiency and effectiveness). The other problem with the measurement choices was the use of input measures about 20% of the time. Input measures are not required under GPRA, but they are easy to construct and do represent some measure of effort for a unit. Thus, they seem to offer an attractive starting point for performance measurement efforts.

An analysis of the pilot project plans uncovered some additional strengths and weaknesses. The strengths seemed to lie in goal linkage and target identification.

Goal Linkage. Several plans were able to directly relate performance measures with overall strategic goals. This is extremely important since the efficient and effective accomplishment of the primary goals of an organization is what the writers of GPRA desired. For example, DeCA arranged its plan such that the goal and measure were identified together; for example (DeCA, 1994, p. 5).

GOAL: MAXIMIZE CUSTOMER SATISFACTION
Objective: Improve customer service at the commissary level.
Performance Indicator: Customer Service Evaluation System (CSES).
Performance Goal: Annual increase in CSES.
Baseline: FY94-average CSES score is 86%.

This allows the administrator to identify the overall corporate goal to which the performance indicator is most closely associated.

Target/Goal Identification: A few agencies found ways to easily articulate the goals and targets for performance indicators. Providing baseline data and targets for the current and future years allows administrators to see trends in the program instead of raw current year workload numbers. This also provides a means for asking intelligent questions about the program's activities and the associated performance. Table 2 is an excerpt from the ARL FY95 plan that shows this arrangement (ARL, 1994, p. 24).

Table 2.   Goal Measure Example

Metric	*Actual FY93*	*Goal FY94*	*Actual FY94*	*Goal FY95*	*Long-term goal (5+ yr)*
Number of invention disclosures	166	100	84*	100	110

Note: * YTD as of 31 May 94.

As can be seen, ARL expected their workload for Invention Disclosures to decline from its FY93 level. The baseline shown in FY93 is considerably higher than the goals set for the next several years. Also indicated is the fact they have completed 84% of this year's goal eight months into the fiscal year. Reviewers might be stimulated to ask questions about this profile.

The plans seemed to have had two primary weaknesses:

1. *Measures Difficult to Capture:* Some plans included measures that would be inherently unmeasurable. These types of measures have goals that simply state "reduce," "minimize," or "develop" some aspect of a program. A prime example of this is the Army Corps of Engineers "Industry delay cost due to unscheduled closures" measurement. The goal associated with this measure is to *minimize* the cost to the navigation industry resulting from unscheduled lock closures (Corps of Engineers, 1994, p. 5). No targets or baseline data were provided beyond this. Several plans took this type of measure only one step farther in that they attached a numerical goal to the measure such as "increase by 10%." One such example comes from the FY95 DeCA plan. The performance indicator in question was the "DeCA regional work force diversity." The goal associated with the measure was to simply "get a 2% increase in categories that have an imbalance."

2. *Bulk:* Several plans were extremely large and discussed items not *directly* related to the performance measures contained in the plan. A couple of plans appeared to be overwhelming in size. The initial

DLA plan was one hundred and twenty pages long. Only forty of those pages dealt directly with the FY94 performance plan itself. The remainder of the plan was used to describe the thirty-plus strategic initiatives currently in progress at DLA. One of the major problems for the budget process has always been information overload and a system which adds even more information to the process risks confusing the decision process with an avalanche of data.

A Case Study: Adapting to the New Performance Measurement System

The Defense Logistics Agency was the first agency chosen within DOD to act as a pilot under the auspices of the GPRA, consequently by 1995 it had two years worth of experience with the new requirements. DLA is the logistics division of the DOD and provides material and logistical services to all the military services. Figure 1 presents the strategic mission statement, vision statement and goals as indicated by the DLA Corporate Plan. DLA began the pilot project on 22 October 1993 and had produced two annual reports on its performance measurement efforts by 1995.

DLA Mission: The Defense Logistics Agency is a combat support agency responsible for worldwide logistics support throughout the Department of Defense. The primary focus of the Agency is to support the warfighter in time of war and in peace, and to provide relief efforts during times of national emergency.

DLA Vision: To be the provider of choice, around the clock--around the world... providing the logistics readiness and enabling weapon systems acquisition at reduced cost... by leveraging our corporate resources against global logistics targets... and finding savings through teams, improved business practices, and technological breakthroughs.

DLA Strategic Goals:
- Put customers first
- Improve the process of delivering logistics support
- Empower employees to get results
- Meet customer readiness and weapon systems acquisition requirements at reduced cost

DLA Customer-Oriented Goals:
- Responsiveness   • Timeliness
- Quality   • Operating Efficiency
- Financial Performance   • Customer Satisfaction

Source: The DLA Corporate Plan (1994).

Figure 1.   DLA Mission and vision statements.

DLA's FY95 performance plan is arranged into three sections, one for each of its major business areas. Each section contains a description of the business area, the budget relationship, the associated performance indicators that apply to the area, and definitions of the various performance measures.

The most important parts of the plan are the performance measures. The GPRA requires that each agency "establish performance goals to define the level of performance to be achieved by a program activity" and "establish performance indicators to be used in measuring or assessing the relevant outputs, service levels, and outcomes of each program activity" (P.L. 103-62, 1993). These measures are provided in the annual performance plan. In order to comply with this requirement, DLA first had to identify the major activities in which it engages. Then it had to arrange these activities by major business area. The next step was to specify performance measures for each activity.

Table 3 presents a comparison of the performance measures contained in the first two DLA performance plans. Starting with the left-hand column, the two DLA plans are represented. The next column is the total number of measures used in the plan. The next five columns represent the percentage of each type of measure used in the plan.

Table 3.   DLA FY94–FY95 Comparison

DLA	Total	Input	Output	Efficiency	Effectiveness	Outcome
FY94	41*	17%	22%	29%	12%	20%
FY95	24	16%	16%	4%	13%	50%

There are three significant results that can be observed in Table 3. First, DLA has shifted from several lower order measures (input, output, efficiency) to more higher order measures in its second plan. The FY95 plan contains a majority of outcome measures. Simple input and output (workload) measures are of limited use; however, when comparing them to standards or costs they become much more useful for managers. This is an indication of DLA's desire to shift toward more customer-oriented type measures.

However, the second result gleaned from this table is the fact that DLA still uses about the same percentage of input measures. This testifies to the extreme difficulty in getting agencies to shift to a result-oriented mentality.

Lastly, DLA significantly reduced the number of measures they intended to use for performance measure reporting. Though many of the FY94 measures had not yet been established, DLA realized that this was going to be far too many measures for purposes of external reporting. Thus, many measures were dropped without ever having been officially included in the plans.

In May 2001, GAO reported on a survey of managers' views on managing for results. Managers from 28 agencies responded that at no more than 7 of the 28 agencies did 50% or more of managers say that they used performance measures "to a great or very great extent" for any of the five key management activities (setting program priorities, allocating resources, adopting or changing approaches, coordinating efforts with other organizations, setting individual job expectations). GAO called these results discouraging. On a more positive note, at 17 of the 28 agencies, 50% or more of the managers responded that they had output measures that tell how goods or services were produced. However, at only 8 agencies did 50% or more of the managers say that they had developed and were using outcome measures to a great or very great extent (GAO-01-592, May 2001, pp. 8, 9). While this may be discouraging, it is certainly no surprise, given the difficulty of the task. What it does re-enforce is the difficulty in establishing performance measures as cited in the pilot studies earlier.

ADVANTAGES AND DISADVANTAGES

Just as with any budget format, performance budgets have many advantages and disadvantages associated with them. Some advantages mentioned by participants in the pilot projects included improved planning, more effective administrative control, decentralized decision making, improved public relations from clearer program information, better focus on the activities of the organization, and provision of more precise quantitative measures, which if pertinent and feasible, are better than vague generalities. Some disadvantages were also noted. Performance budgeting is not equally applicable to all agencies. For example, an agency involved in basic research such as the Army Research Laboratory does not have workload data that is easily quantifiable.

Secondly, efficiency is not guaranteed by using unit cost data. Legislators and administrators can use a performance budget to identify problem areas or wasteful agencies, but this by itself does not increase efficiency. Third, it is very difficult to settle in on an appropriate set of measurements for workload, etc. In practice many indicators have proven to be inappropriate and an agency may have to go through several iterations before a good set of measures is found. Fourthly, the end product of many agencies is not measurable by any known means. Measures of effectiveness and outcome or impacts are extremely difficult to develop. Lastly, this type of budgeting may not be practicable for relatively small agencies. The staffing time and costs associated with monitoring several indicators year-round might inhibit smaller agencies from effectively using performance budgets.

This reincarnation of performance measurement has focused from the start on external relations. Every person interviewed in DLA identified customer satisfaction measures as a major strength of the new performance measurement system. Many also mentioned the value of having a shared sense of vision from the top to the bottom of the organization. These two points alone are significantly different from the performance measurement and budgeting efforts of the 1950s.

CONCLUSIONS

Practitioners involved in developing performance measurement budgeting may wish to consider the following advice:

1. *Agencies should first identify the primary activities in which they engage.* This in turn will help identify the measures of performance to be used in gauging these activities. As DLA did when it created its second plan, deciding upon the primary activities will help clarify just what measures to use.

2. *Agencies should keep the plans simple.* Several examples were given to show that simplicity seems to be the best way to approach GPRA performance plans. Large convoluted measures that would be difficult for an outside administrator to understand are not beneficial in gauging performance. Moreover, verbose explanations of future GPRA implementation plans or of items not directly related to the measures themselves add little value to the plans. The plans should state the mission and vision of the organizations. The measures, their targets, baseline data if available, and perhaps long-term goals as well should be identified. Definitions of the measures should be provided for clarity. Finally, a means for validating the measures as well as their relationship to the budget is also required by GPRA.

3. *Agencies should expect evolution.* Several aspects of performance planning will take considerable time to work out. As shown in DLA, subsequent performance plans created may not look anything like the initial one. DLA changed 66% of its performance measures in the first year alone after realizing the measures were not appropriate. Additionally, the sheer size of its plan was significantly reduced over the two years.

4. *Agencies should concentrate on measures of efficiency and effectiveness.* While outcome measures should be included if possible, efficiency and effectiveness measures are more attainable and should be used as much as possible. Simple measures of output are not nearly as useful as efficiency or effectiveness measures. Input measures are

not required by GPRA and usually are not of interest to outside stakeholders.

5. *Agencies should realize their measures may not be interpreted as expected.* Outcomes were by far the most difficult to capture. Few agencies could include true outcome measures in their plans. An outcome measure at one level could be an input measure at another level. Moreover, outcomes may not even be measurable on an annual basis. Some of these outcomes take years to achieve, depending on the orientation of the agency.

6. *Good accounting and performance measurement systems are required to implement GPRA in an efficient manner.*   DLA already had an Executive Information System in place when it volunteered to act as a pilot project. Agencies with good information systems in place have a significant advantage in developing performance measurement systems. Few agencies have good systems.

7. *Agencies should link together other reform initiatives where synergism is a possibility.*   GPRA fit rather neatly into other DOD reform initiatives in the 1990s, including Total Quality Leadership/Management and the National Performance Review. Most of the pilot projects used GPRA as a means to enhance initiatives already in progress in their organization. For example, the Army Corp of Engineers entered the pilot phase as an extension of its National Operation and Maintenance Program Plan of Improvement. The tools contained within TQL/M were thought to benefit managers as they attempted to create performance indicators and plans.

8. *Agencies should determine how the performance plans would be linked to resource allocation.*   Perhaps the most difficult item to complete in all of GPRA implementation will be to find how the measures can be used to allocate resources. DLA has started this process by creating a performance contract between its field activity managers and the corporate office. Whether this could occur on a federal or even DoD level is still subject to question. The primary stumbling block at the federal level is the object of expenditure base currently used in the federal budget process.

OMB has continued to press for performance information to the date of this writing in 2001. The Director's letters from the midyear review passed back to the agencies provided urgings for more performance information. President George W. Bush has articulated the importance of performance evaluation in public pronouncements. At this point, OMB does not appear to be moving toward a performance budgeting system, but it definitely is emphasizing performance information in the budget process. Some observers note that while many have embraced GPRA and the idea of performance measurement, others are treating it as a short-term phenomenon and waiting for it go away, as ZBB and MBO did, so as to allow them to get on with what they perceive as the "real" work of their agencies. Performance measurement and performance budgeting tie up a tremendous amount of staff time and energy. Unless decision makers are willing to use the information produced from performance measurement, staff and other observers of the process wonder whether the cost is worth the effort and benefit. This perception is magnified when performance measurement and evaluation are viewed as exclusively of interest to the Executive branch, while Congress appears to be ignoring to a great extent the results of the laws it passed. The extent to which this experiment with performance-based budget reform will succeed remains in doubt.

NOTE

1.   The following material is drawn from Wolfgang (1994) and McCaffery & Wolfgang (1998).

CHAPTER XII

BUDGETING, CONTRACTING, AND MANAGEMENT CONTROL

INTRODUCTION

Budget control is exerted by elected officials and other budget decision makers in government in an attempt to assure accountability with respect to the appropriate spending of taxpayer dollars. Management control also should be employed to motivate employees and to improve organizational attainment of objectives. Budgetary management controls are applied in both budget formulation and execution. In this chapter we differentiate between controls applied before and after the budget is approved for spending (appropriated and obligated in the terms used in the federal government) and between control system applications that affect choice with respect to the use of government agencies to provide services to the public versus supply by private contractors. Our focus is more on execution than budget formulation for reasons we explain. Finally, we suggest that, in some cases, as a result of inappropriate choice of control system design and inappropriate application of controls, budgets are simultaneously over-controlled and out-of-control. Inappropriate control system design and wrong-headed application of controls result in a number of organizational pathologies, some of which we document in this chapter.

Perhaps the most challenging task in budgeting is to execute budgets well so that the best program outcomes are achieved with some degree of efficiency and a genuine concern for the proper use of public funds. Budget execution skill is required to respond to inevitable contingencies that arise to complicate the implementation of programs in the manner planned and according to the promises made in budget formulation. Accountability must be maintained and at the same time uncertainty must be accommodated.

Budget execution typically is highly regulated to control what program managers may and may not do. Controllers are driven by the objective of insuring that budget appropriations in total and by legally segregated account are not overspent by programs (Anthony & Young, 1984, Chs. 7–9). However, controllers also must be concerned with under-execution. Department and agency budget officers and program managers do not want to under-spend and thereby lose claim to resources in the following fiscal year. Central executive budget office controllers do not want programs to execute without good cause. From their perspective, money not used in the manner justified in budget formulation or not needed to meet program requirements should be taken back from program managers and reallocated to better uses elsewhere in the organization. Executive controllers want to be able to withdraw funds from programs to protect the integrity of the appropriation process and to reallocate money to areas where it will be spent to achieve results more efficiently and, in theory, in better response to client demand. For these and other reasons, budget execution typically is monitored and controlled carefully both by agency budget staff and central executive budget controllers. Execution also is often monitored closely by legislative oversight committees and their staffs out of a desire to insure that legislative will is implemented faithfully, and also to make sure that benefits are distributed to the clients targeted in the appropriation process (Anthony & Young, 1984, p. 288). Because the electoral fortunes of legislators are tied to some degree to the public perception that they are solving the problems and meeting the demands of their constituents, legislators have considerable interest in budget execution control.

Among the techniques used to control budget execution, variance analysis is probably the most familiar. Controllers and budget officials in government program offices monitor the differences between projected and actual revenues and expenses in total and by account. They monitor revenue and expense rates against allotment controls by quarter, month, week, day—temporal control generally is required by the allotment process. Other variables monitored are purpose of expense relative to budget proposal and appropriation purpose, and location of revenues and expenses by unit and at times by geographical location. Close count is also kept on the number and type of personnel positions compared to the authorized complement in the budget. Monitoring of actual revenue and expense rates as well as program output and demand, where measurable, also is done to compare current spending to proposals made in the budget for the next year that is under negotiation at the same time as the fiscal year budget is expended. Comparisons are made to historical revenue and spending trends in some instances to better understand how current programs are performing. Budget execution monitoring and control is particularly important toward the end of the fiscal year for reasons stated above, to avoid both over- and under-expenditure relative to appropriation.

The purpose of the analysis of budget execution control provided in the following sections is to improve understanding of control dynamics, incentives, disincentives, and behavior of the various participants in the budget execution process. The analysis focuses most closely in this regard on the roles of the central executive budget office controller and the program manager. The other purpose served by this analysis is to ask whether there is cause to change the budget execution process as it operates in most public organizations and, if so, what directions change might take. The analysis delineates alternative types of control applied in executing budgets and the rationale for employing these different methods. A distinction is drawn between budget execution control intended to influence the behavior and performance of managers of government programs from controls applied to affect independent private sector firms that contract to deliver goods or services to the public on behalf of government. The central theme of this analysis is that budget execution control system design should fit the objectives of control and the nature of the entity to be controlled (Anthony & Young, 1984, p. 20).

BUDGET EXECUTION CONTROL CHOICES

Research in public finance has paid considerable attention to budget formulation, but has tended to ignore budget execution (Simon et al., 1954; Schick, 1964, 1982). The reasons for this oversight are understandable. Government budgets are formulated in public, and the issues debated during this stage of the public spending process are dramatic and crucial. On the other hand, budgets are executed in private, and the issues raised in their execution are often mundane. Because of this selective attention, both observers and participants in the public spending process understand program analysis far better than controllership. Consequently, the conduct of program analysis has come to be guided by a fairly coherent set of professional standards. There is agreement on what is good analysis and what is good accounting practice. Although the design and operation of control systems can profoundly influence governmental performance, budget execution controllership is not guided by a coherent set of professional standards. Legal strictures and sanctions exist for fraud, waste and misuse of funds, but they are not enough. By their very nature, they emphasize what not to do, not what to do. Without appropriate performance standards, budget officers cannot be held accountable for performance of this function. Consequently, control systems are not designed to optimize the quality, quantity, and price of goods and services purchased with public money, but "to facilitate the controller's [other] work" (Anthony & Young, 1984, p. 21).

The choice of whom to subject to controls and when to execute those controls is not as easy. The control system designer has at least four options. First, the subject may be either an organization or an individual. Second, controls may be executed before or after the subject acts. The former may be identified as ex ante and the latter as ex post controls (Demski & Feltham, 1967). Ex ante controls are intended to prevent subjects from doing wrong things or to compel them to perform well. Necessarily they take the form of authoritative commands or rules that specify what the subject must do, may do, and must not do. Subjects are held responsible for complying with these commands, and the controller attempts to monitor and enforce compliance. In contrast, ex post controls are executed after the subject decides on and carries out a course of action and after some of the consequences of the subject's decisions are known. Since bad decisions cannot be undone after they are carried out, ex post controls are intended to motivate subjects to make good decisions. Subjects are held responsible for the consequences of decisions, and the controller attempts to monitor consequences and rewards or sanctions accordingly. The control system designer may choose between four distinct design alternatives.

Figure 1 shows some of the variables that influence choice of alternative funding instruments relative to the nature of the product or service supplied as well as the type of controls associated with each method of funding. It contrasts government appropriation or variable type funding with contracting, by type of contract. Where no market exists, there is no advantage to contracting because there is no competitive dynamic to force efficiency in production or supply. Government funding depends in this circumstance on the nature of the product or service supplied. Where products or services are essentially the same, it is most appropriate to fund through appropriations because unit prices and units of products and services can be measured, and measured relatively well. Many of the routine requirements for service provision by government agencies fit into this category, e.g., internal supply of labor and consumables used to provide services. However, where products or services are moderately or highly differentiated, e.g., as with most services delivered by social welfare agencies, it is more appropriate and effective to fund on a variable basis. For example, where the amount of funding fits the demand function, welfare case load, might be funded through a revolving fund or with reimbursable funding. Also, for some accounts, government guarantees the function and pays whatever it costs. The federal government and state governments

Nature of Market and Competition > Type of Product or Service by Attributes (No Differentiation versus High Differentiation)	No Market— One Supplier	Competitive Market— Many Suppliers
Type of Product or Service Homogenous (e.g., identical product or service attributes)	*Less Risk* **Budget Appropriations (Lump-sum, e.g., congressional appropriations to departments and agencies)** **Ex Ante Controls**	*Less Risk* **Fixed Price Contracts (e.g., purchase of X goods for Y price)** **Ex Ante Controls**
Heterogeneous (e.g., differentiated product or service attributes)	**Variable budgets (Budgets based on consumption rates, e.g., revolving/reimbursable funds** **Ex Post Controls** *More Risk*	**Flexible Type Contracts (e.g., Cost-plus Incentive Type Contracts)** **Ex Post Controls** *More Risk*

Figure 1.   Funding, production choice and control alternatives.

often use such procedures to provide funding for small and odd functions (often termed "cats and dogs" by budgeteers).

However, where markets are present, the more efficient method of funding supply of products or services is through contract with the private, nonprofit sector or internally with another government agency. Here the choice between fixed versus flexible type of contract is determined, as for direct government funding, by the degree of differentiation of the product or service to be supplied. Where products or services are standardized, fixed price contracts are most efficient. However, in many cases, product or service attributes are highly differentiated and flexible price, incentive type contracting will be most effective and efficient.

Two other dimensions of this table are critical to understanding our model and the arguments presented in this chapter. Where appropriations and fixed price contracts are employed, the risk of funding product or service production is lower due to the standardized nature of products or services or the absence of market dynamics. Under these circumstances, ex ante controls are generally adequate to achieve management control objectives, given that such controls are applied in the correct manner (more about this in the following sections of the chapter). Alternatively, where risk is higher due to the combination of high product or service differentiation and market competition, ex post controls are necessary because they permit more effective after-the-fact economic and results-oriented evaluation of outcomes and provide opportunity for modification of the incentives of the product or service supplier by government contracting agents, where agents know how to do their jobs, what they want to purchase, and how to contract effectively to exploit the efficiency of markets.

Furthermore, as explained subsequently, choice of funding method involves designation of authority and responsibility for product or service provision decision making and accountability either to individuals or organizations and relates this assignment to the appropriate type of management control method: individual responsibility, ex ante or ex post, and organizational responsibility, ex ante or ex post.

PURPOSES OF EX POST CONTROLS

Ex post financial controls are used to reveal demand. They are executed after operating decisions have been made, after asset acquisition and use decisions have been carried out and output levels monitored. Their subject may be either a freestanding organization, such as a private contractor or a quasi-independent public entity, or an individual manager subordinate to the controller, such as a responsibility center or program manager within a government agency.

In the case of the free standing organization, the structure of authority and responsibility within the organization is assumed to be an internal matter. The controller establishes a price schedule and specifies minimum service quality standards or a process whereby these standards are to be determined. This price or cost schedule may entail all sorts of complex arrangements, including rate, volume and mix adjustments, and default penalties. Where one organization can optimally supply the entire market, the controller may grant it a monopoly franchise, for example, in garbage collection for a small town or neighborhood. The significant characteristic of this approach is that a unit price cost schedule remains in effect for a specified time period (Goldberg, 1976; Thompson, 1984; Thompson & Fiske, 1978). This means that the government's financial liability will depend on the quantity of service provided and not on the costs incurred by the organizations supplying the service.

Where this budget control system design is employed, for example, where a municipality purchases gasoline at the spot-market price or where states commit themselves to pay freestanding organizations such as a university a fixed price for performing a specific service such as enrolling students or treating heart attacks, or where the Air Force buys F-16s for a fixed price, the controller must rely upon interorganizational competition to provide sufficient incentives to service suppliers to produce efficiently and make wise asset acquisition and use decisions. If interorganizational competition is effective, those organizations that do not produce cost-effectively will not survive.

However, even where the declining marginal cost of the service in question makes monopoly appropriate, ex post controls can still be employed. This is done in businesses and businesslike public sector enterprise organizations by holding managers responsible for optimizing a single criterion value, subject to a set of constraints (Anthony & Young, 1984). The principal mechanism through which this control system design is employed at the Federal level is the revolving fund (Bailey, 1967). For example, the manager is given the authority to make spending decisions to acquire and use assets, subject to output quality and quantity constraints determined by clients and is held responsible for minimizing costs. Large private sector firms produce comprehensive operating reports describing the performance of responsibility centers and programs, but their budgets seldom are very detailed. The logic of ex post control is that the purpose of the budget is to establish performance targets that are high enough to elicit from the organization's managers their best efforts. Such budgets might contain only a single number for each responsibility center—an output quota, a unit-cost standard, a profit, or a return-on-investment target.

Under this approach to budget control, the structure of authority and responsibility within the organization is of interest to the financial controller. The effectiveness of this design depends on the elaboration of well-defined objectives, accurate and timely reporting of performance in terms of objectives, and careful matching of spending authority and responsibility. Its effectiveness also depends upon the clarity with which individual reward schedules are communicated to responsibility center managers and the degree of competition between alternative management teams. Finally, under this approach, the financial liability of government depends on the costs incurred in providing the service and not merely on the quantity or quality of the service provided.

EX ANTE CONTROL OBJECTIVES

In contrast to ex post budget controls, ex ante controls are demand-concealing. Their distinguishing attribute is that the controller retains the authority to make or exercise prior review of spending decisions. Ex ante financial controls are executed before public money is obligated or spent, and govern the service supplier's acquisition and use of assets. Examples of ex ante financial controls include object-of-expenditure appropriations, apportionments, targets, position controls, and fund and account controls that regulate spending by account and the kind of assets that can be acquired by governmental departments and agencies. Such controls also govern the behavior of private contracting entities that supply services to government or to clients on behalf of governments.

Execution of ex ante controls requires assessment of the consequences of asset acquisition decisions. This consideration may be implicit, as it is in the execution of the traditional line-item budget and basic research contracts, or explicit, as in the execution of performance and program budgets and systems development contracts. It is often influenced by information on current and past performance, but the consideration of the consequences of spending decisions is always prospective in nature.

The logic of ex ante control is that constraining managerial discretion is the first purpose of budget execution. Since the degree of constraint will depend upon the detail of the spending plan, as well as the degree of compliance enforced by the controllers, these budgets need to be highly detailed. A department or agency budget must identify all asset acquisitions to be executed during the fiscal year and make it clear who is responsible for implementation.

Under ex ante budget control, service-supplying organizations must be guaranteed an allotment of funds in return for continuously providing a service for a specified period. The service provider will assume some responsibility for managing output levels or delivery schedules, service quality, or price to the government customer. Government is directly responsible for all legitimate costs incurred in the delivery of services, regardless of the actual quantity or quality of the services provided.

EFFECTIVENESS OF EX ANTE CONTROLS

Where a manager seeking to increase his budget is subject to tight ex ante controls, the controller can enforce efficiency during the budget period by requiring affirmative answers to the following questions: (1) Will a proposed change permit the same activity to be carried out at a lower cost? (2) Will higher priority activities be carried out at the same cost? (3) Will proposed asset acquisitions or reallocations of savings support activities that have higher priority than those presently carried out? When operating managers are faced with these criteria, they respond appropriately. Controllers approve most changes in spending plans proposed by operating managers because only mutually advantageous changes will be proposed in most circumstances.

However, when line item or lump-sum appropriations have a comparative advantage, to say that ex ante controls are a necessary means of reinforcing the controllers' bargaining power should not imply that tight ex ante controls always must be administered by them. Under certain conditions, authority to spend money, transfer funds, fill positions, etc., may be delegated to subordinate managers. The threat of reimposition of ex ante controls will be sufficient to insure that the manager's behavior corresponds to the controllers' and elected officials' preferences. In order for such delegation to take place, the following conditions must be present: (1) reimposition of controls must be a credible threat; (2) the gain to the manager from delegation must more than offset the associated sacrifice in bargaining power, (the manager of an agency in the stable backwaters of public policy has little to gain from relief from ex ante controls if the price of such relief is a change in business as usual), and (3) controllers must be confident that their monitoring procedures, including post-audit, will identify violations of "trust."

BUDGET CONTROL SYSTEM DESIGN AND CONTRACTING DECISIONS

All long-term relationships with private contractors and government goods and service suppliers rely to some degree on ex ante controls. Even the operation of fixed-price contracts requires prior specification of product quality standards and delivery schedules. But flexible-price, cost-plus type contracts and appropriated budgets require considerably higher levels of reliance on ex ante controls and also on monitoring and enforcing compliance. And the cost of tightly held budget execution control is high.

At the very least, adoption of one of the budget execution control systems described herein means that controllers must take steps to ensure that suppliers fairly and accurately recognize, record, and report their expenses. This, in turn, requires careful definition of costs and specification of appropriate account structures, accounting practices and internal controls, direct costing procedures, and the criteria to be used in allocating overheads. Still, accurate accounting does not guarantee efficiency. Even where the service supplier's financial and operational accounts completely and accurately present every relevant fact about the decisions made by its managers, they will not provide a basis for evaluating the soundness of those decisions. This is because cost accounts can show only what happened, not what might have happened. They do not show the range of asset acquisition choices and tradeoffs the supplier considered, let alone those that should have been considered but were not.

Under line-item or lump-sum budgets and flexible-price contracts, asset acquisition decisions must be made by the contractor, but the contractor cannot be trusted completely to make them efficiently. Consequently, the contractor must be denied some discretion to make managerial decisions. The fundamental question is, how much must be denied? To what extent should government officials or their controller agents regulate, duplicate, or replace the contractor's managerial efforts?

This question must be addressed because oversight is costly both in terms of monitoring and reporting costs, and also because of the benefits sacrificed due to failure to exploit the contractor's managerial expertise. The controller and the government official will very seldom be more competent to make asset acquisition decisions than the contractor. The answer to this dilemma is that controllers and officials should do the minimum necessary, given the incentives faced by and the motivations of the contractor. However, at times, the minimum necessary is a great deal. This decision depends on circumstance and the controller's skill in exploiting the opportunities created by the contractors response to institutional constraints. In other words, all long-term relationships between government officials and contractors must rely on incentives, even those governed by lump-sum budgets and flexible-price contracts. The difference is that when these control system designs are employed, the incentives are deeply embedded in the process of budget/contract execution.

BUDGET MANAGEMENT CONTROL DYNAMICS IN THE "REAL WORLD"

Budget execution control should be matched to circumstances: increasing costs and homogeneous outputs imply one kind of design, while decreasing costs and heterogeneous outputs another. However, what we observe in practice is that this match is not always achieved. Controllers tend to rely on monopoly supply and ex ante controls (Draper & Pitsvada, 1981; Fisher, 1975; Pitsvada, 1983; Thompson & Zumeta, 1981). This combination cannot be appropriate for every service to which it is applied. Evidence can be marshaled to show that a variety of services might be performed satisfactorily by competing organizations, including in air traffic controls (Poole, 1982), custodial services and building maintenance (Bennett & DiLorenzo, 1983; Blankart, 1979), day-care centers (Bennett & DiLorenzo, 1983), electrical power generation (Bennett & DiLorenzo, 1983), fire protection services (Poole, 1976; Smith, 1983), forest management (Hanke, 1982), management of grazing lands (Hanke, 1983) hospitals and health care services (Hanke, 1985, pp. 106–107), housing (Weicker, 1980), postal services (Hanke, 1985, p. 108), prisons and correctional facilities (Hanke, 1985, pp.

108–109), property assessment (Poole, 1980), refuse collection (Bennett & Johnson, 1979; Savas, 1977), security services (Hanke, 1985, pp. 109–110), ship and aircraft maintenance (Bennett & DiLorenzo, 1983, p. 42; Bennett & Johnson, 1979), urban transit (Hanke, 1985, p. 110) and waste water treatment (Hanke, 1985, p. 110). Furthermore, even when controllers eschew monopoly supply, they frequently fail to fully exploit the benefits of competition. In New York City, for example, the municipal social services agency acquires childcare services for its clients from both public and private day-care centers. But public centers are subject to the full panoply of ex ante controls associated with line item appropriation budgets, and private centers to those associated with flexible-price contracts.

To cite another example, Department of Defense (DOD) policy restricts the use of flexible-price contracts to situations characterized by considerable procurement risk (e.g., R&D projects). In other contracts, the degree of incentive is supposed to be calibrated to the project's level of risk. The first ship in a multi-ship construction program is supposed to be constructed under a cost-plus-fixed-profit type of contract, while later editions, in theory, should be built under fixed-price contracts on the assumption that experience permits the contractor to manage to a narrower range of cost outcomes and to assume a greater share of the risk burden. It may be observed that while DOD generally makes the proper transition from cost-plus to award-fee contracts as it moves from design to prototype development, it may not make the transition to a fixed-price contract for downstream production. To be consistent with the logic advanced here, selection of defense system production suppliers should be reduced to a question of cost and price search. Acquisition should be based upon fixed-price contracts, awarded by competitive bidding. Where production volume is sufficient, DOD should try to maintain long-term contractual relations with two or more producers, as multi-sourcing permits price search at each renegotiation of the relationship between DOD and its suppliers. Nevertheless, winning a contract to develop a weapons system continues to be tantamount to winning subsequent production contracts in a high proportion of cases.

BUDGET CONTROL SYSTEM REFORM

Budget controllers often tend to subject government agencies and contractors to a wide array of ex ante controls, and they often hold them to tight output, quality, and service delivery schedules. However, they may employ performance targets that can be met most or all of the time. Such controls are not very ambitious.

What accounts for mismatches between how budgets are controlled in practice and the approach advanced here? One explanation is ignorance of consequences on the part of the controllers and elected officials. Also, some of the empirical data required to employ the control criteria outlined here are often unavailable. The most critical gap in this knowledge is how costs vary with output. Definitions and measurements of service outputs and activities also are often inadequate. Insufficient effort has been made to correct this situation in most public organizations. Of the two tasks, getting knowledge about the shape of cost functions is the more difficult. But if we first answer the question, "Cost to do what?" this knowledge can be derived deductively in a manner similar to the methods used in cost accounting and conventional price theory. Cost and supply analysis can yield highly useful information about marginal and average costs. Finally, experimentation with funding and output levels will increase our knowledge of service supply and cost functions (Cothran, 1981; Larkey, 1979; Wildavsky, 1975a).

The kind of information called for here requires a high level of analytical sophistication both in budget execution and system design, a skill that staff responsible for executing budgets may lack. Indeed, even if controllers had good information on cost and service supply functions, some might not know how to use it. Their experience tends to orient them to the administration of the traditional line-item, object-of-expenditure budget. Effective administration of a lump-sum or line-item appropriation requires no more than a modicum of arithmetical ability combined with a substantial amount of horse sense and bargaining savvy. However, matching control systems design to circumstances requires a practical understanding of applied microeconomics, and financial and managerial accounting. Controllers often fail to understand the ideas outlined here or how to implement alternatives to the line-item appropriations budget—where to exercise judgment and where to exercise specific decision rules. This is demonstrated by the persistent attempt of controllers to employ techniques devised for use within organizations, such as standard costs based on fully-distributed average historical costs, to establish per-unit prices for public organizations such as hospitals and universities.

CONCLUSIONS

Absence of knowledge of control system design options and objectives is not a satisfactory explanation for controller decisions to resist reform. Ignorance can be corrected, and incompetence may be weeded out. If a better match between control system design and circumstances would have a substantial payoff, why isn't this situation corrected? One answer regarding the implementation of reform is explained below.

A large part of the literature on budgeting in the United States is concerned with reform. The goals of the proposed reforms are couched in similar language—economy, efficiency, improvement, or just better budgeting. The President, the Congress and its committees, administrative agencies, even the citizenry are all to gain by some change. However, any effective change in budgetary relationships must necessarily alter the outcomes of the budgetary process. Otherwise, why bother? Far from being a neutral matter of "better budgeting," proposed reforms inevitably contain important implications for the political system, that is, the "who gets what" of governmental decisions (Wildavsky, 1961, pp. 183–190).

If the controllers and elected officials empowered to determine the methods used in executing budgets are rational, this quote implies that they have a strong interest in maintaining the status quo. To explain the persistent mismatch between budget execution control system designs and practice it is necessary to determine who benefits from the status quo and, therefore, who will oppose the adoption of a more appropriate type of control (Zimmerman, 1977). Members of Congress, state legislators, city council members, and any politician with a constituency worth cultivating would appear to lose as a result of reforms proposed. As the collective holders of the power of the purse, legislators clearly have the authority to order budgets to be executed in almost any way they like, including the power to delegate this authority to controllers.

Efficiency implies an exclusive concern with the supply of goods and services to the citizenry with some indifference as to the means used to supply the goods or even to the identity of the suppliers. However, legislators are frequently as concerned about where public money is spent and who gets it as they are with what it buys (Arnold, 1979; Ferejohn, 1974; Fiorina, 1977; Shepsle & Weingast, 1981). Line-item appropriations in general and object-of-expenditure budgets in particular are ideally suited to the satisfaction of legislative preferences with respect to how public money is spent, where it is spent, and who gets it. In addition, some types of contracts provide more political benefit than others despite the fact that options to contracts used would likely result in more efficient supply of services to the public.

CHAPTER XIII

A REVIEW OF RECENT FINANCIAL MANAGEMENT INITIATIVES

INTRODUCTION

This chapter provides a review of major financial laws, rules, and initiatives enacted in the federal government, concentrating on the period beginning around 1980. However, reference is made to measures that were initiated before this time where appropriate. Financial management involves managing the collection of all monies due a jurisdiction and managing the payment of all obligations incurred by that jurisdiction in a timely and accurate manner. It involves managing the systems that enable the jurisdiction to carry out its missions, including procurement, purchasing, personnel, property management, revenue collection, borrowing, and investment of cash balances and pension funds. It involves managing the accounting and budgeting systems so that the mission of the jurisdiction is performed in a manner that avoids fraud, waste and misuse of funds. It also involves management of information systems supporting these efforts in order to produce documents and reports that describe who paid how much for what and what revenues were collected. These documents must conform to generally accepted professional standards, must be understandable by the public and must stand the test of an external audit by disinterested parties. With these provisions in place, the collecting of taxes and the expenditure of funds on program and policy may be assumed to be carried out in an honest and expeditious manner.

In 1985, Charles Bowsher, Comptroller General of the United States (1985 to 1997) said that modern financial management must encompass planning/programming, budgeting, budget execution/accounting, and audit/evaluation. These phases were to be supported by a fully integrated system of data and information and closely linked in a continuous financial management process. Bowsher was critical of federal practices of the mid-1980s, noting that financial management had been practiced as a rather narrow function involving mainly accountants and budget analysts, leading to narrow and isolated analyses and reporting that did not enhance the quality of government decision making. Bowsher laid part of the blame for this state of affairs on the reactive nature of financial management:

> Every so often ... there is a realization that effectiveness in the public policy arena depends in large measure upon the quality of financial management information and procedures. Unfortunately, this realization does not always come soon enough, but rather in the aftermath of a crisis that serves to raise our awareness of the need for sound financial management. In short, we often practice reactive rather than proactive financial management. (Bowsher, 1985).

A local government example illustrates the range of consequences when financial management is neglected. By the middle of 1997, the city of Miami was floundering on the edge of fiscal catastrophe, running an annual deficit of 17.5% of its operating budget when any deficit at all was illegal. Deficits primarily occurred in recurring expenditures, meaning the city was overspending on its regular operations; capital expenditures were approved without knowing where the money was to come from; the city had no reserves, notwithstanding that some fund accounts were legally required to keep some funds in reserve; there was a consistent commingling of enterprise and general revenue funds and a commingling of bond money and general revenue funds; there was a continual underbudgeting of expenditures, interest and pension costs and an overestimating of revenues; some revenues that should have been collected were not; and from 1995 into 1997 payroll costs exceeded budgeted amounts. In 1996, three officials were charged with various forms of financial misconduct, including one member of the city commission, the city manager, and the director of finance. However, the problems continued; elections did not seem to cure the situation; warnings from auditors were ignored and it was difficult to separate corruption from "just plain wasteful behavior." Moreover, "nobody seemed to care very much" if the accounting system provided a correct picture of the city's finances. In fact, the city accounting system could not accurately report the city's fiscal condition and the city had to rely upon its banks to tell it how much money it had on a daily basis. In reaction to Miami's problems, the Governor of Florida appointed a financial emergencies oversight board chaired by the Lieutenant Governor to monitor the situation.[1]

Miami was certainly not the only governmental entity to run into financial difficulty in the 1990s, but when these problems occur the impartial observer is left in a state of amazement, not that difficulties occurred, but that they went on so long, got so bad, involved so many people, programs, and systems, and were not caught by some self-correcting mechanism, embedded in law and routine audit and evaluation stemming from good program and financial management practices. It seems that attention at all levels of government is seduced by the drama of budgeting and assumes that plans will just be automatically implemented correctly and honestly, notwithstanding two centuries of evidence in this country that it is not that easy.

HISTORY OF FINANCIAL MANAGEMENT IN THE FEDERAL GOVERNMENT

Getting financial management right is not a new problem. In 1802, President Thomas Jefferson wrote to his Secretary of Treasury:

> We might hope to see the finances of the Union as clear and intelligible as a merchant's book, so that every member of Congress and every man of any mind in the Union should be able to comprehend them ... I hope ... that by our honest and judicious reformations, we may be able ... to bring things back to that simple and intelligible system on which they should have been organized at first. (Dollenmayer, 1990, p. 2)

This was to be a forlorn hope, where the saving grace was that federal budgets were relatively small and governmental functions narrow, compared to their current shape. The Constitution has little to say about financial management, other than that no spending shall take place except for appropriation by Congress out of the Treasury. Charles McAndrew (1990) suggests that the first major law on financial management controls was the passage of the Dockery Act in 1894. This Act established and strengthened the centralized accounting functions of the government in the Treasury Department by creating a single Comptroller of the Treasury and replacing the several comptrollers then in existence. This simplified the settling of accounts and claims. The Dockery Act also required an annual combined statement of receipts and expenditures. Prior to this, legislation had been passed in 1870 prohibiting federal officials from making expenditures or incurring obligations in excess of available appropriations or in advance of new appropriations. Just as in budget reform, financial management reform played off of developments at other levels of government and in the private sector. The Progressive movement and the good government reforms of the early twentieth century led to local government reform. At the federal level this reform movement eventually resulted in the passage of the Budget and

Accounting Act of 1921, primarily as a result of deficits at the turn of the century and World War I debt. This Act is normally emphasized for its creation of a centralized executive budget procedure for the federal government, but it also created the General Accounting Office as an independent agency under a Comptroller General. McAndrew suggests the purpose of the law was to separate budgeting, accounting and auditing, and to establish an independent audit office as an arm of Congress.

Under the Economy Act of 1932, President Hoover issued an executive order prescribing the installation of accounting forms, systems and procedures, but it was the Budget and Accounting Procedures Act of 1950 which placed the responsibility for establishing and maintaining adequate systems of accounting and internal controls on the head of each executive agency (see McAndrew, 1990, p. 28). The Act required full disclosure of financial results, adequate information for the agency's management purposes, effective control over the accountability of all funds, reliable accounting results to serve as the basis for budget preparation and execution, and suitable integration of the agency accounting structures with those maintained by the Treasury. It required that executive agencies conform to principles, standards and requirements prescribed by the Comptroller General. It also required that the Director of the Bureau of the Budget, the Comptroller General, and the Secretary of the Treasury continuously improve the Federal government's accounting and financial systems. The result of this effort was the creation of the Joint Financial Management Improvement Program (JFMIP) which brought together the Director of the Bureau of the Budget (now the Office of Management and Budget), the Comptroller General of the United States, the Secretary of the Treasury and the Director of the Office of Personnel Management to better coordinate disparate federal management functions. The JFMIP is credited with improving federal accounting, auditing, budgeting, financial management training and education (see Staats, 1981, p. 44), and cash management, e.g., establishing letter of credit financing. As a result of the JFMIP efforts, federal auditing standards were set, Offices of Inspector Generals were established in federal departments and agencies, and accounting standards were evaluated.

The Budget and Accounting Procedures Act was amended in 1956 following the recommendations of the Second Hoover Commission. Perhaps it is best remembered for calling for cost-based budgeting for the Federal government and for including the GAO's agency accounting standards and principals developed from 1950–52. However, after 1956 it appears that GAO turned its attentions from helping executive agencies develop systems to approving systems agencies had designed. The principle embraced was that as specified by the 1950 Act, agencies should be responsible for designing the systems they needed for their purposes, subject to GAO review. In fact, GAO split this review process into three areas: approval of principals and standards, approval of system design and approval of systems in operation (see Steinhoff, Skelly, & Narang, 1990, p. 56). While this was a sensible approach to effecting change, it left the door open for standards and principals to get better while operating reality got worse.

In fact, by 1977, according to Steinhoff, Skelly, and Narang about 98% of the agencies had received approval of their statement of principals and standards with about 60% of the accounting systems being approved. By the end of 1982, 209 of the 332 systems had qualified for approval. However, the 123 unapproved accounting systems accounted for a large part of the government's expenditures, including those in defense, and health and social programs. Some of the unapproved systems could not estimate an approval date and, in addition, approval of a system design did not mean that system would be successfully implemented: sometimes implementation failed. Only with the passage of the Federal Managers' Financial Integrity Act of 1982 would these concerns by addressed. Much of the ferment about financial management reform has to do with the enormous expansion of the federal government role in the 1960s as the federal government addressed itself to a host of social problems. It is worth noting that in the 1980s the systems that were not approved either came from the new growth programs of the 1960s (social service and health) or from defense which was undergoing a rapid buildup in the early 1980s. At the same time a recession and a structural deficit policy left the Federal government with large annual deficits and a quadrupling of the national debt. These factors served to focus attention on fixing Federal financial management systems.

It is also worth noting that the passage of general revenue sharing from the Federal to state and local governments brought with it an increased awareness of good financial management through its emphasis on the independent audit. The 1976 amendments to the General Revenue Sharing Act required all recipients of $25,000 or more in annual revenue sharing to have an independent audit of their financial statements not less than every three years. This meant that all states and about 12,000 local governments were subject to these requirements. The negative side of this was that as Federal grants and aids increased from the 1960s on so did the requirements for audits, thus jurisdictions were subjected to multiple audits and auditors. By the early 1970s there were more than 500 Federal grant programs accompanied with administrative requirements that were "inconsistent, overlapping, contradictory and very burdensome to the grantees" (McAndrew, 1990, p. 35).

OMB circular A-102, issued in 1971, provided a consistent set of guidelines for grant management and reporting for state and local governments. This simplified the auditing and reporting burden of state and local governments and it also paved the way for the Uniform Single Audit Act of 1984. This Act simplified the audit requirement, since it enabled a single audit for all funds received, rather than audits for each grant. This was a step forward in efficiency. More importantly, it made all state and local governments liable for audit: jurisdictions receiving more than $100,000 had to be audited annually; jurisdictions receiving from $25,000 to $100,000 could choose to implement the single audit requirement or continue under the multiple audit profile; jurisdictions receiving less than $25,000 annually were exempt from the audit requirement, but had to maintain records in case a federal agency wished to audit their funds. Moreover the language of the single audit act stated that the audit was to determine and report, "…whether the entity has the internal control systems to provide reasonable assurance that it is managing federal financial assistance programs in compliance with applicable laws and regulations" (McAndrew, 1990, p. 36).[2] What this meant was that acceptance of more than $25,000 of Federal aid allowed the Federal government to pass judgment not only on the proper use of the money, but also on the adequacy of all financial management systems in the jurisdiction.

At the Federal level, the passage of the Inspector General Act of 1978, later amended in 1988, established the Office of Inspector General in departments and Federal agencies. Their charter was to conduct and supervise audits and investigations of executive departments and major independent agencies and provide a leadership role in promoting economy, efficiency and effectiveness and detecting and preventing fraud and abuse in programs and operations. IGs were also given the responsibility of seeing that audit work done by non-federal auditors (on state and local governments for example) complied with Federal audit standards as specified in OMB circular A-73 "Audit of Federal Operations and Programs" (McAndrew, 1990, p. 37). The Inspector General Act is generally considered to have been a landmark piece of legislation; in 1988, at the ten-year mark in its lifetime it was credited with more than $100 billion in savings and cost avoidance measures in federal agencies (Wolf Testimony, cited in McAndrew, 1990, p. 30).

However perhaps the most important piece of legislation on the Federal side in the 1980s was the Federal Manager's Financial Integrity Act of 1982 (FMFIA). FMFIA required each executive agency to make ongoing evaluations and reports on the adequacy of its system of internal accounting and administrative control and to identify weaknesses that could lead to fraud, waste and abuse. Annual reports to the President and to Congress were required. Passage of this Act was part of President's Management Improvement Program (Reform 88) decade long effort to modernize federal financial management, launched in September of 1982, against a backdrop of reports of wasteful spending, poor management, ineffective programs and losses involving billions of dollars. When President Reagan took office in 1981, he and his team found thousands of antiquated, duplicative management systems that could not provide even elementary government-wide management information to the President. Weaknesses in systems made outright fraud more feasible and inadequate, inaccurate, and archaic accounting systems made it difficult to tell the inadvertent from deliberate. While the Federal government had once been a leader in office automation in the early 1950s, it had long since fallen behind the private sector.

Throughout the 1980s, OMB and GAO worked to get the Federal government's financial management systems back on track; their efforts can be seen in a series of OMB circulars and GAO publications during this decade.[3] In his 1988 report on Management of the United States Government, President Reagan criticized the state of Federal financial management systems and outlined a comprehensive plan for modernization and improvement in federal financial management systems, focused on modern, effective accounting systems based on the Federal government's standard ledger system to provide uniform financial information and implement more timely, comprehensive financial reporting. By the end of the decade, serious, comprehensive efforts had been made to improve Federal financial management systems, by law, by OMB Circular, GAO Guidance, and with high-level, high visibility efforts like the Reform 88 initiative, the Grace and Packard Commissions, support from professional groups like the Association of Governmental Accountants, the American Association for Public Administration and the large professional accounting firms with public sector businesses and Presidential Councils on Integrity and Efficiency in Government (PCIE) and on Management Improvement (PCMI). Nonetheless after surveying this history, McAndrew would write in 1990 that, "...financial management remains a pathetic disaster in most federal departments and agencies" (McAndrew, 1990, p. 40). While audit, IG action, and FMFIA reports found many material weaknesses in systems, departments failed to take corrective action and major scandals continued to shake the faith of the public in the Federal government and its handling of money. The title of a 1989 GAO report is indicative of the situation "Financial Integrity Act: Inadequate Controls Result in Ineffective Federal Programs and Billions in Losses" (McAndrew, 1990, p. 40). It is against this background that the Chief Financial Officer's Act was enacted.

In the meantime on the budget side, the 1967 President's Commission on Budget Concepts led to the creation of the Unified Federal Budget in 1968 and important changes in the role of the Office of Management and Budget. The President's Commission also pressed for improvements in Federal receipts and outlay accounting and reporting. And, in 1974 perhaps the most significant single Federal budget reform since the Budget and Accounting Act of 1921 was enacted in the form of the Congressional

Budget and Impoundment Control Act, which reorganized the congressional budget process and established the Congressional Budget Office. However, other less visible efforts to improve Federal financial management have been undertaken. For example, the General Accounting Office (GAO) and Office of Management and Budget have worked over the past two decades to improve and standardize Federal accounting, auditing, reporting, and other financial management procedures.

The Debt Collection Act of 1982 strengthened the Federal government's ability to collect debts owed it. Better management of Federal credit programs became a goal of OMB in the mid-1980s with Circular A-129 Managing Federal Credit Programs. Since the late 1970s Congress had taken an active interest in the timeliness of government payments to vendors leading to passage of the Prompt Payment Act of 1982 which required the Federal government to pay bills within 30 days after receiving an invoice or receiving the goods or services, and prescribed penalties for late payment. In August of 1986, GAO estimated that agencies paid about 24% of their invoices late and about the same amount early (see Steinhoff et al., 1990, p. 51). Continuing effort has been made to improve bill payment. Purchasing procedures have also been improved. Here perhaps the biggest change occurred in DOD acquisition streamlining which involved introducing competitive bidding, decreasing the use of "military specifications" for products that did not need them (e.g., for paper clips as opposed to bombs) and using commercial buying practices rather than cumbersome government contracting practices. This is a long-term effort. By 1997, acquisition reform in pilot programs in DOD had yielded savings of up to 50% by virtually eliminating military specifications and relying on commercially available products. Estimates were that such practices would save DOD, and the taxpayers, about $10 billion annually by the year 2000. These practices were also good for companies that did business with the federal government. In 1996 McDonnell Douglas said acquisition reforms had saved the Federal government about $40 million and the company a similar amount, improving its shareholder value and allowing it to compete more effectively in the marketplace (*Defense Daily*, 1997, p. 408).

What can be seen from all of these efforts is the complexity of the problem and the inertia that a huge fiscal operation generates that has to be overcome. In 1981 Elmer Staats, then the Comptroller General of the United States commented:

> ...financial management is often very low on the list of priorities of many top governmental managers. Financial management deserves its fair share of their time and attention. (p. 54)

In 1985, Charles Bowsher, then the new Comptroller General, recommended a number of changes in Federal financial management, suggesting that,

> For too long "financial management" in the federal government has been seen or at least practiced as a rather narrow function involving mainly accountants and budget analysts. Somehow, the idea of bringing management issues and analyses to bear upon budgeting and accounting questions ... has not taken firm root throughout the [federal] government, in spite of some progress made in this direction over the last two decades. (Bowsher, 1985, p. 11)

Bowsher also cited the need for a more comprehensive and consistent budget and budgetary accounting, better data on Federal agency performance, improved planning for capital investment decision making, increased accountability for costs and results, and refined fund controls. Bowsher concluded, "Action along [these] ... lines would provide the federal government with the tools needed for practicing pro-active financial management ... this cannot be a short-term effort. Although policy makers should feel a sense of urgency about this ... they have to realize that a full implementation would span several years" (Bowsher, 1985, p. 11).

The development, passage, and implementation of the Chief Financial Officer's Act in the federal government underscore Bowsher's insight. The initial step in creating the CFO was made by the Executive branch. In July 1987, OMB director James C. Miller established administratively a Chief Financial Officer for the federal government in OMB (see Riso, 1988). However, efforts to pass a Federal financial management improvement act drafted in the House of Representatives (H.R. 449) during the 99th Congress to endorse Miller's action did not succeed. The chairman of the Senate Committee on Government Affairs also proposed in the same session a "Federal Management Reorganization and Cost Control Act" intended to "...correct the perceived void in financial management information, cash management and credit management practices" (Riso, 1988, p. 55) This legislation would have established an Office of Financial Management headed by a single Chief Financial Officer for the Federal government, defined controller functions in federal departments and agencies, and created the Federal Financial Management Council. However, this legislation also was not passed and neither was the bill (S.1529) sponsored by Senator John Glenn, chair of the Governmental Affairs Committee in the 100th Congress, titled the "Federal Financial Management Reform Act of 1987." Senator Glenn stated that his bill "...would finally make someone in the executive branch accountable for ... a government-wide system ... and financial management improvement plan..." (Glenn statement, cited in Riso, 1988, p. 56).

Despite failure to pass CFO legislation, a number of advances were made in the 1980s in federal financial management including increased compliance with selected provisions (Section 4) of the Federal Managers' Financial Integrity Act (FMFIA), creation of a schedule for adoption of standard general ledger accounting in federal agencies, consolidation of accounting systems, and adoption of uniform core requirements for federal financial systems (initiated by the JFMIP). However, the inability of Congress to pass enabling legislation hindered the effort to systematically improve federal government financial management. Additional attempts were made in Congress in 1988 and 1989 to develop support for comprehensive financial management reform legislation. However, it was not until mid-1990 that this law was enacted.

RECENT INITIATIVES TO IMPROVE FEDERAL FINANCIAL MANAGEMENT

The financial management activities of the Federal government are awesome in scope. OMB and the Treasury Department oversee spending annually an amount equal to one-fourth of the Gross National Product, and they manage a $2 trillion cash flow, $900 million in annual contract payments, a payroll and benefit systems for five million civilian and military personnel, and a budget with 1,962 separate accounts. Altogether, in 1988, the Federal government operated 253 separate financial management systems.[4]

This scope and complexity in financial management systems has created a multitude of problems, some of which have been recognized for some time. For example, OMB concluded that Federal financial management focused inordinately on budgeting to the neglect of other financial management systems. Wright says: "We found federal financial management focused on budgeting and neglectful of cash, credit, and financial management systems."[5] Before reform could take place, considerable groundwork had to be undertaken. For example, as early as 1981, OMB had identified the following problems:

- Failure to establish Federal credit policy for programs totaling more than $50 billion in direct and guaranteed loan portfolios. Total delinquent debt was computed by OMB at $30 billion in FY80 and was projected to grow at a rate of 43.6% annually.
- Absence of a government-wide cash management system. The government could not receive or make payment by electronic funds transfer and 30% of federal payments to firms were late, while 45% were made too early.

- A proliferation of financial management systems. Almost 400 financial systems were in use and many were antiquated, incompatible, and redundant.
- Insufficient awareness of the need for internal controls to prevent fraud, theft, diversion or misuse of funds and federal assets.
- Little connection between budget and accounting data existed and very little management information was available to measure the impact and benefits of spending.[6]

To combat these problems the Reagan Administration introduced Reform 88, a program intended to improve the financial integrity of government. Reform 88 and Congressional efforts in the 1980s led to a number of financial management improvements, including passage of the Prompt Payment and Debt Collection Acts, and improved accuracy of cash management position estimation. A 30-day bill-paying standard was established along with electronic funds transfer and direct deposit capability. Use of credit cards to pay for services provided to government was initiated. Further, 311 accounts in 50 agencies were converted to a nation-wide lockbox system. Annual cash flow through lockboxes increased to more than $26 billion by FY90. Additionally, electronic collection of funds owed the government through the Fedwire Deposit System exceeded $280 billion annually.[7]

Improved credit practices also were instituted, including use of credit reports to screen Federal loan applicants. Federal loan program collection performance was improved through the use of salary and tax refund offsets, private collection firms, and prosecution for delinquent debt by the Justice Department. More than $839 million was collected from the tax refund offset program in three years. Also, an OMB requirement that each Federal agency have a single, primary accounting system addressed the issue of duplicate and redundant systems, and aggressive efforts were made to convince smaller agencies to use systems at larger agencies.

Most of the initiatives noted above were begun in the Executive Branch after consultation with appropriate committees of Congress, the GAO, and department and agency representatives. Initial policy typically was announced by Executive order, OMB circular, or other directive based on Presidential authority. Congress followed up on these initiatives with oversight hearings, the most important of which were convened by the House Government Operations Committee and the Senate Government Affairs Committee. Meanwhile, Federal departments and agencies had an opportunity to experiment with alternative methods of implementation. Congress and the Executive branch evaluated these alternatives, often with the aid of GAO or agency Inspector General audits. A consensus emerged from this process of experimentation in the 1980s that CFO legislation was needed to better co-ordinate and direct financial management reform. However, the decade of the 1980s ended without agreement between Congress and the Executive Branch on the specifics of such legislation.

CONGRESSIONAL ACTION LEADING TO PASSAGE OF THE CFO ACT OF 1990

Testimony given before the Committee on Government Operations in the fall of 1988 focused on three problem areas for financial management reform legislation: management failures and inconsistencies, accounting systems and internal controls, and audited financial statements.

Management failures and inconsistencies. The Committee concluded that decision makers at all levels of the Federal government were not getting the financial information they needed to make policy and management decisions with sufficient knowledge of the ultimate financial impact of those decisions. Too many important decisions were made based on rudimentary cash flow projection and "check book balancing" with insufficient consideration given to the qualitative nature of expenditures and future costs and liabilities.[8] An inevitable outcome of excessive concentration on outlays and cash management was Executive and Congressional struggle over short-term budget targets and outlay rates.

Congressional testimony indicated that the financial decision making process was inhibited because financial management functions were split within the Executive branch between OMB, the Department of the Treasury, and the General Services Administration. Since these control agencies had overlapping responsibilities for oversight and direction of financial management operations, it had been difficult to sustain reform initiatives, despite repeated efforts to assume this responsibility by OMB. Congress concluded, as had the Executive, that a Chief Financial Officer of the United States was needed to provide centralized leadership for federal financial management.

Considerable debate ensued in Congress and within the Executive Branch over whether to locate the federal government's Chief Financial Officer in OMB or in the Department of the Treasury. The final decision favored OMB.

> Ultimately, the Committee decided OMB was the best location; as the management and budget power center for the Federal Government, it is better positioned to establish government-wide policies to achieve financial management reforms. Treasury, on the other hand, with its large staff at the Financial Management Service, was viewed as best suited to continue its operational support role for financial management efforts.[9]

Accounting Systems and internal controls.   As explained by OMB and cited in Government Operations hearings, "Once a leader in the early days of automation, the government's financial systems and operations have eroded to the point that they do not meet generally accepted accounting standards."[10] Congress concluded from testimony that the Federal government was managing today's financial challenges with yesterday's technology and that without modern accounting systems; financial managers could not perform their jobs well. Costs associated with servicing, upgrading and replacing antiquated systems were estimated in the billions of dollars. While accounting systems and internal controls had been strengthened somewhat, continued deficiencies still had serious consequences. For example,[11]

- In making multimillion-dollar program funding decisions, Congress had to rely on Selected Acquisition Reports that may not have provided an accurate or timely reflection of program costs and schedule variances for major weapons systems.
- Weaknesses in agency debt collection systems were significant and delinquencies in non-tax debt owed the Federal government grew by 167% from 1981 through FY87 to $32 billion.
- For 10 years DOD had not been able to account adequately to Congress and GAO for hundreds of millions of dollars of advances made by foreign customers for weapons system purchases.
- Financial audits routinely uncovered weak controls, which permitted, for example, more than $50 million in undetected fraudulent insurance claims at the Federal Crop Insurance Corporation, or excessive rate charging by the Rural Telephone Bank.
- In reports required by the Financial Integrity Act, 17 of 18 agencies disclosed significant weaknesses in financial management and associated areas.
- Between 1982 and 1988, DOD received about $55 billion more for anticipated inflation than was warranted by the inflation that subsequently occurred. According to the Department of Defense, for example, most of the inflation dividends were cut by Congress, spent on defense programs, or lapsed and returned to the Treasury. Since these funds had not been fully monitored and accounted for, the full disposition of inflation funds could not be determined by Congress.

The Committee on Government Affairs concluded that the absence of timely, relevant, and comprehensive financial information, and persistent internal control weaknesses compounded the difficulty of controlling government operations and costs. One approach presented in hearings suggested that the government adopt the same accounting principles employed by businesses and many governments—Generally Accepted Accounting Principles, or GAAP (see Mautz, 1991).

The Federal government employs a cash basis budgeting and accounting system to measure spending. It was argued that instituting GAAP rules would move the process toward capital budgeting and accrual accounting. GAAP had been developed to provide users of financial documents with improved understanding of financial data for reporting and decision making. "Most importantly, GAAP recognizes liabilities as they are incurred and associates the cost of assets with the period during which they are utilized or consumed."[12] Under GAAP assets such as Federal buildings or equipment would be recognized as capital items with specific values and rates of depreciation. The advantage advocated in Congressional hearings from using GAAP was that decision makers would be given a more complete and accurate picture of government finance then they currently received from the cash-basis snapshot. For example, on a balance sheet using GAAP, the construction of a new building would not appear as a one-time debit with no future benefit, as it does now on a cash basis. Instead, the full value of the building over its entire life would be recognized by budget decision makers.

GAAP also would make it more difficult for OMB, Federal agencies (and Congress for that matter) to manipulate budget entitlement accounts. For example, trust fund accounts in surplus often were added into the unified budget to offset deficits in other areas of the budget. Other practices such as the shifting of pay days from one fiscal year to the next to meet outlay ceilings would not be necessary under accrual accounting. Under GAAP financial statements, such "games" would be unnecessary and implausible because liabilities appear on the balance sheet, regardless of when they must be paid.

Audited financial statements. The Committee was impressed by testimony indicating that a key element of financial management reform would be strengthened with expanded financial reporting through the development of audited annual financial statements. Financial statements provide a scorecard for an agency and subjecting them to the rigors of an independent audit would, it was argued, instill discipline in financial systems and strengthen accountability. Bowsher testified that financial statement audits ensure that "accounting transactions, accounting systems, financial statements and financial reporting to Treasury, OMB, the Public, and the Congress are properly linked."[13]

Audited financial statements have been used and have proven successful at the Federal agency level as well as in state and local governments. The Social Security Administration published its 1988 annual report including audited financial statements that attempted full disclosure of financial information on agency-administered programs. These financial statements attested to the financial soundness of the Social Security system. In another instance, audited financial statements were said to have proven their worth by detecting serious financial problems. When GAO audited the Federal Savings and Loan Insurance Corporation using accrual-based accounting, it showed a $13.7 billion deficit. The cash-based audit for the same period reflected a substantial surplus.[14]

Notwithstanding all the ferment about financial management reform in the 1980s, much remained to be done. In 1989 President Reagan said that while the Federal government had once been a leader "the government's financial systems and operations have eroded to the point that they do not meet generally accepted standards" (Steinhoff et al., 1990).

COMPREHENSIVE REFORMS ENACTED

The decade of the 1980s was a turbulent period for financial management in the Federal government, which culminated in the passage of the Chief Financial Officer's Act of 1990.[15] While the Savings and Loan rescue had drawn attention to one set of federal financial management oversight mechanisms, other problems existed which, though less apparent, were very real: GAO and the Office of Management and Budget (OMB) studies of "high risk" programs in 1989 identified as many as 78 different problems which posed potential federal liabilities reaching into the hundreds of billions of dollars.[16] Other problems identified by Congress included failure of the IRS to collect $63 billion in back taxes, an alleged $30 billion in unnecessary inventories bought by the Department of Defense and losses at the Federal Housing Administration estimated at more than $4 billion. The identification of these problems led to passage of the CFO Act and other recent financial management reforms.

In 1990 Congress passed the Chief Financial Officer's Act (CFOA) to improve federal financial management.[17] Subsequently, Congress enacted the Government Performance and Results Act (GPRA, 1993), and the Government Management Reform Act (GMRA, 1994)[18] to extend the mandate for financial management reform in the Federal government and accelerate its implementation. These three pieces of legislation together with the Federal Managers' Financial Integrity Act (FMFIA)[19] and the Inspector General Act[20] establish a framework for improved accountability and provision of better, and more timely information for Congress, the President, and the public. This structure may lead not only to improved financial management, but also to better decision making, a more responsible government and a public better informed about the actions and resource capacity of its government.

The Chief Financial Officer's Act (see Jones & McCaffery, 1993, 1992) created the critical leadership and mechanisms to integrate all of these reforms and to keep the process of financial management reform moving. It established a Chief Financial Officer (CFO) for the United States in the Office of Management and Budget and twenty-two CFOs in the major agencies. The Chief Financial Officer (CFO) position was established to provide leadership, policy direction, and oversight of federal financial management and information systems, including productivity measurement and improvement, credit and asset management, cash management, and internal controls. While some of this structure had been created by administrative directives prior to 1990, the passage of the statute gave this reform effort a statutory basis and a life beyond the particular policies of any particular Presidential administration or Congress.

The CFO of the United States is appointed by the President, with the advice and consent of the Senate. As Deputy Director for Management, the CFO is charged to "provide overall direction and leadership to the executive branch on financial management matters by establishing financial management policies and requirements, and by monitoring the establishment and operation of Federal Government financial management systems." Essentially, the CFO is tasked to provide the framework and guidelines indicating how the government should implement financial management improvements. This is to be done by specifying the type and form of information that will be produced by the government's financial management systems, identifying projects that will accomplish systems integration, and estimating the costs of the plan. The Act requires that OMB submit annual reports to Congress on the status of Federal financial management.

With regard to the rest of the Executive, in accordance with the CFO Act, CFOs were appointed and confirmed by the Senate for 24 major departments and agencies. CFOs also have been appointed for major agencies within large departments. Deputy CFOs have been appointed as well and a CFO Council was established to determine objectives and policy, and to oversee implementation. Within individual agencies, CFOs report directly to the head of the agency regarding all financial management matters. CFOs oversee all financial management activities relating to programs and operations of the agency and they develop and maintain integrated agency accounting and financial management systems, including those for reporting and financial controls. CFOs direct, manage, and provide policy guidance and oversight of financial management personnel, activities, and operations. They are also charged with monitoring the financial execution of the budget.

One CFO observed that he had not thought that there was anything wrong with Federal financial management until he discovered that in many programs it was difficult to tell the results of outlays, the location and value of inventories, the wear and tear on buildings, the aging of receivables, and the souring of loan and loan guarantee portfolios. He noted that on the OMB high-risk list were some $14 billion in delinquent loans at the FHA, $13.7 billion in Department of Energy contracting that was inadequately managed and Medicare and Medicaid mis-estimates of $21 billion and $9 billion respectively. He further observed that in some cases the financial numbers were not known on an auditable basis, due diligence was not taken in extending the nation's credit and credit guarantees and that the results of expenditures and investments often was not measured and when it was there was little assurance that the measures were accurate and comparable across programs (Hodsoll, 1992).

In 1985, former Comptroller General Charles Bowsher had recommended a number of changes in Federal financial management, suggesting that "for too long" financial management in the Federal government had been practiced as a rather narrow function involving mainly accountants and budget analysts and that the idea of bringing management issues and analyses to bear upon budgeting and accounting questions had not "taken root" throughout the Federal government.

The CFO Act is intended to knit the budget and accounting functions together and to centralize all financial management functions at the department and agency level with a Chief Financial Officer reporting to the head of each agency or department. The centralizing bias of this Act was further revealed in the official creation of a Chief Financial Officer for the Federal government as an Executive Deputy Director in the Office of Management and Budget whose task it is to take the lead on concept creation and development of systemwide efforts to improve federal financial management. Passage of the Budget Enforcement Act compromise in the Reconciliation Act of 1990 during the same time period tended to obscure the importance of the CFO Act, but now enough time has passed to allow for the full impact of this piece of legislation to be recognized. Its goal is to dramatically change the shape of Federal financial management, relying, like the Budget and Accounting Act of 1921 before it, on financial management practices prominent and proven in the private sector. Among these are the requirement for one Chief Financial Officer responsible for all financial functions reporting to the head of the agency, an annual financial statement that is understandable in generally accepted accounting terms and which will bear the weight of an annual audit and Inspector General certification, and a reduction in the number of separate department/agency accounting systems. The Act also has mechanisms for continuing modernization of financial systems.

The major initiative of the CFO Act is preparation of auditable consolidated financial statements for departments, agencies and the Federal government as a whole. Audit responsibility has been assigned to the Inspectors General (IGs) of each department and agency. IGs have performed some audits on their own. GAO has provided assistance and oversight in this effort. IGs may contract with outside private sector accounting firms to assist or to conduct audits and GAO also has authority to outsource audits when appropriate.

Underlying both the CFOA and GMRA is the need for a comprehensive set of Federal accounting standards and principles. The Federal Accounting Standards Advisory Board (FASAB) was established by a Memorandum of Understanding among the three principal agency heads concerned with overall financial management in the federal government: the Secretary of the Treasury, the Director of OMB, and the Comptroller General. The federal government has never had a body of "generally accepted accounting principles."[21] Recognizing that such standards were needed, and that compliance must be measured on a regular basis, FASAB was tasked to develop financial and cost accounting standards.

Congressional oversight for implementation of the CFO Act and the other Acts continues to be provided by the two oversight committees that sponsored much of this legislation: the House Government Reform and Oversight Committee and its subcommittee on Government Management, Information and Technology, and the Senate Governmental Affairs Committee. However, substantial responsibility for oversight has been delegated to the General Accounting Office (GAO). Under the guidance of former Comptroller General Charles Bowsher and Comptroller General David Walker, the GAO has been a driving force behind much of the implementation effort,[22] as is OMB.

Pursuant to the CFO Act, in the mid 1990s auditable financial statements were prepared for selected departments and agencies. The GMRA extended the audit requirement from 10 to 24 departments and agencies and for all types of accounts, required auditing within five months of the close of the fiscal year to make data available in a timely manner for the budget process, and directed an audit of the government-wide financial statement for FY 1997. Departments and OMB have made substantial efforts since this time to enable preparation of these statements and to improve and consolidate agency accounting systems. Considerable investments of time, money and energy have been made to reengineer and refine agency accounting procedures and processes. In addition, OMB has expanded the scope of initiatives to improve Federal financial management under the authority of the CFO and other Acts. However, initial progress was slow.

For example, in December 1996, the Department of the Navy (DON) submitted its first Annual Financial Report required by the CFO Act and the GMRA. The report was reviewed by the Office of the Secretary of Defense (OSD) Comptroller and by the Naval Audit Service prior to its publication in 1997. Information was obtained from financial and functional managers throughout the Department of Navy and from the Defense Finance and Accounting Service (DFAS) to produce the DON Principal Statements that provide the foundation for the Annual Financial Report. This report included an overview of the DON, outlined its history, mission, and programs and included the Principal Statements and their related footnotes and a supplemental information section. This information was meant to be used by managers within the DON, Congress and the public.[23] However, audit of the information submitted was highly critical and found many errors. The objective of achieving a "clean" audit report (i.e., with no errors) was not met. As of this writing it still had not been met for the Navy or for the Department of Defense as a whole.

Underlying both the CFOA and GMRA was the need for a comprehensive set of Federal accounting standards and principles. The Federal Accounting Standards Advisory Board (FASAB) made responsible for achieving these goals is staffed by the three principal agents concerned with overall financial management in the federal government: the Secretary of the Treasury, the Director of OMB, and the Comptroller General. The federal government has never had a body of "generally accepted accounting principles."[24] Recognizing that such standards were needed, and that compliance must be measured on a regular basis, FASAB was tasked and subsequently developed a set of financial and cost accounting principles and standards. By fiscal year 1999, auditors for 21 of the 24 CFO Act agencies reported that those agencies' financial systems did not substantially comply with FFMIA's requirements. The three agencies in compliance were the Department of Energy, National Aeronautics and Space Administration, and the National Science Foundation.

The inability of many Federal agencies to accurately record and report financial management data at the end of the year and on an ongoing basis for oversight and for decision making purposes is a serious weakness. Without reliable data on costs, decision makers cannot control or reduce costs, effectively evaluate programs' financial performance or direct additional resources to underprovided programs. In addition to requiring annual audited financial statements, the CFO Act sets expectations for agencies to build effective financial management organizations and systems and to routinely produce sound cost and operating performance information throughout the year. While progress seems slow, the key is to take steps to continuously improve internal controls and their underlying financial management systems. A clean audit opinion is important, but it should not be seen as the ultimate goal. The ultimate goal is a government that delivers more for less, where the outcomes of governmental action benefit its citizenry and where the costs to achieve those outcomes can be seen, understood, and tracked. The Federal Financial Management Improvement Act helps promote this goal by creating a process for continuous improvement in financial management systems and ensuring that those systems routinely provide reliable and useful information on a timely basis: "With such information, government leaders will be better positioned to invest scarce resources, reduce costs, oversee programs, and hold agency managers accountable for the way they run government programs."[25]

CONCLUSIONS

The Federal Financial Management Status Report and Five Year Plan for 2000 noted that with the majority of agencies attaining a clean audit opinion, the emphasis on financial management reform would switch to improving financial management systems (p. 7). It is useful to review the size of this task. In 1997, the agencies covered by the CFO Act reported that they had 751 agency financial management systems that consisted of 1,117 applications in operation and 123 agency financial management systems under development or phased implementation.[26] In 1992, the Federal government operated 878 systems with 1306 financial management systems.[27] In the five-year period the number of systems and applications have both decreased somewhat (about 15%), but the Federal government financial management apparatus remained large and diverse. There is no trend toward one system or just a few applications, nor should such a trend be expected. Rather environmental complexity must by met with appropriately diverse, but effective systems. In 1997, on average, the 24 CFO agencies operated 31 systems with more than 46 applications and had 5 under development. The two tables below adapted from the 1998 OMB Status Report further illustrate the diversity, complexity and churn (continuous system development and replacement) in the CFO agencies. Table I indicates the range in the two simplest agencies and the four most complex.

**Table 1.   Financial Management Systems and Applications:
Simplicity and Complexity**

Agency	FM Systems	FM Applications	In Development
DOE	1	7	1
OPM	1	8	1
DOD	156	156	0
TREASURY	97	112	37
HUD	84	84	6
USDA	69	140	13
TOTAL (for all 24)	751	1117	123
AVERAGE (for all 24)	31.3	46.5	5.1

Source: Adapted from the Federal Financial Management Status Report and Five Year Plan, OMB, 1998.

Table 2 indicates the diversity of financial management applications in five sample agencies. Again, a relatively simple agency is used (DOE) and the four most complex are included for contrast. The applications range from acquisition, through payroll, to systems tailored to carry out the agencies own special needs built up over decades before the push to financial management reform gathered steam, thus the large category of "other" systems. A zero in a cell means an agency either uses a government-wide system (there were 21 of these in 1997) or has its own compound system, included in the "other" category. It is worthwhile to remember that building a system for specific needs has its uses; it usually fits that client better. However, this results in many different information systems and when decision makers attempt to gather data to enhance the policymaking process, complexity defeats clarity. Moreover, all systems need maintenance; otherwise, they fall prey to malfunctions. When money is involved, the malfunctions may range from costly mistakes to outright fraud and abuse.

Financial management systems follow the mission of the organization. DOD had 16 payroll systems because it hires permanent and temporary employees and pays their salary and benefits. For temporary employees the systems differ somewhat among the services. Agriculture is complex because it is a mixture of Federal employees and functions, grants and aids to various entities, and direct payments to individuals. This complex environment is not evolving toward a steady state: in September 1997, agencies indicated that they intended to plan to replace or upgrade 71% of their operational applications![28] This means that the environment will continue to be turbulent as new systems are developed and implemented and old systems become obsolete and are replaced. Since no perfect end state exits, this cycle of obsolescence and rebirth may continue almost forever. More-

Table 2. Financial Management Applications by Type in Five Agencies

Application Type	DOE	DOD	TREAS	HUD	USDA
Acquisition	0	0	6	0	11
Budget	1	0	1	1	2
Core Financial	5	93	32	15	31
Travel	0	4	7	1	3
Pay (civilian)	1	7	13	3	12
Pay (other)	0	9	0	0	2
Labor	0	0	0	0	0
Inventory/property	0	22	15	2	7
Inventory held for sale	0	0	0	0	0
Revenue	0	0	9	0	8
Loan	0	0	0	6	18
Exec. Inf. System	0	0	2	3	4
Other	0	21	27	2	42

Source: Adapted from data in the Federal Financial Management Status Report and Five Year Plan, OMB, 1998.

over, the possibility exists that the rate of system development may lag behind system obsolescence. The 1998 Status Report (pp. 15–16) observed that agencies expected to upgrade 708 of their applications within five years, but that 891 would reach the end of their useful life span in that period. The obsolescent systems could still be operated, but inadequate financial management systems might lead to costly errors. The departments to watch for this sort of turbulence include Defense, Transportation, OPM and the Small Business Administration. The number of systems and the applications within them indicate the size and complexity of the Federal government efforts.

Those who chafe at the lack of speed with which reform is progressing must understand the tremendous complexity of the task at hand and must accept that these financial management reforms do not envision applying one perfect system and/or one application to the Federal government. The goal is systems that accurately report data in understandable ways on a timely basis according to generally accepted professional standards. This may continue to be an evolutionary and turbulent process as agency missions change, new ways of doing business are tested and innovations in hardware/software occur. The 2000 Five Year report states that ten years earlier, before the passage of the CFO Act, Federal agencies could not answer the most basic questions about the state of their finances, could only offer guesses at how much they had spent the previous year, did not gather financial data automatically and consistently and could not report their finances in accordance with accepted professional standards because no such standards existed for the federal government.[29] All of this has changed. The 2000 Five Year plan basically declared that the battle for clean audit statements had been won and the battleground would now shift to improving financial management systems.[30]

By the year 2000, the following achievements had been made:

1. All 24 agencies covered by the CFO Act issued annual audited financial statements in 2000.
2. More than 60% of them received clean audit opinions.
3. The Treasury Department issued a consolidated financial statement for the U.S. Government for the first time in 1998.
4. A complete set of government-wide basic accounting standards was issued in 1996 by the Federal Accounting Standards Board (FASAB), itself created in 1990.
5. In October of 1999, the Institute of Certified Public Accountants, an internationally acknowledged authority, recognized FASAB's standards as generally accepted accounting principles (GAAP).[31]

These efforts have led to visible payoffs in modernizing financial management practices and saving taxpayer dollars. For example, in 1999 the Federal government made almost 1 trillion payments electronically, about 80% of all non-tax payments. Small purchase bank card use had increased fourfold since 1995, saving taxpayers $450 million in administrative costs. Streamlined processes led to the reduction of delinquent debt owed the federal government from $60 billion to $53.3 billion. Agencies continued to work on modernizing and replacing their financial management systems and applications. OMB continued to help by ensuring that these efforts were carefully planned and adequately funded.[32] These are major achievements. More remains to be done, however. Fifteen of the 24 CFO agencies had clean audit opinions (62.5%), but nine did not. Moreover, the budget authority for these nine agencies amounted to more than 65% of Federal government discretionary budget authority in 1999. This means more than $380 billion was executed in 1999 without the guarantee of a clean audit opinion. By any measure, this is a substantial amount of money, thus it is perhaps more accurate to suggest that the battle is being won, but it is not over.

This chapter traced the development of financial management reform in the 1980s and summarized some of the testimony that led directly to the CFO legislation. The provisions of the CFO Act were described and some of its outcomes detailed. The next chapter assesses the status of these financial management measures in terms of what more needs to be done to fulfill the potential of reform with particular attention to the Government Performance and Results Act.

NOTES

1. "Crisis in Miami discussed at ASPA Gathering." *PA TIMES*, 20(3, March), 1997, pp. 1–2. In the 1970s, the cities of New York, Detroit, and Cleveland had had serious financial difficulties; these helped focus attention on improving government and financial management. In the 1980s, attention would turn to the federal government.

2. These requirements were further clarified in OMB circular A-128 to explicitly include internal accounting and "other control systems," meaning administrative controls, which had previously been off limits for independent auditors. (See, McAndrew, 1990, p. 36).

3. For example see GAO Title 2, *Policy and Procedures Manual for Guidance of Federal Agencies* issued in November of 1984 and *OMB Circular A-127 Financial Management Systems*, December 1984 and the follow on guidance in May of 1985 of M-85-16 *Guidelines for Evaluating Financial Management and Accounting Systems;* GAO's *Controls and Risk Evaluation Audit Methodology* issued in July 1985; OMB's Circular A-130, *Management of Federal Information Resources* issued in December of 1985 and so on. GAO issued a series of guidances on internal control guidelines (1982) standards (1983) and evaluation (1987) and in 1988 issued a comprehensive revision of the 1981 government auditing standards, called the 1988 *Yellow Book Revision* originally issued in 1972, for government and for organizations that receive funds from government, including contractors, not-for-profit organizations and other non-governmental organizations. OMB reinforced these standards with Circular A-73 *Audit of Federal Operations and Programs.*

4. Statement of Joseph R. Wright, Jr., Deputy Director, Office of Management and Budget, *Hearings on Improving Federal Financial Management*, House of Representatives, Committee on Government Operations, Sub-Committee on Legislation and National Security.100th Congress, 2nd Session, September 22, 1988. Washington, DC: U.S. Government Printing Office, 1989, p. 150. (Hereafter cited as "*Hearing 1988.*)

5. Wright, *Hearing 1988*, p. 136.

6. Wright, *Hearing 1988*, pp. 136–137

7. Wright, *Hearing 1988*, p. 140. The estimate for 1988 was $286 billion.

8. Statement of Hon. Joseph J. DioGuardi, N.Y. *Hearing 1988*, p. 38. Representative DioGuardi had been a CPA for 22 years and a Congressman for four at the time of this hearing.

9. House of Representatives Report no. 101-818, 101st Congress, 2d Session, pt. 1, Chief Financial Officer Act of 1990, p. 16.

10. Statement of Charles A. Bowsher, Comptroller General, *Hearing 1988*, p. 58.

11. Bowsher, *Hearing 1988*, pp. 59–60. See also Financial Integrity Act: Continuing Efforts Needed to Improve Internal Controls and Accounting Systems. GAO/AFMD-88-10, December 30, 1987.

12. DioGuardi, *Hearing 1988*, p. 45.

13. Bowsher, *Hearing 1988*, p. 69.

14. Statement of Hon. Rep. Larry E. Craig, Idaho, *Hearing 1988*, p. 25.

15. For example, other legislation designed to improve financial management at the federal level included the Federal Managers Financial Integrity Act, the Inspector General Act, the Debt Collection Act, the Prompt Payment Act, the Single Audit Act, the Federal Grant and Cooperative Agreement Act, the Competition in Contracting Act, the Debt Collection Act and the Intergovernmental Cooperation Act. Statement of John L. Lordan, p. 216. *Hearings on Improving Federal Financial Management*, House of Representatives, Committee on Government Operations, Sub-Committee on Legislation and National Security, 100th Congress, 2nd Session, September 22, 1988. Washington, DC: U.S. Government Printing Office, 1989.

16. House of Representatives Report no. 101-818, 101st Congress, 2d Session, pt. 1, Chief Financial Officer Act of 1990, p. 14

17. Previous research has reported on the objectives and initial steps taken to implement this Act. See Jones and McCaffery (1992, 1993).

18. PL 103-356 1994, also referred to as the Federal Financial Management Act of 1994.

19. This Act requires each agency to establish internal controls which provide reasonable assurance that obligations and costs are in compliance with applicable law; that fund, property and other assets are safeguarded against waste, loss or abuse; and that revenues and expenditures are properly recorded. See Schick, Keith, and Davis (1991, p. 187).

20. P.L. 95-452, Oct. 12, 1978. The Inspector General Act of 1978 is the legal foundation of the IG Community. It has created more than 60 IGs in federal agencies and given them wide authority to conduct audits, investigations and inspections in their agencies. The purpose of the IGs is to promote economy, efficiency, and effectiveness, and to prevent and detect fraud and abuse. The Act gives the IGs independence of action by providing for separate administrative authority, direct reporting to Congress, and protection against removal. Another major reform not addressed in this article is the Information Technology Management Reform Act of 1996 (P. L. 104-106, February 10,1996).

21. See "FASAB Standards Completed and Signed by Principals," *JFMIP News*, 1996, 8(2, Summer), p. 2. The FASAB newsletter notes that the new standards signal the beginning of the creation of a reliable and meaningful database to better report on the financial condition of federal government entities and mark the first time cost accounting requirements will be imposed to help measure the cost of outputs as called for under GPRA. Developing the standards took about five years. Former standards were not accepted because they were based on private sector standards and the "for profit" reporting model. The new accounting standards have been "uniquely designed" to provide useful information for those interested in analyzing the financial condition and cost of government programs. See the June 1996 *FASAB Newsletter*, p. 1.

22. Researchers interested in this area are directed to the following sources: the *Federal Financial Management Status Report and Five Year Plan* produced each July by the Office of Management and Budget; annual JFMIP reports, for example, *Report on Financial Management Improvements*, 1993.; records of Hearings held by the Senate Governmental Affairs Committee and the House Committee on Government Reform and Oversight and its subcommittee on Government Management, Information and Technology; various GAO publications and reports. For example: *Executive Guide: Effectively Implementing the Government Performance and Results Act.* Washington, DC: GAO/GGD-96-118. June, 1996. *Managing for Results: Achieving GPRA's Objectives Requires Strong Congressional Role.* Washington, DC: GAO/T-GGD-

96-79. See also GAO reports GAO/T-GGD-AIMD-95-187; GAO/GGD-95-20,GAO/ GGD-95-22,GAO/T-GGD-95-187,GAO/T-GGD/AIMD-95-158 and GAO/AFMD-93-4. See also reports issued by OMB for, example, OMB Circular A-11, OMB Memoranda 95-05, 95-19, 96-18, 96-22. See also OMB *Primer on Performance Measurement,* February 28, 1995. The CFO Council issues reports from time to time as do JFMIP and FASAB. Financenet on the internet is an excellent clearinghouse for citations to many of these vehicles; it also has reports, testimony and briefs which may be downloaded; there are also subscription lists that will distribute electronic mail on various topics and to which one may post questions. Lastly, the federal budget carries various summary schedules including the list of federal financial high risk entities and financial management reports OMB recommends be discontinued; in the FY 1997 budget, there is a carefully written explanation describing the development of a framework for evaluating the stewardship of resources, somewhat similar to a business balance sheet. This framework requires three charts and five tables to explain what would normally be presented in a business balance sheet. See "Stewardship: Toward a Federal Balance Sheet": 15–31, *Analytical Perspectives, Budget of the U.S.* FY97. See also Vice President Al Gore, *Reaching Public Goals: Managing Government for Results.* Resource Guide. National Performance Review. October 1996.

23.   See "DON CFO Statements Issued," *DC Connection*, Issue 15 (January), 199, p. 3.

24.   See "FASAB Standards Completed and Signed by Principals," *JFMIP News*, 1996, 8(2, Summer), p. 2. The FASAB June newsletter notes that the new standards signal the beginning of the creation of a reliable and meaningful database to better report on the financial condition of federal government entities and mark the first time cost accounting requirements will be imposed to help measure the cost of outputs as called for under GPRA. Developing the standards took about five years. Former standards were not accepted because they were based on private sector standards and the "for profit" reporting model. The new accounting standards have been "uniquely designed" to provide useful information for those interested in analyzing the financial condition and cost of government programs. See the June 1996 *FASAB Newsletter,* p. 1.

25.   Testimony of J. Christopher Mihm, Associate Director, Federal Management and Workforce Issues of the General Government Division of the U.S. General Accounting Office, before the House Committee on Government Reform, Subcommittee on Government Management, Information and Technology, July 20, 2000.

26.   Federal Financial Management Status Report and Five Year Plan. prepared by the CFO Council and OMB, October, 1998. This series of reports is referred hereafter as the OMB Five Year Plan.

27.   OMB Five Year Plan, 1995, Table 2.

28.   OMB Five Year Plan, October 1998, p. 5.

29.   OMB Five Year Plan, November, 20, 2000, p. 1.

30.   OMB Five Year Plan, November, 20, 2000, p. 7.

31.   OMB Five Year Plan, November, 20, 2000, p. 1.

32.   OMB Five Year Plan, November, 20, 2000, p. 1.

CHAPTER XIV

CONTEMPORARY FINANCIAL MANAGEMENT CHALLENGES

INTRODUCTION

Reviewing the experience across the Federal government, given its focus on strategic planning, customer involvement, and performance and outcome measurement, Government Performance and Results Act (GPRA, 1993) has drawn great attention within the Federal government and even from abroad. Visitors from New Zealand, one of the leading nations in the integration of performance and outcome measurement, have stated that the United States is a better example of reform than their nation (Scott, 2001). However, the core of Federal financial management reform is the Chief Financial Officer's Act, because all improvements in financial management rest on the existence of accurate financial information. Government Management Reform Act (GMRA, 1994) extended the requirements of the CFOA across the Federal government. If accurate financial data, reported consistent with the requirements of the CFOA, were linked to the budget planning and review process through GPRA, taxpayers and government managers would, in theory, be better able to see what they are paying for and what they are getting for their money, i.e., transparency would be vastly improved over current practice. This chapter assesses some of the requirements of these reforms and attempts to evaluate how well they are being implemented.

A key implementation assumption is, of course, that the information produced through these reforms will be used to make decisions. There is reason to question this assumption given that any comprehensive reform in government is difficult to implement and manage, and that resources are not easily obtained to support implementation. These problems, combined with institutional preferences for the status quo, make successful reform very difficult to achieve, as we explain in this chapter. However, there is some evidence to suggest that real progress is underway. For example in the case of GPRA, the President's Office of Management and Budget (OMB) reported that for the first time, the Department of Veterans Affairs budget shows performance plans and resource requirements in the same alignment (see Rodriguez, 1996, pp. 2–4). OMB official Justine Rodriguez saw this as a distinct improvement over previous reporting, characterized as a clutter of tiny accounts in the budget mixed with large accounts that are not homogeneous and lack systematic alignment with programs:

> ...resources used [presently] to achieve results are not charged to the programs' budget accounts. Salaries and expenses are often entirely or partially paid centrally; there is no charge for some accruing benefits; many support services are provided free or at a subsidized price; and fixed assets may be paid centrally. ... Resources are not linked to results in budgeting, and managers have no incentive to maximize results with a resource limit. (Rodriguez, 1996, p. 3)

It is this potential to link data produced in compliance with CFO Act standards to the performance and results measures deemed necessary by the GPRA that could lead to provision of accurate and meaningful information for decision makers in both the Executive branch and Congress. If achieved, this would represent a highly significant reform of Federal budgeting, accounting and reporting.

The CFO Act initially created the Office of Federal Financial Management (OFFM) in the Office of Management and Budget to spearhead implementation. The organizational status of this office within OMB has been modified since its inception to integrate it within OMB rather than to have it operate as a semi-independent entity within OMB as was initially the case. This office is directed by a Controller. The functions of OFFM established before organizational changes made in the late 1990s have continued as OFFM was integrated into OMB. This part of OMB also became responsible for implementation of a large part of the GPRA,[1] GMRA and FMFIA.

IMPLEMENTATION ISSUES AND PROBLEMS: AN INTRODUCTION

The goals of the Government Performance and Results Act are far broader than those established in the CFO and GMRA Acts. GPRA expressed congressional will that performance measurement and reporting be introduced throughout the government. GPRA required Federal agencies to complete a strategic plan incorporating performance measures and submit to it to OMB by September 1997.[2] Reports were submitted, although some were late. Problems with these submissions are treated in a later section of this chapter. The issues associated with implementing GPRA are highly complex, particularly because the law calls for output, outcome and performance measurement linked to costs. This ties the purpose of GPRA to CFOA implementation. Without accurate accounting information, the types of analysis required by GPRA are impossible to perform so as to have any confidence that the data reported are valid and reliable.[3] More on this issue is reported below.

CFOA and GMRA require preparation of auditable financial statements. However, with the passage of GPRA, the financial management reform mandate grew to encompass a much more ambitious set of goals. The purpose of reform, according to former Vice President Gore, was to report to American taxpayers what "bang" they were getting for their buck. He predicted unrealistically, undoubtedly influenced by his anticipation of using success as an element of his bid for the Presidency, "...by 1998, the Federal government will have its first financial statement. Americans will soon know for the first time whether they are getting what they pay for" (Gore, 1995, p. 5). Alas, as with so many rosy political statements, Gore's politically motivated prediction was terribly optimistic. Neither act was implemented fully, and in many cases only marginally or not at all by 1998. Within six months after the elections of 2000, the Bush administration had adopted a much more realistic view of implementation, i.e., that it is needed but will require a long time and great effort to achieve.

Preparation and auditing of financial statements generally fall under the scope of responsibility of accountants and auditors. However, reengineering financial systems requires the talent and experience of seasoned financial managers, often assisted by knowledgeable external consultants. Relation of costs to outcome measures to influence budgets requires the skills and participation not of just accountants, auditors and financial managers; it demands the close attention of policy and budget decision makers. It is perhaps an understatement to observe that the task of improving Federal financial management has become much more complicated than proponents of the CFO Act initially envisioned. Fundamentally, GPRA makes the critical and necessary connection between costs and policy and program; it recognizes the necessity to make financial data relate to program in a timely and useful manner.

Former Comptroller General Charles Bowsher stated that, "...financial management is finally becoming a top priority of Federal managers." Annual preparation of financial statements and the independent audit opinions required of them are "...bringing greater clarity and understanding to the scope and depth of problems and needed solutions. These annual public report cards are also generating increased pressure to fix long-standing problems."[4]

In assessing the potential impact of the CFO Act and GPRA and the other laws noted, the intent is that in the future budget numbers will accurately relate to audited statements of government assets and liabilities. Better information should indicate to decision makers where to focus additional efforts to improve financial management. Better financial management also is intended to lead to more informed public policy decisions.

In assessing the longevity of GPRA reform, OMB Controller Joshua Gotbaum noted that those who thought GPRA would simply fade away were wrong. Moreover, said Gotbaum, "…we have accomplished much. Almost a hundred Federal agencies developed strategic plans. They followed up with three sets of annual performance plans and this past spring (2000) completed the first-ever set of annual performance reports."[5] He claimed that many agencies did an excellent job of developing useful, informative FY 1999 performance reports and mentioned two in particular.

First, the Department of Transportation linked program decisions to results by linking its various air, rail and highway programs to department wide objectives such as safety, economic growth and mobility. They then tracked performance by these measures, which Gotbaum, suggested were heavily oriented toward outcomes (i.e., reduction in transportation related fatalities and injuries), rather than intermediate measures of program performance or output measures. Gotbaum suggested that DOT was clearly using strategic planning and performance management to steer programs and set priorities. And when it needed to redirect its efforts, or shift priorities, it did so, using these tools.

Gotbaum also praised the Department of Education for working hard to develop measures of effectiveness and for being honest about measures limitations. Many Education programs involve grants that operate by funding the work of nonprofits, states, and local governments. While Education keeps track of the ultimate outcomes (e.g., nationwide literacy), they also recognize that these are affected by many factors beyond the particular grant program. Gotbaum noted that many Federal agencies face this challenge.[6]

In 1996, the General Accounting Office (GAO) warned that the issues associated with implementing GPRA were highly complex. First, as noted earlier, *unclear goals and missions* have hampered the targeting of program resources and caused overlap and duplication. Secondly, agencies often do not quickly and easily *shift their focus* in response to consumer demand and congressional directives because major changes in services and processes are required. Further, *outcomes are difficult to define and measure*. However, GPRA provides a mechanism for assessing agency mission and program while downsizing and increasing efficiency, at least in theory. More Federal agencies are recognizing the benefits of focusing on outcomes rather than activities or outputs to improve program efficiency and effectiveness. However, we may note that Australia has never attempted to measure outcomes because the task is too difficult from the perspective of the Department of Finance, and New Zealand, which initially led the charge to measure outcomes began to shift back to outputs in 2001 for the same reason.

GAO also warned that strong and *sustained congressional attention* was needed to ensure GPRA success. According to GAO, Congress needed to hold periodic, comprehensive oversight hearings and to gather information on measurement of outcomes. Congressional leadership was urged to determine how GPRA performance goals and information drive daily operations, how agencies use performance information to improve their effectiveness, to review progress in improving financial and information systems and staff training and recruitment, and to pay attention to how agencies are aligning their core business processes to support mission-related outcomes.[7]

In summary, beyond CFOA and GMRA, with the passage of GPRA, the financial management reform mandate has grown to encompass a much more ambitious set of goals. As Congressman Dick Armey put it in July 2000:

> The Results Act we passed eight years ago recognizes that government must be held accountable. Used properly, the Results Act is a powerful tool by which agencies can measure their performance and root out the waste, fraud and abuse of taxpayers' money. ... our Federal government exists for the people. Federal agencies are and should be expected to spend tax dollars efficiently and to implement the laws Congress passes as they are intended—to achieve results. [However] The most brilliant laws can fail to make America a better place when the execution is mishandled.[8]

How well is execution being managed? To this question we turn in subsequent sections of this chapter.

THE ROLES OF OMB AND DEPARTMENTS AND AGENCIES

OMB has responded with a number of initiatives to the challenge posed by simultaneous implementation of these ambitious pieces of legislation. To understand the priorities for change emphasized by the Clinton administration, it is useful to review OMB's eight-point program for improving financial management:

1. *Financial Management Organization.* To establish a government-wide and agency level organization structure to support financial management improvements and foster communication and cooperation among financial management personnel.

2. *Financial Management Personnel:* To improve financial management education, training and career development programs for Federal financial management employees.

3. *Accounting Standards:* To establish clear and comprehensive accounting standards and performance measures.

4. *Financial Systems:* To develop and operate agency-level systems that process, track and provide accurate, timely information on financial activity in the most cost-effective manner.

5. *Internal Controls:* To design and operate management structures that ensure accountability for achieving results, complying with laws and regulations, and safeguarding assets.

6. *Asset Management:* To design loan programs, collect taxes and other debts owed to the Federal government and to manage Federal cash.

7. *Federal Assistant Management:* To provide management guidance for grants to state and local governments, colleges and universities, and not-for-profit organizations.

8. *Audited Financial Statements:* To create and maintain a systematic means for disclosing information that enables decision makers to understand the financial implications of budgetary, policy, and program issues and for strengthening agency accountability for sound management performance (Steinberg, 1996, p. 57).

In issuing five year plans for improving Federal financial management, OMB has attempted to integrate the tasks required by each of the individual Acts in a consistent manner. Former Director Alice Rivlin asked departments and agencies to prepare financial statements and to develop performance standards and measures that could be reported both in financial statements and in budget proposals submitted to OMB. Spring reviews of strategic and performance plans including performance measures developed by departments were conducted by OMB as early as 1995 and 1996.

In September 1995, OMB issued two important documents, a memorandum on strategic planning and a new part two to the budget guidance circular A-11. In the strategic planning memo, the Director stated that the A-11 revision was to be the first step in a larger effort to link various GPRA requirements to the budget process. The addendum to A-11 provided instructions for preparation and submission of strategic plans.[9] OMB intended that performance measures be used in budget review. As former OMB Director Alice Rivlin observed, "Given today's questioning of government, we must work harder: GPRA gives us a set of tools, an excuse to do what we should be doing anyway" (Rivlin, 1995, p. 3). This supports the OMB stewardship role to ensure that departments and agencies prepare both auditable financial statements as stipulated by the CFO Act and performance measures as demanded by the GPRA. Budget examiners in the five Resource Management Offices in OMB were designated as the principal points of contact responsible for analysis of agency budget submissions.

OMB reviews agency strategic plans, performance plans and measures, and where possible attempts to use audited financial statement information to improve the integrity of budgets examined. Performance measures were required from agencies for FY 1999, but they were included in some budget submissions for FY98. Pursuant to a new part 2 of OMB Circular A-11, OMB staff has assisted agencies in developing measures and comprehensive plans for improving their financial systems and management practices. Strategic plans prepared by departments and agencies are intended to indicate what initiatives need to be taken and in what order of priority.[10] Department and agency strategic plans are not identical in that each organization has its own definitions of mission, performance plans and measures, and priorities.

In his testimony in the summer of 2000, Joshua Gotbaum emphasized that GPRA had been a high priority for the Clinton Administration: "The Administration created a set of Priority Management Objectives: after Y2K, GPRA was ranked the next most important objective for the first several years. Now the Administration's number one priority management objective is to 'use performance information to improve program management and make better budget decisions.'" Gotbaum noted that OMB's work implementing GPRA had been intensive and long-standing. He pointed out that OMB staff helped draft the original legislation and each year OMB has worked to improve and use agency performance information in its internal discussions on agency funding levels. He said that at the same time OMB had worked actively with agencies to improve their performance plans and to increase their own use of GPRA information. Within OMB he observed that the same analysts who work on a particular agency's budget and management issues every day also reviewed the agency's performance reports and worked with the agency on GPRA implementation. This was certainly one of the major goals of GPRA and one that some who were skeptical of GPRA implementation felt might not be achieved. Gotbaum added that each year in developing the President's Budget, OMB employed more performance information and made better use of it. He said that for the FY 2001 process, OMB asked the agencies to provide performance information as part of their budget submissions and, using that information, OMB was better able to analyze what performance could be achieved at different levels of investment. Relevant performance information was used for every agency budget review. For FY 2002, Gotbaum noted that OMB was asking agencies to submit an integrated Annual Performance Plan with goals based on current services levels and, to the extent feasible, develop budget estimates associated with each goal. This integrated document would be used to provide a succinct description of each agency's mission and goals, based on the strategic plans that agencies send to OMB and the Congress in the fall. The document presents the agency's recent performance results, and discusses any external factors outside of the agency's programs that affect its outcome goals.

In looking ahead, Gotbaum observed that one idea OMB was pursuing was helping agencies to realign their budget accounts to follow programmatic lines. He noted that the budget structure is, in most cases, distinctively different from the groupings of program performance goals set out in individual plans. While historical and logistical reasons explain why this happens, the fact is that this divergence makes it harder to compare program results accurately with program costs. One OMB goal is to examine how better alignment would contribute to better integration of performance plans and budgets, and how OMB could better account for the cost of individual programs and activities. Gotbaum noted that another ideal would be to use performance measures more actively as an incentive to better management. He said: "...rewards could increasingly be tied to program performance goals and their achievement. Similarly, distribution of grants could consistently be tied to past performance and promised performance. Rewards for contractors could also be tied to performance targets. Good information and appropriate incentives are powerful drivers toward achievement of performance targets..."[11]

Reviewing the experience of one department with respect to GPRA, in 1994 John Hamre, then Under Secretary of Defense (Comptroller), noted that Act was not just a comptroller's program; rather, it was meant to help the larger defense community in getting essential outcomes for a given level of resources.

> GPRA implementation should evolve to present performance information on the most important aspects of Defense. It should facilitate the development of how to best measure critical Defense outputs and outcomes. And, to be more than another layer of reporting, the process must be integrated with and reflect the expectations of the planning and budgeting process and the Future Years Defense Plan. It is not a "Comptroller Program." Rather, it is a methodology to engage the DOD community at large in focusing on essential outputs and results at given resource levels. (Hamre, 1994)

The GPRA effort within DOD was intended to be carried out at two levels, including a DOD-wide implementation process and a set of pilot programs in specific commands and agencies.[12] With the Planning-Programming-Budgeting System in place, DOD already had a mechanism to focus on strategic planning prior to the passage of GPRA, thus DOD has been going forward melding the two conceptual frameworks of PPBs and GPRA. In August 1994, an internal working group representing all OSD offices, the Military Departments, and the Joint Chiefs of Staff was created to study how to refine the PPB system to meet the requirements of GPRA and to strengthen DOD internal management processes. The group set out to study how to integrate GPRA into the PPBS, how to make GPRA a meaningful Secretary of Defense level report and how to develop corporate level goals and corporate level performance measures for DOD.

In its deliberations, the working group analyzed a number of existing DOD strategic planning documents, including the Bottom-Up Review, the National Security Strategy, the National Military Strategy, the Defense Planning Guidance, the Chairman's Program Assessment and key DOD Congressional testimony. The group extracted the DOD GPRA "corporate level goals" from these existing documents, along with the DOD mission and vision statement that were published in the 1996 Defense Planning Guidance. Next, the group attempted to determine key performance measures that would indicate progress toward meeting the corporate goals, concentrating on the selection of performance measures that would be meaningful to the Secretary of Defense. Subsequently, draft sets of corporate level performance measures were provided to the Office of Program Analysis and Evaluation, Office of the Secretary of Defense (OSD/PA&E) to serve as a starting point for further development within the programming phase of PPBS.

In the PPBS process, with "owners" having been assigned GPRA responsibilities in strategic planning, program analysis, evaluation, and budgeting, DOD anticipated that the FY 1998–2003 PPBS cycle would satisfy GPRA requirements one year in advance of the legislative requirements. (For more detail on this effort, see Maroni, 1996, pp. 23–26.) In sum, in the mid-1990s DOD seemed well on its way to integrating GPRA into its PPBS and other systems. Subsequently, to manage the extensive reporting requirements of the GPRA, DOD leadership decided and then persuaded Congress to allow GPRA reporting to be integrated into the congressionally mandated Quadrennial Defense Review (QDR) under the Clinton administration. By the late 1990s, GPRA was subsumed under the QDR and did not appear to have a high priority within the department as a distinctly independent reform.

Much of the failure to push GPRA more assertively during the Clinton administration was reportedly due to the absence of support from the top-level of DOD leadership in the Office of the Secretary of Defense, and particularly from Hamre himself who was rumored to have asked his staff never to even mention either reinvention or GPRA to him. Hamre left DOD in 2000 and his successors have been more supportive of efforts to comply with Congressional intent on GPRA and other reform acts. Through the QDR, and through other initiatives, GPRA appears to have been integrated successfully into portions of DOD acquisition and into a variety of programs in the individual service branches. However, it is still too early to tell whether GPRA will disappear as a priority in DOD or if it will sustain some momentum.

STANDARDS FOR FINANCIAL AND COST ACCOUNTING

As noted, the Federal Accounting Standards Advisory Board (FASAB) recommended and adopted a framework for Federal financial reporting and the basic standards needed to implement it. By June 1995, FASAB had completed work on the eight basic concept statements, accounting standards and cost standards,[13] all of which were approved by OMB, Treasury, and GAO. In addition, approval of the Revenue Accounting standard by the three principals marked the completion of the basic accounting and cost accounting standards called for by the National Performance Review.[14] As issued by OMB, these standards become GAAP (Generally Accepted Accounting Principles) for Executive Branch agencies. By issuing the standards, OMB fulfilled its responsibility to prescribe the form and content of agency financial statements by modifying its existing *Form and Content of Financial Statements* guidance to incorporate the new standards.

While it took a long time for FASAB to complete its tasks of developing standards for financial and cost accounting, a number of very contentious issues including appropriate means for accounting for depreciation of Federal assets had to be resolved. Furthermore, as is always the case with modification of standards, FASAB had to spend a considerable amount of time putting draft standards and guidelines out for review and comment and responding to comments prior to their promulgation. GAO played a very strong role in assisting FASAB, pressing for closure in part as a result of Bowsher's desire to see standards issued prior to the completion of his tenure as Comptroller General in September 1996.

To assist agencies with implementation of new accounting methods, the Center for Applied Financial Management and FASAB jointly sponsored workshops on Federal Financial Accounting Standards and Concepts. Two-phase workshops were delivered in Washington, DC and other areas. The first workshops covered the concepts (objectives, entity and display), new reporting formats and their effect on OMB form and content requirements, and standards for managerial cost accounting and supplementary stewardship reporting. The second workshops provided instruction on standards for selected assets and liabilities, direct loans and guaranteed loans, inventory and related property, liabilities, revenues and property, plant, and equipment.

EDUCATION AND TRAINING INITIATIVES UNDER THE CFO COUNCIL

The Human Resources Committee (HRC) and the GPRA Committee that serve the CFO Council defined and developed the criteria and standards needed for education and training to enable executive departments to implement the CFOA, GMRA, and GPRA. The HRC developed competency-based guidelines for financial management personnel position classification, and education and training career paths for Federal financial management employees. Core competencies for the Federal financial management community were defined and published over the 1996–1998 period, documenting the appropriate knowledge, skills, and abilities necessary for financial personnel to succeed in their careers. These core competencies were central to the development of CFOs Council human capital strategies in professional development, recruitment, and qualification standards.[15]

For accounting and financial management education and training, efforts were made successfully to define how educational and training experience outside of formal classroom instruction could be factored into provision of credit for career enhancement. To supplement departmental initiatives, whether formal education or on-the-job training, plans were made and executed to develop curricula for education and training. Given that the financial resources needed become available, if sufficient education and training opportunity cannot be provided by departments, universities and colleges or private contractors may be and have been called upon to develop and deliver what is needed. A comprehensive needs assessment of financial management education and training in the Federal government was completed.

The HRC and staff wanted to avoid duplicating education and training that departments already were providing. The idea of consolidating existing departmental training and curricula to save education and training dollars was rejected because the existing need for training far exceeds supply. The HRC and CFO Council attempted first to define the status of FM educational opportunity in the Federal government, because no comprehensive catalog of departmental education and training existed. Subsequently, where gaps or deficiencies are found, a variety of options have and are being assessed to fill them. It has not been assumed that educational and training programs ought to be developed and provided exclusively by government. Cooperation with alternative service suppliers, including universities and the private sector, has been emphasized.

The need for increased attention to better definition of educational opportunities for Federal FM employees and to development of career paths within departments and across the government has been recognized.

The most promising outcomes of HRC efforts may be better counseling and advising of FM employees on what they need to do to get ahead in their careers, and department support for the career path approach. However, the issue of the provision of adequate funding for employee education and training remains. Other partially or completely unresolved issues include quality assessment of education and training programs and improved valuation of non-traditional educational experience.

As of this writing a comprehensive Federal financial managers certification program and examination process had been implemented and a number of Federal employees had taken the exam and had received certification. This represented a successful outcome relative to the intent to comply with the requirements of the CFO Act and other financial legislation passed in the 1990s. Moreover, some very innovative approaches have been taken to find and develop human capital, including a CFO Fellows program to provide career development for promising financial managers within the CFO community, a CFO Careers program aimed at attracting well-qualified applicants to financial management disciplines, a CFO Internship Program to provide structured on-the-job experiences to undergraduate and graduate students that may lead to permanent career opportunities and a CFO Scholars program in cooperation with the Association of Government Accountants to provide competitive scholarships for outstanding Federal financial managers to pursue degree programs and professional certifications.[16] This is a very creative and broad-gauge set of measures to attract, develop and keep talented individuals within the financial management community.

With respect to implementation of GPRA it has become increasingly clear that (a) significant education and training are needed to enable skillful development of performance measures, (b) the demand for GPRA education overwhelms the supply, (c) training on strategic planning and performance measurement, (d) executive and staff devising performance plans and measures have to learn the ropes of GPRA on the job. Greater emphasis on education and training is essential to effective implementation of GPRA.

At a training symposium sponsored by the HRC and GPRA Committee held at the Bureau of Labor Statistics in October 1996, then OMB Director Franklin Raines, former Comptroller Edward DeSeve and other OMB officials indicated strong support for the GPRA, sending a clear message that OMB expectations were high with respect to department strategic and performance plans. It is clear that OMB will use performance plans and measures in budget review. Director Raines stated that he would not attend budget hearings for departments or agencies where strategic and performance plans were absent.[17] Such resolve has remained in OMB into the new millennium.

GPRA IMPLEMENTATION ISSUES

The strategic plans and the performance measurement initiatives required by GPRA were implemented in a two-step sequence under OMB's intention to integrate the results to the greatest extent possible through what were termed "Accountability Reports" in conformance with the National Performance Review in the 1990s. Accountability reports were supposed to integrate audit and financial statement data with information contained in strategic and performance plans, including performance measures.[18] OMB thus responded ambitiously to the formidable agenda provided by Congress and the Executive, and it has been up to departments and agencies to produce financial reports, strategic plans and performance standards and measurement methods to satisfy OMB and Congress. One example of the many problems faced in implementing the CFO Act is provided in the case study in Appendix C.

Departments have moved forward to complete the financial statements required by the CFO Act so as to eventually produce reports that receive clear audits. And, as noted, OMB has to an extent intended to integrate financial statement data into budget review and accountability reports. Thus, the primary goal of the CFO Act appears to be obtainable as departments refine their accounting and reporting methods. However, the issue of major accounting systems improvement remains unresolved.

While all departments and agencies are responding to both Acts with financial statements, strategic and performance plans and performance measurement, executives and staff wonder about the extent to which Congress and OMB are willing to provide the resources needed to implement the Acts effectively. This is a significant issue given that many agencies are operating under conditions of fiscal stringency due to the budget squeeze on discretionary spending resulting from efforts to reduce the deficit and an Executive and Congressional decision in 1994 to further downsize the Federal workforce by 272,900 employees by 1999.[19] This latter issue is particularly important. The size of the personnel reduction was based on the logic that half of the 700,000 Federal financial management and related positions estimated to be engaged in "overseeing" work (managers, supervisors, and specialists in personnel, procurement, budget, and audit) could be eliminated if up-to-date information systems were put in place. It also was estimated that 100,000 new positions would need to be created and filled by new people with new skills, or by retrained employees, thus leaving a net reduction of 250,000 equivalent full time employees. This number was increased as the bill passed through Congress.[20] By 1999, Federal full time equivalent employees had been reduced from 3.017 million in 1992 to 2.686 million, a reduction of 331,000. In the narrower category of civil service employees, the Federal government was reduced from 2.174 million employees in 1990 to 1.778 employees in 1999, a reduction of 396,000 employees. The year 1990 was chosen as the base year because the CFO Act was passed then, and because it allows for benchmarking of the "peace dividend" from the end of the Cold War. Most civilian personnel reductions came from Defense which was downsized from 1.006 million civilian employees in 1990 to 681,000 in 1999, a reduction of 325,000 or 82% of the total Federal reduction. Military personnel were reduced from a high of 2.213 million in 1987 to 1.386 million in 1999, for a total 827,000 positions or more than 37%.[21]

As these reductions were made, departments and agencies faced a dilemma in that they were asked to do more and to perform more efficiently while also developing and implementing major financial systems improvements with fewer people. Moreover, the new systems demanded skills the current employee cohort did not have. In the mid-1990s this tension was clearly apparent. Scott Fosler commented:

> The problem is that the position reductions have begun, but in very few instances have the new systems been developed or the new employees and skills put into place. Consequently, throughout the government one finds fewer employees attempting to operate cumbersome old systems, while simultaneously designing and implementing new systems, but without the training or access to skills required to do either.[22]

To help remedy this situation, Fosler advocated a larger investment in training. He observed that top-rated businesses commonly invest as much as 10% of their payroll in training and development, while the Federal government, by contrast, spends less than 1% of payroll costs for these purposes.[23]

Ron Young, Executive Director of the FASAB, observed that while agencies are actively pursuing changes needed in their financial management systems, progress is not as rapid as envisioned under the CFO Act and by some members of Congress. Young concluded that, "…much of the slowness is due to the significant cutbacks in funding of government financial management and the resulting inability to attract and retain highly regarded financial management specialists."[24]

Many department and agency officials believe they have been asked to do too much, too quickly. In some cases, the view has been expressed that while Congress and OMB have mandated very laudable objectives and ambitious implementation schedules, agencies having to do the real work to fulfill the promises made to the American public for a more efficient and effective government complain that they are under-resourced for this task. Officials lament that neither branch of government or political party appears willing to defend them against this onslaught of ambition. In the 1990s, the Clinton administration attempted to drive implementation of the National Performance Review and OMB pushed implementation of the financial management reform acts passed by Congress. The Republicans in Congress either wanted more efficiency for less money or elimination of programs, and in some instances cuts of entire agencies. Many Democratic members shared their views on efficiency, while differing on means, but not on significant program elimination.

Department and agency administrators have been placed in the difficult position of having to support rapid and ambitious change while accommodating budget reductions and organization-wide reinvention and reengineering initiatives that culminated in the effort termed the 'revolution in business affairs,' i.e., to cause government to be efficient compared to best practices in the private sector. Change is taking place fast, but morale has suffered as line managers and employees have been confused by the magnitude of change and the intermingling of various downsizing and reform initiatives. In some departments and agencies, staffs have been uncertain about what is expected from them and which initiatives have had highest priority. These issues continue to be problems that confront implementation.

Federal staffing reductions were achieved by 2001 and the grand reform agenda mandated by the CFO Act, GPRA and FFMIA has continued to move forward. Thus, the surprise should not be that sometimes the pace of change is slow or that missteps are taken, but that change happens at all, given staffing and training and funding shortfalls, and the power of inertia.

OVERCOMING BARRIERS TO REFORM

In a *Counterpoint* essay concluding a symposium on Federal financial management reform that appeared in the journal *Public Budgeting and Finance* in 1993, it was argued that the Chief Financial Officers (CFOA) and other financial management reforms might not achieve their objectives due to a number of barriers to implementation (Jones, 1993). The potential impediments identified were (a) accounting system weaknesses, (b) that Congress passed the Act for the wrong reasons, (c) inability of Congress to use financial statement data for decision making, (d) executive branch incentives to avoid scrutiny, (e) incapability within the management component of the President's Office of Management and Budget, (f) weaknesses of financial statements, (g) inability to successfully implement performance measurement in budgeting, (h) budgetary incentives to avoid identification of full program costs, and (i) unachievable requirements for agency cooperation and compromise in implementation.

In addition, the essay concluded that President Bush (1988–92) had not taken a high profile stand in support of the CFOA. One reason offered to explain this was the judgment on the part of presidential advisors that the CFOA was not interesting to voters and taxpayers relative to other initiatives. Therefore, it appeared that an important impediment to Federal financial management reform was absence of strong support personally from the President. The following portion of this chapter evaluates progress in implementing the CFOA and the Government Performance and Results Act of 1993 relative to the potential impediments noted above.

ACCOUNTING SYSTEM WEAKNESSES

Accurate and reliable accounting systems are critical to successful production of auditable financial statements. *Counterpoint* (Jones, 1993, p. 88) suggested that departments and agencies might not invest sufficient effort to improve accounting systems to produce accurate data upon which financial statements would be based. This absence of investment was not predicted because departments would not want to make such investment, but because they would lack the money.

What we have found is that departments and agencies have invested to a considerable extent in improving their accounting systems. They also have in some instances provided detailed estimates of the costs of substantial improvement and consolidation. The President and Congress initially made an effort to address these funding demands. For example, the President's Budget for 1992 requested $647 million for funding financial systems upgrades and Congress appropriated $628 million.[25] However, since this time significant amounts have not been appropriated specifically for improving accounting systems with the exception of funding for the Internal Revenue Service and the Department of Defense.[26]

With respect to the total cost of implementing the CFO Act, OMB and the CFO Council issued the following statement:

> The CFO Act … requires … an estimate of the cost of implementing this government-wide five-year plan. For fiscal year 1995, these 24 agencies estimated that maintaining, operating, and improving financial management activities will cost an estimated $7.5 billion.[27]

Annually in the fall, agencies are directed by OMB to budget sufficient resources to support their five-year CFO plans. Hearings are held between OMB and the agencies to review agency plans and identify the impact of potential changes on the budget.[28] Thus, departments must report the costs of accounting system improvements, but these reports in no way require OMB support for the funding shortfalls that impede improvement of systems in accordance with the intent of the CFO Act.

Weaknesses in accounting systems still abound and some cases cause large-scale problems. For example, current statutes dictate that excise taxes be earmarked for certain purposes, but according to GAO the IRS accounting system does not have the capability to segregate these funds by type. Consequently it is possible that the Superfund Trust Fund and the Highway Trust Fund may be receiving more or less than is due them. Another example is the inability of the IRS to match social security wage information and actual tax payments. The Social Security Administration receives payments based on wage information reported to IRS, even if the taxes are ultimately not paid. This results in amounts going to the Social Security Fund from other tax sources, and while the IRS knows there is a discrepancy, it could not identify the amount in 1995.[29] Other IRS problems included consistent underestimation of loss reserves in farm loans, in student financial aid, and in housing guarantees, more than $100 million of Medicare receivables under contractor supervision where collectibility was questionable, and liability for known environmental cleanup requirements that could range from $200 to $400 billion, not counting estimates for items like groundwater pollution where reliable data to solve existing problems do not exist.[30]

Insufficient funding to make improvements to accounting and related systems is still a significant problem in 2002 as it was in the 1990s. In the 1995 *Federal Financial Management Status Report*, agencies identified 436 financial management systems currently in operation that need to be replaced or upgraded in the next five years. However, the report states, "...agencies lack the funds to replace or upgrade many systems that need it, and consequently have no plans to improve them. Funding, personnel, and technology constraints make it difficult to implement all of the systems improvements that are needed."[31]

Improving financial systems, developing financial statements and accounting standards, and the implementation of the Government Performance and Results Act (GPRA) are the top three priorities of the Chief Financial Officers Council established by the CFO Act to guide financial management reform. From 1992 to 1994, the total number of accounting systems was reduced by 7% and the number of applications by 9%, but the Federal government still operated 816 financial management systems, and used 1183 financial management applications.[32]

While more than half of the applications met agency computer standards, only 10% of the applications used off-the-shelf computer software packages. By 1997, this had increased to 13%. In 1998 JFMIP established an office to test and certify commercial systems. Many large private sector firms use off-the-shelf packages and are satisfied with them.[33] This is not currently a powerful option for the Federal government. Federal government systems appear either to be too dissimilar or to demand too many agency specific routines to use off-the-shelf software. The continuing effort to modernize systems holds out hope that at some point in the future com-

mercial packages may also serve government needs, especially with the
JFMIP office tasked to oversee and certify commercial systems.

In 1984, OMB Circular A-127 on financial management systems directed
agencies to meet two goals: single, integrated, accounting systems and a
reduction of the number of administrative subsystems performing the
same function. The General Services Administration introduced an off-the-
shelf software schedule to help meet these goals, and in 1986 a government-wide standard general ledger was established.[34] By 1992, about 34%
of the applications met the standard general ledger requirement. Also
interesting is that 61% of these applications are less than ten years old, i.e.,
have been designed and implemented since Circular A-127 was issued.
According to the 1992 OMB Five Year Plan, "Until the mid 1980s duplicative, inconsistent, inefficient, and antiquated financial systems were the
rule not the exception."[35] The fact that more than 60% of these systems
were less than ten years old illustrates the pace of financial management
reform in the 1980s and 1990s. With steady growth of plans to replace
applications, a higher usage of off the shelf software would seem an important goal.[36]

These numbers may paint too pessimistic a picture, but it is clear that
much work remains to be done and a significant investment in modernizing
systems, upgrading procedures (e.g., data entry), and training people has to
be made. Initial estimates were that the cost of financial management
reforms covered by the CFO Act would be about $7.5 billion per year. This
number has remained stable throughout the decade. For 2000, it was estimated at approximately $7.6 billion.[37] In a decade of fiscal pressure, stu-
dents of these reforms were correct in worrying where the money was going
to come from and if it would be sufficient, but Congress and the Executive
branch thus far have found the funds to carry out the reforms. Whether or
not that money found its way to the most appropriate places is still not clear.
Reporting on a survey on financial managers and Inspectors General in
1995, Mr. William Phillips of Coopers and Lybrand commented:

> The financial managers and the IGs were clear [that] the downsizing and
> budget cuts are affecting their operations. Only one-third of the financial
> managers reported that their offices received additional funding to imple-
> ment CFO act requirements. However, nearly two-thirds of the financial man-
> agers and the majority of the inspectors general noted that downsizing and
> the National Performance Review's emphasis on streamlining administration
> was hampering their implementation of the Act.[38]

Additionally, Phillips suggested that Congress needed to provide
resources and protect those implementing the Acts from 'excessive downsizing':

It is important … that Congress protect the offices of the CFO and the offices of the inspector general from excessive downsizing cuts while still holding them accountable for improved financial management and reporting, customer service and cost-effective operations. These improvements are both necessary and important. Investing a few million now to implement the CFO act will yield billions of dollars of savings in the future.[39]

How much the CFO's were protected, if at all, from downsizing is unclear. In fact, the 2000 report states the past decade had seen the downsizing of administrative financial management functions in government, along with a marked increase in the number of employees eligible to retire, and a highly competitive job environment for people with pertinent skills.[40] Thus, substantial achievements have been made under difficult conditions. It is clear that the promise of saving billions of dollars in the future with reformed financial management systems has been a very attractive goal.

CONGRESS PASSED THE ACT FOR THE WRONG REASONS

Counterpoint argued that the CFO Act was a product of the competition for power in Congress between oversight and appropriation committees.[41] The oversight committees in question—the House Committee on Government Reform and Oversight and its subcommittee on Government Management, Information and Technology, and the Senate Committee on Governmental Affairs—have not wielded substantial power in the past over funding decisions made by appropriations committees in the budget formulation process. The CFO Act was viewed as having created a mechanism for these committees to gain additional leverage over appropriators. Thus, much of the impetus for approval of the CFO Act appeared to be to strengthen one set of committees against another.

What we have found is that chairs and members of appropriations committees still are not particularly interested in having financial statements to help them make budget decisions, nor are they knowledgeable about the implications of the CFOA or GPRA. However, OMB and many members of Congress not serving on these powerful committees still appear to want appropriators to use financial reports and GPRA performance data. Pressure from the oversight committees has not lessened in the transition to and from a Republican controlled Congress. In fact, in 1995 and 1996, Senators Ted Stevens (chair) and John Glenn (minority chair) of the Governmental Affairs Committee, who along with Senator William Roth (Senate Finance Committee Chair) was an original sponsor of the CFO and GPRA Acts, continued to press for implementation and results. In the House, Rep. William Clinger, Committee Chair, Rep. Collins and subcommittee chair Rep.

Steven Horn among others, applied similar pressure. Consequently, it appears that while overall Congressional interest in implementation of the CFO Act, GPRA and GMRA is low, these Acts have a few strong advocates whose resolve has not lessened. Senator Fred Thompson, former chair of the Governmental Affairs Committee is highly informed and enthusiastic about implementation of the CFOA and GPRA. In the House, former Speaker Newt Gingrich and his staff embraced the CFOA and GPRA. As Speaker, Rep. Gingrich sponsored a series of training sessions for Republican House members and staff on the implementation and implications of financial management reform legislation, particularly the GPRA.

This support notwithstanding, the view still prevails in some quarters that Congress passed the CFO Act and GPRA as well for the "wrong" reasons, despite all of the lofty rhetoric about the need for financial management reform. Eventually, the critics may be a minority in Congress in an era when much more emphasis is placed on increasing government effectiveness and efficiency. The CFO Act and following legislation,[42] the Government Management Reform Act (GMRA) and the Government Performance and Review Act (GPRA) appear to be in tune with current Congressional preferences. Does this mean that appropriator behavior will change? It is too early to tell, but they probably will face more pressure from oversight committee members, from more of their colleagues and from OMB to use financial statement and performance information in appropriation decision making. The task at hand presently for reform advocates in Congress is to better educate members and staff about the CFOA and GPRA as some still know little, if anything, about the legislation.

INABILITY OF CONGRESS TO USE FINANCIAL STATEMENT DATA FOR DECISION MAKING

Counterpoint speculated that even if Congress wished to implement the CFO Act for the "right" reasons (i.e., to stimulate needed financial reform), *and* even if financial statement data were accurate, Congress is institutionally incapable of making long-range financial decisions based upon information in financial statements.[43] The same observation may be made with respect to the use of performance measures and strategic plans mandated by GPRA. It was argued that financial statements would not replace the annual budget as the primary methodology for resource decision making in the nation's capitol because the budget provides the money that keeps the wheels of politics rolling and financial reports do not provide budget justification. What members of Congress and their staffs care most about in budgeting is winning and losing battles over programs and money to operate them. Further, it was argued that in many instances, Congress appears not to have much interest in costs.

Evaluating behavior relative to these criticisms, it appears that, in an era of budget balancing, Congress has become more cost conscious and strongly inclined to pressure departments and agencies to cut costs.[44] If members of Congress come to perceive the CFO Act, GPRA and GMRA as helping them to demonstrate to the American public their commitment to budget balancing and cost cutting, then it seems they may be more likely to embrace the products of these Acts.

OMB staff are attempting to deal with how to use data in audited financial statements and performance reports once they are available. Former OMB Director Franklin Raines, and former Comptroller Edward DeSeve and other officials made clear when they were in office the intention to use department financial and performance data in budget proposal examination and, perhaps, in budget execution control. While it is still true that neither OMB staff nor Congressional oversight staff yet know exactly how they are going to use financial statement and performance data, OMB is well on its way to integration of data so that it can be used. However, neither the President nor OMB can force Congress to use data as they wish. Congress will have to be persuaded that it is in its interest to do so before any significant change in congressional practice will occur.

Some observers clearly view use of financial statement data in the appropriation process as critical to the ongoing implementation and utilization of the CFO Act, the GPRA, and GMRA. For example, drawing on their study of CFO implementation Mr. William Phillips of Coopers and Lybrand observed:

> ...it's important that Congress use the financial statements when deliberating that organization's budget request. This would visibly integrate the intent of the act into the budget process and address one of the questions that we've heard a lot from them (program managers) when their concern is if the financial statements don't help us somehow, some way in terms of budget requests, it becomes difficult to put the full force and intent of the efforts that you need to meet those acts in place.[45]

In this regard it is useful to review testimony from the period when the CFO and other reform acts were assessed in Congressional hearings in the 1990s. Concern was expressed by members of Congress about the nature of the data in audited financial statements. Senator Hank Brown emphasized that summary data might not be useful to the appropriation committees in a remark to Edward DeSeve during a Government Affairs hearing on the CFO Act:

...It's fine to have a summary like this. Your chairman (Sen. Stevens) is also one of the very senior members on the appropriations committee. When he's over there trying to put an appropriations bill together and supervise all of the subcommittees and all of that kind of stuff, they can't operate on a summarized view of things. They have to have specific line items, dollar figures, dollars and cents to put in the appropriations. They can't do it just on generalized figures. If this summarizes those other things in enough detail, they can do that; then this is a big step forward. If not, if this is a summary that isn't useful to him, then it doesn't seem like it does much.[46]

Mr. DeSeve responded:

This is ... if you will, the audited financial statement and the summary of performance of results. What we need to do is spend time with this Committee (Senate Committee on Governmental Affairs), with OMB, and then with the appropriators to find out how to create a similar document on the front end of the appropriations process.[47]

Mr. DeSeve went on to say that he was uncomfortable with the idea that,

...the administration requires departments to submit to the President budget information. They then have to resubmit different information to the Congress. Well, if it's good enough for the Congress, it ought to be good enough for the President. We'd love to find a way to have a seamless transmission, working with the appropriators, of detailed performance information and financial information that meet their needs, and we need to spend some time working with them to find out how to do that.[48]

This would, of course, make a dramatic change in the budget process insofar as the appropriators are concerned. Given the dictates of appropriation process history, DeSeves' view seemed very optimistic. Nonetheless, Senator Stevens, then Committee Chairman, expressed a need for consistency in the use of data from financial reports in the entire Federal budget process:

In my opinion, I think we ought to have what the comptroller general says that Australia has ... We ought to have the ability to look at the reports you've got and analyze them before you come up, and we ought to be dealing with the same numbers ... We ought to have the same printout available to us, the same computerization available to you, and we ought not to have this constant bickering about what the numbers are. We need just one set of numbers.[49]

Mr. DeSeve agreed with this comment and suggested some of the complexity that prevented the Federal government from having a more uniform system.

When you look at corporate America, there are really two different models. The Wal-Mart model is a single integrated firm that does essentially the same kinds of things within the firm. The other model for firms is what I'll call the General Electric model, the holding company model, where the large steam turbine generator division, where General Electric Credit Corporation … (they) are very different kinds of enterprises. They require very different kinds of information coming up to a consolidated reporting framework at the management level. What we've decided to do in the Federal government is begin the process by designing for each of those enterprises, each of those entities, as GE does, an accounting system that meets management's needs. That's the process that is undergoing now…[50]

Mr. DeSeve concluded that the challenge in the next three years was to integrate all financial statement and budget information so it would be useful across government and then use these data (and the systems that produce financial information) without unduly interfering with the operability of agencies:

That's the strategy we've chosen rather than a one-size fits all, to allow 24 entities to design one just for them, and then to find the commonalties … [then to] take the best system and migrate to that system, and we believe that is an appropriate step, but it's a process that's got three or four steps to it. Unfortunately, moving to a single system, we think, would blur some of the utility for particular agencies.[51]

In response to DeSeve's testimony, Senator Stevens indicated that the Federal government was closer to Wal-Mart than GE. He then asked DeSeve why he had picked GE as a model. DeSeve answered that there were great differences among agencies:

I think the GE model was picked because of the great differences among the agencies in their roles and missions. Again, even setting aside the Defense Department, which is very large, the mission of the Department of Housing and Urban Development is very different from the mission of the Environmental Protection Agency. One serves the public directly by providing housing and other services through state and local government. The other is a regulatory entity that regulates and monitors and establishes liabilities over time, so that's very different. And then you throw the State Department into the mix which is a direct service agency. There are really—and I don't mean to belabor this—different accounting issues. One of EPA's big problems is how do we value Superfund sites and the liability for those sites? … A system that doesn't monitor income eligibility doesn't help HUD. One that does doesn't help EPA. So that's really the reason we started with that strategy.[52]

Senator Stevens then commented,

> ...my eyes are appropriator's eyes, and I see all of those entities out there doing two things: Either spending taxpayer's money or bringing in taxpayer's money.[53]

Senator Glenn reinforced and elaborated on the perspective of appropriators:

> ...I've been preaching for years that there are three parts of the budgeting process. One is the revenues, one is the expenditures, and the other is the efficiency, and we never get around to efficiency. And that's the reason for CFO and all the rest of these things here.[54]

Elsewhere in testimony, Senator Glenn asked a representative of the accounting firm of Coopers and Lybrand if he could identify the dollars saved as a result of efficiency-oriented audits. The representative replied that the ratio was approximately $10 saved[55] for every dollar spent. He added that application of activity-based costing (ABC) in the private sector is critical to achieve savings. Implicitly supporting the core of the GPRA, he also noted that ABC,

> ...tells you what it costs to really do something as opposed to the way that we traditionally manage in terms of payroll lines, travel lines, training lines, budget lines. Those are the kinds of things that we need to get to so that we know what we're paying for. And measures with focus on ... customers will allow you to determine if in fact agencies are doing what they're supposed to be doing.[56]

In discussing the use of the standard general ledger, Senator Brown made the following comment with respect to achieving cost savings as a result of audits of financial statements.[57]

> What I was concerned about is, you go through this process of trying to find areas to control expenditures. Where I've run into it is the fact that, given the number of expenditure areas, we didn't have a standard account that would reveal, for example, how much a department had spent on travel or how much had been spent on printing, or how much had been spent on rent, or so on. Is there a way your office could forward to us a breakout of what might be thought of as the overhead accounts and their description? ... It's one of the intriguing things, because at least in business ... I found the kind of things I would have looked at first in business to cut, we didn't even have a way of ascertaining how much was spent on it.[58]

Mr. DeSeve responded that it was easier to analyze costs within departments than to make cross department comparisons.

All of this discussion indicates that some members of Congress are interested in using data from financial statements and performance reports to examine the costs and efficiency of executive agencies.[59] As revealed in the testimony of Congressman Richard Armey, the promise of cost savings continues to lure legislators: "The Results Act has created a paradigm shift in Washington, D.C. Today, agencies are judged on results out instead of dollars in. Yet eight years after the Results Act was enacted, our government is still too big and spends too much. We need to hone government's ability to use this tool to receive information from agencies about the size and location of inefficiencies, waste, duplication and mismanagement within the executive branch."[60] However, it may be misleading to assume that Senators Stevens, Glenn, Brown and Congressman Armey accurately represent the views of the majority of members of Congress or the appropriations committees in particular.

EXECUTIVE BRANCH INCENTIVES TO AVOID SCRUTINY

Counterpoint suggested that departments and agencies may not want to aid Congressional oversight committees in micromanagement of the Executive, nor do they want to assist Congress in gaining its programmatic priorities over those of the President and his Cabinet appointees. Therefore, they would be unlikely to want to wash the "dirty linen" of departmental mismanagement before Congress under the legislative and media spotlight in review of financial statements and performance measurement reports.[61]

Thus far, it is too early to determine an outcome relative to this criticism. Until financial and performance data are provided to OMB and made public, we cannot tell what they will show. Moreover, until Congress receives this data, we cannot define what they will do with it. However, what can be said at this point is that OMB will use financial and performance information directly in examining agency budgets. This supplies strong incentive for agencies to respond to OMB requests, but the incentive to "oversell" or to "strategically represent or misrepresent" budget data would seem to be unchanged. And, as observed with respect to Senator Brown's comments above, the proclivity of Congress to micromanage is omnipresent. In our view, it seems that Congress may use more and better financial and performance information to further "micromanage" the Executive branch. Neither OMB nor departments want this to happen, yet how to avoid it is not clear. The approach apparently now favored by OMB at the time of this writing is to provide Congress with full financial data in accordance with the CFO Act but only summary performance data in compliance with GPRA.[62] Thus, the prospect exists that OMB and executive departments may use one set of performance measures and Congress another.

CAPABILITY OF THE MANAGEMENT COMPONENT OF THE PRESIDENT'S OFFICE OF MANAGEMENT AND BUDGET

Counterpoint observed that the "M" in OMB (the Management side) might not have sufficient capacity to fully implement the CFO Act. By making a commitment to use of financial and performance report data in budget review, OMB has implicitly recognized the validity of this criticism.[63] Budget examiners and OMB senior officials will provide the incentive for departments to comply with the CFOA and GPRA through budget review. OMB use of budget financial and performance data is intended to be part of a comprehensive process of review, from policy development through program implementation and evaluation. To serve the President well, these responsibilities should be carried out in an integrated rather than fragmented manner. On this point, an OMB official suggested that:

> Recent evidence from both here and abroad suggests that integrating budget and management responsibilities, not separating them, is the most productive and effective approach. At a recent symposium of the Organization for Economic Cooperation and Development (OECD), ministers responsible for public management from the 26 OECD countries identified common features of successful governance reforms. What became apparent was that reform efforts are likely to fail if management considerations are seen as distinct from budgetary policies. Countries moving toward public sector reform are building alliances between these efforts and see them as mutually reinforcing. Indeed, important aspects of many reform agendas are inherently budgetary in nature. These include controlling the costs of direct Government operations, providing financial flexibility to permit resources to be used more effectively, financing essential training, reallocating tasks to the private or voluntary sectors and assessing performance.[64]

A General Accounting Office's report entitled *Changes Resulting From the OMB 2000 Reorganization*[65] analyzed the results of the reorganization under former Director Alice Rivlin intended to better integrate OMB's budget analysis, management review, and policy roles. GAO found that:

> ...there was greater attention to agency management issues in the fiscal year 1996 budget process (after OMB 2000 was implemented) than in the fiscal year 1995 process. A greater variety of management issues were presented in more depth in the fiscal year 1996 documents than in the previous years' documents ... OMB's initial experience with the OMB 2000 approach during the 1996 budget process showed the clear support of top OMB officials and staff to enhance the treatment of certain management issues in the budget. Even though this was a particularly difficult budget cycle, there was a noticeable increase in the attention OMB gave to management issues that transcended immediate budgetary concerns.[66]

It is clear that former OMB Director Rivlin recognized these issues. In 1993 as a part of this reorganization, OMB decreased the size of the Office of Federal Financial Management. OFFM personnel were assigned at least part of the time to the Resource Management Offices (budget analysis offices) where they work side by side with the budget examiners and analysts.

These changes did not go unnoticed by Congress as questions from Senator Glenn to Mr. DeSeve illustrated:

Sen. Glenn: …the OMB 2000 [initiative on reorganization] … resulted in the shrinking of the statutory office you had, OFFM, from a staff of 41 down to 20, and I know they're supposedly working off here in other places and things. Do they report back to you or how do you do that? I guess the basic question is, are you still able to do your job with only 20 people?

Mr. DeSeve: One of the criticisms of the management side of OMB is that it never talked to the budget side, so we sent our agents out into the budget side. We have them burrowed into the budget side. Whether it's cash management or whether it's debt collection or whether it's getting budget people for the first time to look at an audited financial statement, understand and interpret it…

Sen. Glenn: …when they first proposed this thing … I didn't see how you were going to put people out [there] without getting them preempted out there, wherever they are, and you have to have absolute trust that these people are feeding you back all the information you need or the system doesn't work right, it seems to me. Is it working?

Mr. DeSeve: Yes, sir. I think it is. Yesterday we had a need—very quickly—within a couple of hours to prepare some answers to some legislative questions. I called on the people who formerly had been in our organization, for example, asking questions about IRS. They used to be in our place. I said, "how are they doing?" Within 10 minutes I got a response back from an individual, giving me chapter and verse of what was going on there. And we had other situations that were very similar to it yesterday.

Sen. Glenn: Since these people are supposedly reporting to you but they're being paid out there, have you had any cases, so far, where their boss … has said … "I'd just as soon you didn't tell all this stuff up there, because … I don't think he should know this." Any cases like that?

Mr. DeSeve: None that I know of. In fact, it's actually been the reverse. Our folks have affected, we believe, the budget side of the

> House with the need for better financial management, giving us a
> lot of leverage. Instead of losing 20, we think we've probably
> gained 200 [analysts].[67]

This testimony demonstrated that Mr. DeSeve was confident in the capability of OMB to fulfill the requirements of CFOA and GPRA. The then
new Director of OMB, Franklin Raines, indicated that OFFM and the budget staff appeared to be moving in the same direction to implement the
Acts. Furthermore, department financial and accounting staff opposed to
the CFOA and GPRA had not been able to convince their top leadership
that what OMB wants under the Acts is unreasonable or unobtainable. Still,
departments argued convincingly that some changes requested by OMB
(e.g., significantly redesigned accounting systems) are presently unafford-
able. Finding the dollars necessary to improve financial systems in the current climate may be a significant barrier to reform despite acceptance of
the goals of the Acts. Absence of funding also could provide an excuse for
departments that fail to obtain clean opinions (i.e., no errors) in audits of
their financial statements. Nonetheless reform continues and the integration in OMB of budget and management tasks appears to be working.

WEAKNESSES IN FINANCIAL STATEMENTS

Counterpoint observed that financial statements for one year may confirm
facts already known by department financial managers but, to use financial
statement data effectively, trend data from multiple years is needed and
that most departments do not possess reliable trend data outside of budgetary accounts. And even here, data bases are weak in some departments.[68]

It is too early to draw a conclusion on this criterion, but financial statements have been prepared and audited for selected agencies. All agencies
prepared statements for 1997 and there is every intention to build reliable
data bases that will enable trend analysis. OMB's 1995 *Federal Financial
Management Report* indicated steady progress in producing and auditing
financial statements. As of July 1995, 100 entities had been audited and
58% were given a clean opinion, meaning that their statements were presented fairly in accordance with the basis of accounting adopted by the
agency. Forty-three percent were reported by auditors as having no material weakness in internal controls, meaning that the design or operation of
one or more of the internal control elements reduced to a relatively low
risk any errors or irregularities occurring in amounts material to the financial statement. If any errors or irregularities occurred, they would be
detected in a timely manner by employees performing their assigned func-

tions. In contrast, only three entities were audited and only one had a clean opinion in 1990.[69]

While this is an indication of substantial progress, many issues remain. Some experts have proposed a selective, rather than comprehensive audit approach, urging that attention be focused on what can be audited and what is most important to audit. As explained by Mr. Edward Sheridan of the Federal Executive Institute in testimony before Congress:

> ...rather than look at DOD as a huge entity, it's so big, it's so complex, that you can never get your arms around; if you go down to the legal entity basis, find those entities that we can audit and are auditable; do them first and have a program of systematic audits so there would be a score card that will say, okay, there are some issues out here that are going to be so difficult to deal with ... In the meantime, you go to those entities that are part of the cutting edge delivery of services and make sure that they're working. I'd far rather know that the air combat command is doing its job well. It's got its financial house in order, then trying to account for some bombs that have been out in the deserts for 20 or 30 years.[70]

Mr. Phillips of Coopers and Lybrand offered two recommendations to Congress regarding the use of financial statements and performance data.[71] First, he suggested that Congress should be observed using financial statements and performance data when deliberating over budget requests. Second, if financial and performance statements are not viewed as helping agencies in the budget process, he felt that agencies might become discouraged and not put forth the effort needed to meet the requirements of the CFOA and GPRA.

The CFO and GPRA initiatives appear to have increased attention markedly to how financial and performance statement data may be used in detecting and resolving financial problems, e.g., identifying previously unidentifiable disbursements and eliminating overpayment of contractors in DOD, or defining unspecified revenues and identifying pending liabilities in Treasury. However, what must be guarded against is promising too much from financial statement data. Financial statements do not provide enough of the right kinds of data to support budget anaalysis for example. Even if departments and OMB are able to integrate financial and performance data in a way that relates to budget accounts, caution must be exercised to avoid sweeping claims of success. The road to Federal government financial management and budget reform is littered with similar, politically motivated promises that tend to turn off Washington insiders who have watched as the various initiatives have blossomed and withered with the passing of Presidential regimes.

INABILITY TO SUCCESSFULLY IMPLEMENT PERFORMANCE MEASUREMENT IN BUDGETING

Counterpoint predicted that performance measurement as required by the GPRA might not be implemented well or at all by departments and agencies. It also suggested that performance measurement is expensive to perform properly. If performance measurement were affordable and easy to accomplish, it already would have been done, since the Federal government has attempted to implement performance budgeting in one form or another from the late 1940s through the 1950s when Maurice Stans was Director of the Bureau of the Budget under President Eisenhower.[72]

In reviewing the evidence thus far, more than 70 pilot performance measurement projects were submitted by twenty-seven agencies in 1995 in response to OMB's request for proposals to conduct performance measurement experiments[73] under the authority of the GPRA. It is apparent that few agencies wanted to be left out of the performance measurement initiative. Given that the budget will eventually be the primary leverage point available to OMB to enforce the requirements of the CFOA, GMRA, and GPRA, agencies apparently have perceived that they needed to be viewed as willing and eager to play in this new game.

What will result from these experiments is uncertain. A repackaging of measures already in use is one alternative. Preliminary reports from a diversity of agencies demonstrate successful implementation of portions of the GPRA mandate. These agencies include the Department of Transportation's Office of Budget and Program Performance, The Defense Logistics Agency, The Office of Strategic Planning in the Department of the Treasury, the Office of Policy and Strategic Planning, National Oceanic and Atmospheric Administration (Department of Commerce), and the Bureau of Reclamation, Department of the Interior.[74]

The GAO has issued reports to help agencies implement GPRA in which understandable instructions on how to define missions and outcomes and to develop performance measures are provided.[75] The experience of these agencies shows that strategic and performance plans including measurable indicators of performance can be prepared successfully. Moreover, agencies reported that they benefitted from the experience—the goal was not mere compliance with GPRA and OMB directives. Strategic and performance planning enabled review and reformulation of agency missions, achieved greater clarity of objectives, and resulted in a better understanding of relationships between missions and outcomes.

OMB envisions eventual development of definitive performance measures linked to accurate cost accounting with results issued in "Accountability Reports" in conformance to National Performance Review imperatives. This is a worthwhile goal, one shared by many governments worldwide, and real progress has been made in some venues, e.g., New Zealand.[76] OMB recognizes that the leap from performance measurement as required by GPRA to performance budgeting, which is not required, is fraught with problems, not the least of which is the need for accurate cost accounting data. Since FASAB produced and OMB issued accounting principals and standards for the Federal government in 1996 and departments and agencies are training employees in compliance with these, it will be awhile before we can determine the result of all this activity. The intent to do it well is present in OMB, and there is no doubt that congressional oversight committees want the data. We still maintain that appropriators will resist what they perceive as "budgeting by formula" because it will reduce their discretion and power.

The risk that OMB will tilt at windmills in attempting to implement performance measurement under a single template in Federal organizations tremendously diverse in mission and operation seems to be low. OMB policy guidance appears to circumvent this problem. OMB wants to avoid creating a blizzard of paper containing useless information of the type that helped kill zero-based budgeting, and such a goal is probably obtainable. Nevertheless, the utility of performance data will continue to be subject to interpretation. Experimentation with performance budgeting pilot projects began in 1997 for FY 98 and beyond, but all parties involved in GPRA implementation were cautious about the outcome of the pilot projects. In the end, Congress bears the responsibility for determining whether performance measurement and budgeting pilots reveal sufficient promise to cause wider application across the Federal government.[77]

BUDGETARY INCENTIVES TO AVOID IDENTIFICATION OF FULL PROGRAM COSTS

Counterpoint concluded that the CFO Act may fail to meet its goal of causing the full costs of programs to be considered from a financial management perspective at the point of decision due to the fact that some agency budget analyst and decision makers might not be skilled enough to apply net present value to determine appropriate discount rates or to carefully weigh benefit—cost ratios of alternatives from a long-range financial perspective.[78]

The point of this criticism was that decision makers and program advocates in some instances do not want the full costs of decisions to be assessed in budgeting. Alteration of this incentive structure through implementation of CFOA, GMRA, and GPRA is unlikely. There remain very real incentives for departments and agencies to hide the full costs of comprehensive social welfare, national defense, public land management, transportation, energy and other programs in the Federal budget decision process. This tactic that rewards full cost concealment in the budget process was identified long ago by Aaron Wildavsky (1964, pp. 111–113) as the "camels nose" strategy.

The manner in which Congress makes decisions in the annual budget cycle at times stimulates the concealing of full costs. However, in considering the budget from a long-term perspective to achieve balance, and in attempting to insure the financial stability of entitlement programs including Social Security, Medicare, and Medicaid, both Congress and the Executive demonstrate an increasing ability to use more sophisticated analytical methods in budgeting. Appropriations committees now deal with some budget requests based on present value estimates, especially in credit programs and for major capital acquisitions. Appropriators are also particularly sensitive to full cost disclosure in this era of capped domestic discretionary spending. Congressional staff suggest that appropriators do not seek to hide full program costs, but rather have led the fight against "coercive deficiencies." They also note that appropriators are not so much resistant to using financial statement data, but rather have never been given clear examples of how and why such broadly aggregated and dated information ("quite dated" in the words of one staffer) should be used in the appropriations process. Moreover, congressional staff support our previous assertion that aggregated data is generally inconsistent with the congressional appropriation budget structure and cycle.[79]

Philosophically, some members of Congress and staff are likely to resist performance-based budgeting as a mechanistic approach to resource allocation because it assumes certain linear cause and effect relationships, while "very little of the Federal government is so innocently linear."[80] However, whatever the virtues of the appropriators, Congressional resource allocation decisions in the 1990s have typically involved "end games" of continuing resolutions, government shutdowns, omnibus appropriation acts and reconciliation bills where pursuit of macro goals often requires dysfunctional side payments that confound logical approaches to resource allocation, such as performance indicators tied to costs.

UNACHIEVABLE REQUIREMENTS FOR AGENCY COOPERATION AND COMPROMISE IN IMPLEMENTATION

Counterpoint observed that implementation of the CFO Act [and GPRA] requires extensive cooperation and coordination between OMB, the Department of the Treasury, GAO, 24 departments and agencies, two oversight committees of Congress, authorization and appropriations committees, the CFO Council, the Federal Accounting Standards Advisory Board and other entities. It was noted that the track record for cooperation, coordination and compromise of this magnitude between and among Federal government entities in attempting broad scale reform was mixed at best.[81]

We are pleased to report that the necessity for cooperation, coordination and compromise does not appear to present a substantial barrier to implementation of the Acts. This is due to the determination of OMB, Congress, GAO and others that reform will succeed and will provide an example that government can be made to "work." OMB is determined that traditional defenses of turf will not dominate efforts to implement the various provisions of the Acts. Differences on technical issues have been and continue to be addressed by OFFM and other OMB staff, by GAO, and by departments and agencies. Issues such as accounting standards and inventory valuation methods have been addressed responsibly by FASAB and GAO. This is not to say that all departments agree with the results. Several departments have expressed reservations over some of the financial and cost standards. Most departments remain somewhat skeptical about whether performance measurement is worth the cost and effort. The extent that their skepticism is validated by experience will tend to slow the implementation process. However, it seems clear that it will not stop it.

GPRA IMPLEMENTATION: 2001–2005

Review of CFO and GPRA and their associated vehicles as of 2001 suggests that steady progress is being made, albeit slowly. GPRA seemed to have attained a higher level of visibility with its broad bipartisan support, its emphasis on government accountability and performance and its focus on the actual results of government actions, outcomes rather than outputs. Its insistence on the requirement that agency results be integrated into the budget process makes it rare among governmental reforms as does the fact that much of it has been carried out in a climate of downsizing, reinvention, and privatization of government functions. Moreover, GPRA is law; unlike other reforms that were the whim of one administration or another (Carter and zero-based budgeting; Nixon and management by objectives), GPRA has statutory underpinnings for its performance measurement requirements.[82] Moreover, GPRA has been marked with the steady deployment of a more and more complex set of apparatus, with the Strategic Plans due September of 1997, Performance Plans in 1998 submitted with each budget and revised to reflect actions in the President's budget and the Performance Reports first due in March 2000 and annually thereafter. This steady cascade of key implementation measures would give the appearance that progress was being made even if it were not. Let there be no mistake, progress is being made and progress of an impressive nature. Documents posted on the Internet trace this progress. A compilation of Better Features of Annual Performance Plans for FY99 are cited in Exhibit 1.

EXHIBIT 1
Better Features of FY1999 GPRA Implementation Plans

Department of Agriculture

Agricultural Research Service—Aggregate display of total funding by goal by program activity.

Animal Plant Health Inspection Service—Presentation of related performance information at different levels of detail from general goal to annual workload indicators.

Agricultural Research Service—Specific performance goals for research over a multi-year period.

Agency for International Development

Presentation of outcome goals.

Commerce

Performance goals presented in a multi-year array; several performance indicators for each goal. Performance goals linked to strategic goals and objectives.

Table of cross-cutting programs and activities grouped by agency, and cross-walked by Department of Commerce component and activity.

Education

Integrated presentation for an objective distinguishing between budgetary and non-budgetary strategies.

Environmental Protection Agency

Display of resources by appropriation account for each objective; resources displayed are specific to the objective since appropriations fund more than one objective.

Health and Human Services

Office of Child Support—Performance goals for a state-administered program with brief description of the use and value of the measure; Description of means and strategies.

Office of Refugee Resettlement—Performance goals (including outcome goals) for a program administered by states and voluntary agencies. Description of external factors that could effect achievement of the performance goals.

Interior
Cascade of strategic goal, strategic objective and annual goals.

Labor
Crosswalk of Strategic Goal Area by Congressional Committee.

National Science Foundation
Descriptive statement of a successful program and a minimally effective program.

Transportation
Cascade of goals from Department-wide to component to grouping by strategic goal area.

Integration of information by goal.

Prevalence of Outcome goals.

Description of means and strategies.

Cross-cutting strategies.

Treasury
Tabular array containing actual performance levels for FY95–97, planned performance levels for FY97; estimated levels for FY98; projected levels for FY99.

Veterans Affairs
Crosswalk by agency, illustrating scope of cross-cutting VA activities and programs.

(Other features were cited, but this list of best practices illustrates the complexity of the effort to comply with GPRA as well as the progress being made.)

The FY 2000 plans were critiqued in a series of letters sent to the 24 major Federal departments and agencies in August of 1999 by Senator Fred Thompson, then Chairman of the Senate Government Governmental Affairs Committee which has major oversight responsibilities for GPRA. These letters were based on committee staff work and GAO evaluations of each FY 2000 GPRA implementation plan. In general, Thompson praised each agency for the progress it had made over the last year and identified the most important work to be done in implementing its FY 2000 plan. Most agencies were characterized in the letters as having made moderate improvements from the previous year. The Department of Education is a typical example. It was praised for making moderate improvement in addressing the weaknesses of the FY 1999 GPRA implementation plan. The major strengths of the FY 2000 plan were cited as "(1) its performance objectives and indicators are generally objective and measurable; (2) it includes baseline or trend data for most performance indicators; (3) it discusses the role of external factors on the Department's ability to achieve its objectives; (4) it describes the limitations of its data and measures to verify the reliability of performance measures; (5) it describes specific validation and verification efforts; and (6) it shows how evaluations will be used to mitigate performance measurement shortcomings."

GAO found that the Department of Education FY 2000 implementation plan had four key weaknesses: "(1) some performance measures do not sufficiently cover key aspects of performance; (2) it does not discuss coordination of specific programs with similar programs in other agencies; (3) it does not include separate discussions of how capital assets, mission critical management systems, or human capital will support achievement of program results; and (4) it does not indicate how some data limitations will be resolved."

Thompson concluded by saying that overall GAO had found Education's plan to be among the more useful of the 24 agencies included in the GAO evaluation and closed by commending the Secretary and his staff. In general, this was how most of the letters unrolled.

USAID was urged to develop "clearer linkage between broad development goals and specific USAID country program goals and results." USDA strengths were that it used goals and measures that addressed program results and performance; used intermediate outputs to show progress toward intended results, and explained how proposed capital assets and management systems supported achievement of program results. However, GAO found that the Agriculture FY 2000 plan had three key weaknesses: it did not consistently include strategies for mitigating external factors; it did not adequately describe efforts to verify and validate data; and it did not consistently discuss the impact of data limitations. The Department of Commerce was criticized for the absence of complementary performance goals and measures for the many crosscutting programs and activities in which Commerce shared responsibility with other Federal agencies. Thompson warned that this shortcoming was particularly serious in view of the fact that Commerce was essentially a "holding company" composed of numerous disparate missions, programs, and activities.

Thompson also warned that performance goals for management problems should be included in the performance plan. Moreover, Thompson noted, Commerce's FY 2000 performance plan addressed only two of the ten high risk problem areas identified in the Department by GAO and the Department's Inspector General.

Of DOD, Thompson wrote that he continued to be concerned with the financial managment problems that continued to plague the Department: "Weaknesses in DOD's financial management operations continue to hinder its ability to effectively manage its $250 billion budget and $1 trillion in assets. GAO wrote recently that DOD's Biennial Financial Management Improvement Plan lacks critical elements necessary for producing sustainable financial management improvement over the long term. Specifically, the Plan's discussion of how DOD's financial management operations will work in the future—its concept of operations—does not address: how its financial management operations will effectively support not only financial reporting but also asset accountability and control; and budget formulation." Thompson noted that this was one of approximately 50 open GAO recommendations made to improve the credibility of DOD's financial reporting and financial statement preparation.[83] Thompson then enclosed a number of recommendations made by the Inspector General and GAO. In sum, the tone of these letters was positive and it was clear that significant improvements had been made and more could be expected. It was also clear that significant problems remained for all agencies as they attempted to envision concrete ways to affect outcomes and particularly for those agencies with complex missions. All of this needs to be reevaluated by 2005.

CRITICISM OF GPRA

Criticism of GPRA has focused on the complexity of its mission, credibility of the data produced, and its focus.[84] GAO has pointed out that performance measures chosen by agencies do not meet Congressional needs for oversight data and that agencies have problems producing credible performance data. These two points were eminently predictable from the start of GPRA. What was perhaps not as easily foreseen was the complexity of government and the grandiosity of the GPRA intent. GAO has noted that virtually *all government results are produced by two or more agencies* and, as a consequence, mission fragmentation and overlap are widespread and cross-cutting programs are poorly coordinated, resulting in wasted dollars, customers who are confused and frustrated and the undermining of overall effectiveness. The best features list above shows the attention paid to cross-cutting goal identification, both those that exist within Departments but between or among agencies, and between and among Departments. Unfortunately identifying cross-cutting goals does not mean that problems of coordination and focus and unity of effort are solved. GAO further notes that many stated goals are outside the control of Agencies, Departments and even government. For example, those agencies that would improve the economy or the environment or an ecosystem, do not really have the capability to do so. They may have some impact on those targets, but events totally unrelated and outside the control of the agencies may dilute, reverse or overturn their efforts. The attempt to specify outcomes—

the move to some desirable end state—may always risk setting up a goal that is not realistically attainable solely through government action. Yet to stop at output measures is inherently self-defeating. GPRA may be used as a cost-cutting measure as it encourages government to operate more efficiently, but it is inherently very optimistic in its specification of outcomes that improve government and the life of the governed. Perhaps the bottom-line is that outcomes must be plausibly seen to be impacted favorably by government action. In this sense a carefully crafted statement is far superior to an exaggerated statement of what might happen, in the sense that to reduce the effect of evil is plausible when ridding the world of evil is not plausible and only calls into question the amount of resources used to pursue an unobtainable goal.

The structure of American government also poses a problem for GPRA. Very few public service provision functions are performed by the Federal government alone. Even defense relies on state level components like the National Guard or cooperation from private sector contractors to produce weapons systems at acceptable prices. For agencies who pass money through to states and local governments in grants and aids or who pay nonprofit corporations for health or welfare delivery services, the problem of cross-cutting complexity and goal specification and attainment are equally difficult. Block grant agencies who pass money to states have problems specifying outcomes because they cannot bind states to pursuing those outcomes; states may have other items on their agenda than Federal goals. Following a 1999 survey, OMBwatch said that GPRA is being taken seriously by the Federal government, but that its influence over Federal agencies and programs was small at that time, however "GPRA coordinators believe its influence will grow."[85]

OMBwatch suggested that GPRA's influence over nonprofits may likewise grow, although the rate of growth will be slow because of the layers of state and local governments lying between Federal, state, and local governments and many nonprofit service delivery agencies. OMBwatch observed that the nonprofit community was only dimly aware of GPRA and that Federal agencies whose money ultimately went to nonprofits were similarly unaware of nonprofits. OMBwatch warned that this would be a problem for goal setting and for goal achievement, for measures that are not correctly chosen can end promoting outcomes that are undesirable. OMBwatch advocated more nonprofit interest and involvement in GPRA by nonprofits and a reaching out to all stakeholders by those implementing the law at the Federal level, including both Congress and the executive branch agencies. In 2000, Ellen Taylor of OMBwatch observed that GPRA success still depends on government's commitment to it and that there was considerable uncertainty about whether GPRA was working.

Taylor observed that there was not a lot of public awareness of GPRA. She warned that GPRA should not be used as a partisan tool, e.g., by either the executive or Congress to attempt to score political points off the other, and concluded that performance was not the whole story. She noted that surveys had found that satisfaction with specific government services was rising measurably and nearly on a par with the private sector, but that trust in government had only slightly increased and remained low, still not rising to the level of trust obtained in surveys taken in 1988. In her testimony she urged Congress to focus on successes in government and on the way its services are improving, rather than to maintain a focus on failures.[86] She also urged that public access to information used to develop performance measures be improved and suggested that public knowledge in itself may lead to corrective measures. As a case in point, she observed: "Although EPA never identified specific amounts of reduction in emission of toxic chemicals, the public accessibility of the Toxics Release Inventory helped create a 45% decline in the release of those chemicals."[87] This again suggests the great optimism which underlies GPRA efforts, reminiscent of the 'If you build it, they will come,' line from the movie *Field Of Dreams*, only with GPRA the premise is '…give them the right information and they will do the right thing.' At this point the reader might want to consider theorists who perceived the world in darker hues—Hobbes, for example—and suggest that much of government has to do with the coercion necessary to get people to do the right thing.

CONGRESS AND CROSS-CUTTING PROGRAM PROBLEMS

Cross-cutting programs pose a special problem for Congress because it is not set up to review, fund, or exercise oversight of cross-cutting programs. Chris Mihm of GAO re-enforces this point:

> Unfocused and uncoordinated crosscutting programs waste scarce resources, confuse and frustrate taxpayers and program beneficiaries, and limit overall program effectiveness. Our work in over 40 program areas across the government has repeatedly shown that mission fragmentation and program overlap are widespread, and that crosscutting Federal program efforts are not well-coordinated. For example, we have reported on 50 programs for the homeless that were administered by 8 Federal agencies. Housing services were provided under 23 programs operated by 4 agencies, and food and nutrition services were under 26 programs administered by 6 agencies.[88]

Mihm argued that the government-wide performance plan and the agencies' annual performance plans and subsequent performance reports should provide Congress with information on agencies and programs addressing similar results. Once these programs have been identified, then Congress can consider the associated policy, management, and performance implications of crosscutting programs as part of its oversight over the Executive branch. Mihm notes that this will present challenges to the traditional committee structures and processes and observes that Congress has no direct mechanism to use in providing a Congressional perspective to the President's government-wide performance plan or to agency goals, missions and alternatives, particularly for mission areas and programs that cut across committee jurisdictions. It seems that the logical outcome of oversight of GPRA efforts will have to change the structure of Congress, itself, an effort not lightly undertaken or easily accomplished.

Building, maintaining, and marshaling human capital seems to still be problematic. Mihm concluded that most of the fiscal year 2000 performance plans do not sufficiently address how the agencies will use their human capital to achieve results:

> Although the plans often discuss human capital issues in general terms, such as recruitment and training efforts, they do not consistently discuss other key human capital strategies used by high-performing organizations. For example, few agencies discussed how they would build, maintain, and marshal the human capital needed to achieve their performance goals. This suggests that one of the critical components of high-performing organizations—the systematic integration of human capital planning and program planning—is not being adequately and uniformly addressed across the Federal government.[89]

Although the need for specific training in the elements of GPRA is necessarily not as great as it was in the early years of the Act, human capital problems still remain.

CONCLUSIONS

Most financial management reform is neither exciting nor high profile. It is complex and no one discipline has a monopoly on the skills needed to accomplish it. Reform must be concerned with a myriad of small but important issues in addition to the big questions, because little issues often add up to important matters of Federal policy and practice—and perhaps to billions of dollars either saved or lost through inefficiency and misguided reform.[90] Further, Federal financial management reform advocates are concerned with prospects for obtaining sufficient funding to implement needed reforms. This concern is legitimate given the certainty of tight domestic budgets from the President and Congress.

The attraction of some aspects of reform remains persistent: Speaking of GPRA Congressman Dick Armey noted:

This tool gives Congress the ability to identify what's working, what's not, what's wasted, what's duplicative, and to end wasteful and unnecessary spending. These laws are not ends in themselves; rather they are a means to obtain systematic, credible information about the operations of the Federal government, while holding government accountable to the taxpayers. The core tenet of the Results Act is '...you get what you measure.'

Armey observed that the "urgent," too often crowds out the time for issues that are merely "important," that too much time is spent on fighting fires and not enough on preventing them. Said Armey: "GPRA forces us to take the long view: to consider our goals and measure our results."[91]

With respect to progress on implementation of the CFO Act, early returns were very positive. In 1995, Coopers & Lybrand and the Association of Government Accountants polled nearly 100 Federal agencies to assess the implementation of the CFO Act and related legislation. The sample consisted of 124 senior financial managers, CFOs, and deputy CFOs; 26 Inspectors General, and 150 program managers. Seventy-five percent of the senior financial managers, 81% of the Inspectors General, and 66% of the program managers noted broad leadership support for the CFO Act at the Secretary, Deputy Secretary, and Assistant Secretary levels. All three groups agreed that the benefits of the annual financial statements justify the initial cost and effort. The Inspectors General overwhelmingly agreed that the CFO Act has contributed to improved financial operations, with 80% reporting improved financial systems; ninety-six percent noted improvement in financial data, and, most significantly, 100% recognized that, as a result of the CFOA and GPRA, internal control procedures were improving. Both the financial managers and the IG's suggested that the process of developing statements was more valuable than the actual statements themselves because the process contributed to a better understanding of program costs and what drives these costs.[92]

To gauge agency progress on financial reporting, the survey analysis of responses from senior financial managers, including the CFOs and deputy CFOs, and the 26 IG's revealed that nearly 80% were preparing most of the documents and reports required by CFO Act and GPRA. Although much work remained in developing the performance measures, 86% reported at least partial progress. Progress also was reported in integrating financial statement information into the budget process by about half of the respondents. The bottom line was that 70% of the financial managers and 62% of the IGs believed that their organizations would have auditable financial statements by the March 1, 1997 deadline.[93] While these conclusions are most optimistic with respect to financial statements versus the full panoply of requirements of CFOA and GPRA, they do indicate satisfaction with progress in implementing the key provisions of both Acts. Our research reinforced the findings of this survey. Implementation of the CFOA was proceeding to produce the outputs required by law, although large complex agencies were moving predictably more slowly. With regard to the GPRA we are far less confident that the results desired when the legislation was passed will be realized. Furthermore, we are not sure that much of what this Act requires should be implemented beyond the agency and department level where it appears to have strengthened strategic planning and linkage between plans and budgets in many instances. Given the difficulties of full implementation of results-oriented budgeting detailed previously in this book, we are skeptical that Congress is able to handle or is willing to use the analyses produced as required by the law. The arguments we have advanced in favor of output-oriented budgeting are compelling, but they require institutional reform in Congress and the Executive in order to be implemented successfully, and the likelihood of adoption of such comprehensive reform seems slim.

It is apparent that absence of strong support from the President, OMB and Congress would retard the effort to implement the CFOA and GPRA and the new Federal financial management structure supported by this and other financial management reform legislation. However, Presidents Clinton and Bush have supported implementation of these reforms. OMB has been steadfast in its determination to move ahead with resolve. Sean O'Keefe, Deputy Director, OMB, in a letter of May 11, 2001, reviewed the GAO report on a survey of Federal managers regarding results-oriented agency climates, measurement of program performance, and use of performance information to make decisons in high performance organizations. O'Keefe said, "It is encouraging that significantly more managers overall reported having performance measure (both outputs and outcomes) for their programs. But it is disappointing that you found a significant decrease in the reported use of performance information from your last report" (in 1997). O'Keefe continued that these findings were "consistent with our view that while many agencies have made substantial progress implementing the Government Performance and Results Act (GPRA), many others are still simply going through the motions. While all are in full compliance with the law—preparing strategic and annual plans and finalizing performance reports—most are not yet at a stage where they are truly 'managing for results.'"

O'Keefe added that systematic inclusion of performance into budget decisions had yet to occur, that GPRA "has not been fully harnessed to improve management and program performance." He then promised that OMB was going to formally integrate performance with budget decisions and that program managers would be held accountable for managing to targets. His letter indicates that these plans would come to fruition in the FY 2004 budget where detailed performance and budget data will establish a strong public link between agency budget requests and performance measurement in the President's budget.

It appears that this implementation effort will not fail to garner support under the Bush administration. Whether this support will result in more funding for departments for accounting system improvements, employee training, and other necessary ingredients to enable real reform remain key issues.

NOTES

1.   Responsibility for GPRA is placed in the hands of the Director of OMB. Under the 1993 reorganization (OMB 2000) the Director placed responsibility for implementation with each of the five Resource Management Offices (RMOs) and responsibility for coordination with the Budget Review Division (BRD). This structure may be changed at the discretion of the Director.

2.   See the Committee Report accompanying GPRA, Senate Report 103-58, especially 18-19. See also Genevieve J. Knezo, *Government Performance and Results Act, P. L. 103-62: Interim Status Report: Revised.* CRS Report for Congress. 95-713 SPR. June 15, 1995.

3.   "Managing for Results: Achieving GPRA's Objectives Requires Strong Congressional Role" (Testimony, 03/06/96, GAO/T-GGD-96-79), p. 5.

4.   Charles Bowsher, Comptroller General of the United States, *Statement,* before the Committee on Governmental Affairs of the U.S. Senate, December 14, 1995, p. 2.

5.   Joshua Gotbaum. Executive Associate Director and Controller, Acting Deputy Director for Management, U.S. Office of Management and Budget in Testimony before the House Committee on Government Reform, Subcommittee on Government Management, Information and Technology, July 20, 2000.

6.   Gotbaum, 2000.

7.   "Managing for Results: Achieving GPRA's Objectives Requires Strong Congressional Role" (Testimony, 03/06/96, GAO/T-GGD-96-79), p. 5.

8.   Rep. Dick Armey in Testimony before the House Committee on Government Reform, Subcommittee on Government Management, Information and Technology, July 20, 2000.

9.   See part 2, OMB Circular A-11, *Preparation and Submission of Annual Budget Estimates,* and the memorandum from the Director, Alice Rivlin titled *Strategic Plans, Budget Formulation and Execution,* OMB, Washington, DC, September 1995.

10.   GMRA accelerated the adoption of auditable financial statements and increased the number of CFOs and required a government-wide financial statement by 1998. See Al Gore (1995, p. 86), *Common Sense Government: Works Better and Costs Less. Third Report of the National Performance Review.* Washington, DC: U.S. Government Printing Office.

11.   Gotbaum, Testimony (2000).

12.   Starting in 1993, DOD established seven GPRA performance measurement pilots: Defense Logistics Agency (DLA); Air Combat Command (ACC); Army Research Laboratory (ARL); Defense Commissary Agency (DeCA); U.S. Army Corps of Engineers Civil Works National Operation and Maintenance Program; Army Audit Agency, and a CINCLANTFLT Carrier Battle Group.

13.   These included: Objectives of Federal Financial Reporting; Entity and Display; Accounting for Selected Assets and Liabilities; Accounting for Direct Loans and Loan Guarantees; Accounting for Inventory and Related Property; Managerial Cost Accounting Concepts and Standards; Accounting for Liabilities of the Federal Government; Accounting for Property, Plan, and Equipment. "Form and Content of Agency Financial Statements," *OMB Bulletin,* pp. 94–01.

14.   Financial and cost accounting standards for the Federal government are provided in FASAB, *Managerial Cost Accounting Concepts and Standards for the Federal Government,* Washington, DC, June 1995. These standards were promulgated by OMB: *Statement of Federal Financial Accounting Standards,* Number 4, 1996.

15.   *Federal Financial Management Status Report & Five Year Plan,* July 2000. Washington, DC: U.S.Government Printing Office, p. 6.

16.   Status Report (2000).

17.   Franklin Raines, Keynote Address, GPRA Training Symposium, Bureau of Labor Statistics, October 7, 1996.

18.   By June, 1996, five agencies had issued pilot Accountability Reports for fiscal year 1995. These included the Social Security Administration, General Services Administration, National Aeronautics and Space Administration, Department of Veterans Affairs, and Nuclear Regulatory Commission. The reports consolidated data from the CFO Act financial reports, performance information required by the GPRA, and reviews of management controls under the Federal Managers' Financial Integrity Act (FMFIA). See "Financial Management Status Report and 5-Year Plan Issued," *JFMIP NEWS,* Summer 1996, 8(2), p.1.

19.   See The Federal Workforce Restructuring Act (FWRA) of 1994 (P. L. 103-226) that made these cuts was enacted March 30, 1994. See also P.L.103-130, 1994, (*Congressional Quarterly,* 1994, p. 2872); also *Statement* by Alice Rivlin, Director of OMB before the Senate Committee on Governmental Affairs, May 17, 1995, p. 4.

20.   See *Statement* of R. Scott Fosler, President of the National Academy of Public Administration before the Senate Committee on Governmental Affairs May 17, 1995, *Federal News Service* (FNS), p. 193. By the end of 1994, Federal employment had already been cut by 100,000 positions. Rivlin *Statement,* May 17, 1995, *FNS,* p. 176.

21.   From *Historical Statistics of the U. S. Budget, FY2002.* Table 17.5, p. 284.

22.   Fosler, *Statement,* May 17, 1995, *FNS,* p. 93. Fosler also adds that there is some evidence that the most experienced and capable people were leaving government, sometimes enticed by buyouts, just at the time their special knowledge was needed.

23.   Fosler, 1995.

24.   See "FASAB Standards Completed and Signed by Principals," *FASAB Newsletter,* June 1996, Issue # 35, p. 2.

25.   *Federal Financial Management Status Report & Five Year Plan,* July 1992. Washington, DC: U.S. Government Printing Office, p. 16.

26.   The IRS has been criticized by the GAO for its poor performance in redesigning and reengineering portions of its accounting systems. See GAO, *IRS Compliance Initiative,* AIMD/GDD-95-220, August 1995, and GAO, *Financial Audit: Examination of IRS FY94 Financial Statements,* AIMD-95-141, August 1995. See also GAO financial audits of IRS for FY 92, FY 93, and FY 95 (AIMD-93-2, 94-120, 96-101). The Department of Defense also has experienced difficulty in consolidating and redesigning its mammoth accounting system, partly due to the large number of individual systems operated by the Office of the Secretary and the three Military

Departments. Responsibility for DOD system redesign and consolidation rests with the Defense Financial and Accounting System.

27.   "Foreword," *Five Year Plan*, 1995, p. iii. This estimate is required each year.

28.   *Five Year Plan*, 1995, p. 9.

29.   Bowsher, *Testimony*, Committee on Governmental Affairs of the U.S. Senate December 14, 1995, p. 5.

30.   Bowsher, *Testimony*, Committee on Governmental Affairs of the U.S. Senate December 14, 1995, p.10.

31.   *Five Year Plan*, 1995, p. 5.

32.   *Five Year Plan*, 1995, p. 4. Table 1 was derived from Table 1 Financial Management Systems on page 4. Five (DOD, HUD, USDA, DOT, and Treasury) of the 24 CFO agencies account for 67% of the Federal financial management systems and 53% of the applications, e.g., DOD has 259 systems and 259 applications; USDA has 72 systems and 125 applications. See *Five Year Plan, 1995*, Table 2, p. 5.

33.   The advantage of off the shelf software is that it is generally cheaper than custom tailored applications, training costs are generally lower and transferability is easier and cheaper, including the ability of employees to move from one agency to another with reduced training needs and costs in the new agency.

34.   *Five Year Plan*, 1992, p. 14.

35.   *Five Year Plan*, 1992, p. 14.

36.   Making better use of off the shelf technology is an explicit goal of the 1995 *Five Year Plan*; an ongoing responsibility is cited to "promote sharing of information on off-the-shelf software for various financial management applications. "The responsibility for this goal is shared among the CFO Council, JFMIP, and OMB. See *Five Year Plan*, 1995, p. 10. Another use of software in this area is as an efficiency multiplier using technology to capture data at the outset of a transaction stream and reduce errors now multiplying in the system through clerical errors in repeated entry of the same data into different systems. To quote Ted Sheridan, President of Sheridan Management Corp. and Chairman of the Financial Executive Institute's Committee on Government Liaison: "A lot of the problems are data entry problems. You have all of those clerks out in Columbus and Cleveland, shuffling pieces of paper. The technology exists now. Use image scanning to get it into the system or require that your vendors use electronic commerce so that it's all in digital form. Then, with this, you have the integrity of the data going in. You utilize advanced telecommunications and relational data bases to keep track of it, then you can do exactly what you want ... including unit level reports that you could roll up into total unified statements." *Hearing* of the Senate Governmental Affairs Committee, 12/14/95, *FNS*, 12/15/95, p. 56.

37.   *Federal Financial Management Status Report & Five Year Plan*, November 2000, p. 16.

38.   Mr. Phillips, *Hearing*, 12/14/95. *FNS*, 12/15/95, p. 52.

39.   Mr. Phillips, *Hearing*, 12/14/95. *FNS*, 12/15/95, p. 53.

40.   *Federal Financial Management Status Report & Five Year Plan*, November 2000, p. 6.

41.   *Counterpoint*, pp. 88–89.

42.   John Mercer, Keynote Address "Congressional Perspective on GPRA Implementation," GPRA Training Symposium, October 7, 1996.

43.   *Counterpoint*, p. 89.

44.   Evidence of this is provided by the Federal Workforce Restructuring Act (FWRA) of 1994 (P. L. 103-226) enacted March 30, 1994, in which Congress made substantial cuts in Federal employment.

45.   William Phillips, *Hearing*, 12/14/95. *FNS*, 12/15/95, p. 52.

46.   Sen. Hank Brown, *Hearing*, 12/14/95. *FNS*, 12/15/95, p. 44.

47.   Mr. DeSeve, *Hearing*, before the Senate Committee on Governmental Affairs, 12/15/95. *FNS*, p. 44.

48.   Mr. DeSeve, *Hearing*, Senate Committee on Governmental Affairs, 12/14/95. *FNS*, 12/15/95, p. 44.

49.   Sen. Stevens, *Hearing*, 12/14/95. *FNS*, 12/15/95, p. 43.

50.   Mr. DeSeve, *Hearing*, 12/14/95. *FNS*, 12/15/95, p. 45.

51.   Mr. DeSeve, *Hearing*, 12/14/95. *FNS*, 12/15/95, p. 45.

52.   Mr. DeSeve, *Hearing*,12/14/95. *FNS*, 12/15/95, p. 46.

53.   Sen. Glenn, *Hearing*,12/14/95. *FNS*, 12/15/95, pp. 45–46.

54.   Sen. Glenn, *Hearing*, 12/14/95. *FNS*, 12/15/95, p. 62.

55.   William R. Phillips, Partner, Government Consulting Practice, Coopers and Lybrand L.L.P. in *testimony* before the Senate Governmental Affairs Committee 12/14/95. *FNS*, 12/15/95, p. 61. Phillips adds that the ratio had been $6 to $1 for "probably 15 or 20 years" in his office, but a reorganization had increased the ratio to 10:1 for the last two years.

56.   William R. Phillips, *Testimony* before the Senate Governmental Affairs Committee 12/14/95. *FNS*, 12/15/95, p. 62.

57.   Sen. Brown asks Deseve "Where are we with regard to the concept of standardized accounts; that is, an account meaning the same thing in the Department of Energy as it means in the Department of Commerce and having some basic accounts which are fairly descriptive across the board." *Mr. DeSeve*: "I think the implementation of the standard general ledger has been—the implementation of a standard general ledger has been our benchmark so far for that, and we are at about ... at about 60% across agencies, in systems which implement the standard general ledger. And that's the first step, as you indicate, to having a code of 503.5 mean the same here as it does there. All of the agencies are moving in that direction, and every new system that is being built implements the standard general ledger. The question of migration and how quickly we migrate towards that; that standard is very clear and agencies are moving towards that standard general ledger very quickly." *Hearing*, Senate Governmental Affairs Committee, 12/14/95. *FNS*, 12/15/95, p. 49.

58.   Sen. Brown, *Hearing*, Senate Governmental Affairs, 12/14/95. *FNS*, 12/15/95, p. 49.

59.   Interview with OMB official, Washington, DC, October 7, 1996.

60.   Armey, *Testimony*, July 20, 2000.

61.   *Counterpoint*, pp. 89–90.

62.   Interview with OMB official, Washington, DC, October 7, 1996.

63.   *Counterpoint*, p. 90.

64.   Quotation from review of a working draft of this paper by OMB staff, March, 1996.

65.   See statement of L. Nye Stevens, Director, Federal Management and Workforce Issues, GAO, before the Subcommittee on Government Management, Information and Technology of the Committee on Government Reform and Oversight of the House of Representatives, on February 7, 1996 titled *OMB 2000: Changes Resulting From the Reorganization of the Office of Management and Budget*. GAO/T-GGD/ AIMD-96-68. GAO, USGPO. Washington, DC, 1996.

66.   Stevens, *Statement*, pp. 4–5.

67.   Mr. DeSeve and Sen. Glenn, *Hearing*, Senate Governmental Affairs, 12/14/95. *FNS*, 12/15/95, pp. 46–49.

68.   *Counterpoint*, pp. 90–91.

69.   *Five Year Plan*, 1995, p. 16.

70.   Mr. Sheridan, *Hearing*, 12/14/95. *FNS*, 12/15/95, p. 56.

71.   Phillips, 1995 (see note 45).

72.   Maurice H. Stans served as deputy director of the Bureau of the Budget for six months in 1957 and then was appointed Director in March 1958, holding the position until 1961. Stans spearheaded efforts to develop performance measures in the Federal budget while in OMB. See also Seckler-Hudson (1978, pp. 80–93). Seckler-Hudson points out that the National Security Act Amendments of 1949 made presentation of performance budgets by the Department of Defense mandatory. The Budget and Accounting Procedures Act of 1950 also is cited as having required performance budgeting in the Federal government (p. 83).

73.   Under the law, performance budget experiments are slated to begin in 1998 and 1999.

74.   Joint Financial Management Improvement Program, *Report on the GPRA Training Symposium* (October 7–8, 1996), CFO Council, Washington, DC.

75.   See Effectively Implementing the Government Performance and Results Act. GAO/GGD-96-118, June 1996.

76.   For an excellent description of New Zealand initiatives, see *Toward Better Governance: Public Service Reform in New Zealand and its Relevance to Canada*. Office of the Auditor General of Canada. Ottawa, Canada, 1995.

77.   See Joyce (1993, p. 46), in its entirety and conclusions. See also Joyce (1993, pp. 3–17; 1996, pp. 70–75). See also Wholey and Hatry (1992, pp. 604–610).

78.   *Counterpoint*, p. 92.

79.   Review of earlier draft of this chapter by Congressional staff, March 1996.

80.   Congressional staff, 1996.

81.   *Counterpoint*, p. 93.

82.   OMBWATCH, *GPRA Basic Information*. GPRA 2000.

83.   The data from this section is taken from a series of letters from Sen. Thompson, Chairman, Senate Governmental Affairs Committee, August 1999.

84.   Recent GAO reports evaluating GPRA include: *Managing for Results: Barriers to Interagency Coordination*, GGD-00-106, March 29, 2000 (23 pp.); *Managing for Results: Challenges Agencies Face in Producing Credible Performance Information*, GGD-00-52, February 4, 2000 (19 pp.); *Managing for Results: Views on Ensuring the Usefulness of Agency Performance Information to Congress*, GGD-00-35, January 26, 2000 (35 pp.); *Managing for Results: Measuring Program Results that are Under Limited Federal Control*, GGD-99-16, December 11, 1998 (24 pp.); *Managing for Results: Opportunities for Continued Improvements in Agencies' Performance Plans*, GGD/AIMD-99-215, July 20, 1999 (124 pp.); *Managing for Results: Analytic Challenges in Measuring Performance*, HEHS/GGD-97-138, May 30, 1997 (44 pp.).

85.   OMBWATCH, *GPRA Study*, 1999.

86.   Ellen Taylor, "Seven Years of GPRA: Has the Results Act provided Results?" Testimony before the House Committee on Government Reform, Subcommittee on Government Management, Information and Technology, July 20, 2000.

87.   The data is taken from the EPA "1998 Toxics Release Inventory Data Summary," EPA-745-00-001, May 2000, p. 4, but the data is so carefully qualified that it is difficult to judge what the real outcome is.

88.   Christopher Mihm, Associate Director, Federal Management and Workforce Issues, General Government Division, GAO, Testimony before the House Committee on Government Reform, Subcommittee on Government Management, Information and Technology, July 20, 2000.

89.   Mihm (2000).

90.   William Phillips of Coopers and Lybrand in Testimony before a *Hearing* of the Senate Governmental Affairs Committee, 12/14/95 in FNS 12/15/95 said "Investing a few million now to implement the CFO Act will yield billions of dollars in savings in the future." *FNS*, 12/15/95, p. 53.

91.   Armey, *Testimony,* July 20, 2000.

92.   See Coopers and Lybrand and the Association of Government Accountants. *Chief Financial Officers Act Survey Results,* September 1995.

93.   William Phillips "Testimony" before a *Hearing* of the Senate Governmental Affairs Committee, 12/14/95. *FNS,* 12/15/95, p. 51.

APPENDIX A

BUDGETING AND FINANCIAL MANAGEMENT CURRICULUM AND COURSE DESIGN

INTRODUCTION

Over the past several decades, graduate programs in public affairs have evaluated whether and how to expand course offerings in public financial management. In part this effort has responded to student and market demand. However, it also has been motivated by faculty recognition that students need better instruction in financial management concepts and practices, and need improved skills training to perform effectively in the contemporary public sector work environment. In some cases, faculty responsible for teaching budgeting, financial management, and related courses have become aware of the need to modify the traditional public affairs curriculum in the area of finance as a result of interaction with financial management practitioners. The absence of instruction in the basics of accounting and the lack of exposure to financial management concepts and analytical techniques other than those for budgeting have been recognized as weakening the competitiveness of MPA graduates in the employment market.

As new courses in public financial management, government accounting, applied microeconomics, cost/benefit analysis, and related topics have been added to public affairs curricula, the importance of course content and sequencing also has become more evident. In response to the perception of the need for change, the Association for Budgeting and Financial Management of the American Society for Public Administration (ASPA/ABFM) selected a distinguished group of practitioners and academics to serve on a National Task Force on curriculum reform. The Task Force published a final report, "Graduate Curriculum in Budgeting and Financial Management-Recommendations for Reform," dedicated to the memory of Ken Howard. The report was a culmination of the efforts of five working groups: core skills and skill concentrations, curriculum design and institutional constraints, information systems and computer applications, current curricula and course design, and reconceptualizing the role of the budget in the political process. The National Task Force final report recommended a set of thirteen financial management skill concentration areas of expertise as potential components of MPA curricula rather than specifying one particular set of courses. The report did not recommend a single curriculum design. Rather, it stressed that there is not one best way to design a public financial management specialization. Instead, there are multiple approaches and, therefore, the Task Force's specific recommendations on curriculum design permit a fair degree of flexibility across programs. This flexibility is intended to encourage alternative emphases, teaching methods, and course designs.

Prior to issuance of the Task Force's final report, a study by Alexander indicated that major financial management categories could be articulated into various dimensions, subfunctions, and analytical categories: for example, the dimension of budget execution includes cash flow and capital management subfunctions, and expenditures/revenue forecasting analytical foci. Alexander indicated that decisions on curriculum reform should be based upon asking the right questions regarding conceptualization of the context within which financial management functions such as budgeting are performed. Further, he raised the question of content and sequencing of financial management concepts and skills as curriculum design issues as follows.

Which subfunctions in each dimension should be considered part of the core concentration and which considered elective? And at what level of sophistication? How could these be effectively and efficiently organized into courses and many? Which subfunction must be treated and at what level of sophistication before other subfunctions; can be introduced?

MANAGEMENT CONTROL FRAMEWORK

The approach to design of a financial management curriculum presented in this study is based on the recommendations provided by the ASPA Task Force Report and Alexander's study. It assumes that the sequencing of courses and course content topics are important to facilitating student learning. Further, it asserts that a good curriculum integrate as the courses within the context of some unifying framework that relates the parts to the whole. The framework suggested here to accomplish this task is that of the management control cycle. The rationale for using this framework is based upon the assumption that the principal objective of financial management in public organizations is achievement of management control. Furthermore, the management control cycle systematically integrates the functional components of organizational action in the sequence needed to achieve strategic objectives.

The management control cycle has been defined generally as programming, budgeting, control of operations, reporting, and audit. Management control is achieved in public sector organizations to a considerable extent through the development and deployment of financial management systems. Instruction in public financial management concepts, functions, and systems may be provided in consonance with the sequence of management control tasks performed by public and private sector organizations. The concept of controllership as the ordered means for implementing strategic planning provides the theoretical basis for this approach. Design of a public financial management curriculum within the context of controllership is a departure from public administration formulations that tend to view financial management and analysis as institutional support functions, or solely as inputs to policy formulation and decision making.

SEQUENCING AND CONTENT OF COURSES IN THE PUBLIC FINANCIAL MANAGEMENT CURRICULUM

The National Task Force report recommended a six-course financial management component within a two-year, eighteen course MPA program. The Task Force advised that course requirements be flexible across programs to facilitate adjustment to existing MPA curricula that vary widely in emphasis and content. The report also emphasized the importance of building skill concentration areas through the integration of core and elective courses, and recommended that different courses could be offered for a concentration in budgeting versus financial management. For example, core courses for a budgeting concentration suggested in the report included theory and politics, operating budgeting, financial management (including debt management), government accounting, public finance and revenue administration, and forecasting. A financial management concentration would include core courses in financial management, economics (cost/benefit and pricing), government accounting, public finance, budgeting and advanced financial management. Six elective courses also were recommended for each concentration.

The curriculum presented in this appendix offers only one of many potential approaches that might be taken in responding to the ASPA/

ABFM National Task Force recommendations. The concentrations recommended in the task force report are augmented and ordered here into a sequence that is intended to be cumulative so that each course builds skills and understandings that lead to better quality instruction and learning at the next level. As noted, the course sequence is organized according to the management control cycle. The curriculum includes four core courses to be taken by all MPA students and four electives, two of which would be required for all financial management concentration students. All four electives could be taken by MPA students concentrating in financial management. The six-course core requirement conforms to the number recommended by the Task Force. Additional elective courses also are listed as potential substitutes or augmentations to the basic eight-course financial management program. Detailed course descriptions are provided, indicating content covered and sequencing of topics.

Introduction to Management Control

The initial core course in the financial management curriculum is an introduction to management control for government and nonprofit organizations. The management control cycle of program planning, budget preparation, budget execution, operations control, performance measurement, financial reporting, performance evaluation, and audit presented initially and then followed by a step-by-step exploration of each component of the cycle. Also included is an introduction to cost accounting, pricing, output measurement, systems design, and program implementation concepts applied to public sector organizations. The practice and purpose of dividing organizations into centers of revenue, expense, cost, and investment for purposes of measurement and evaluation is explained. Part of the objective of this course is to demonstrate how accounting, budgeting (operating and capital), cash management, and asset acquisition/management systems are used by government to implement controllership objectives. Also emphasized is the point that management control takes for granted the mission and goals of the organization. Thus, strategic planning is identified as a precursor to, rather than a component of, management control. The management course concludes with an overview of the sequence of courses to follow so that students understand the purpose and organization of the curriculum.

Nonprofit Accounting

The second and third courses in the sequence concentrate on accounting, to provide students with the basic skills necessary to understand and perform financial analysis and to manage financial systems effectively. Training in accounting also is intended to enable public affairs program graduates to compete better in the public-sector job market with MBA degree recipients and CPAs.

The second course is an introduction to financial, managerial, and nonprofit accounting concepts and practices. Some faculty and students might prefer that these topic areas be taught as separate courses, and this option may be attractive if such courses are offered adequately by another academic unit (e.g., a business school). However, in the self-sufficient public financial management curriculum outlined here, a single course incorporating financial, managerial, and nonprofit accounting instruction would be developed for public affairs master's degree students. This would be accomplished in much the same way as applied microeconomics courses have been developed in some public policy schools to meet the needs of master's degree students.

This core course introduces students to key concepts and practices employed in financial and managerial accounting, including transaction identification and recording, the accounting cycle, double-entry bookkeeping, the money measurement concept, and the preparation of basic financial reports-the balance sheet, the income statement, and the statement of sources and uses of funds. An introduction also is provided to generally accepted accounting practices (GAAP) and governmental accounting and financial reporting standards (GASB) for public-sector entities. This helps students understand, for example, the peculiarities of applying the matching concept to tax-supported entities. Additional concepts presented include historical cost and other approaches to estimation and use of depreciation in nonprofit organizations. This required course introduces students to cost concepts: fixed and variable, direct and indirect, incremental and average, discretionary and uncontrollable. It covers basic propositions about cost behavior and explains the rudiments of cost finding and breakeven analysis. Perspectives on "creative" government accounting and reporting practices, such as those identified by Anthony, that misrepresent the actual financial position also may be presented in this course.

The nonprofit accounting course provides an introduction to government fund accounting, account structure design, and financial and budgetary account monitoring and control. It familiarizes students with the substantial variation in accounting system designs and practices in different types of public organizations-schools, universities, hospitals, utilities.

Analysis of actual financial reports of public organizations is performed to approximate "real world" experience with public-sector accounting procedures. The course identifies three basic public-sector fund categories (general government, enterprise, and trust funds) and explains the purpose for the different funds that are commonly employed in each general category-the general fund, the capital projects fund, the internal services fund. The course concludes by demonstrating how the fund structure articulates with annual budgetary accounts and the permanent chart of accounts using examples from different types of public organizations.

Management and Cost Accounting

The third course, an elective that precedes the public financial management and budgeting courses, is management and cost accounting. Cost accounting is taught at this point in the sequence on the assumption that knowledge in this area is necessary to understand instruction in financial management, budgeting, cash management, investment, auditing, and other skill concentrations that follow in the curriculum. This course builds on the nonprofit accounting skills established earlier in introducing cost finding and allocation procedures, full versus direct costing approaches, job and process costing systems, statistical and financial forecasting, and cost estimation techniques. Basic cost accounting procedures are illustrated using examples and cases. Case-based instruction is employed to indicate the relationship between cost accounting and the development of unit cost-based budget formulas, external prices and internal transfer prices, and standard cost/expense variance analysis. Explanation of the use cost information in forecasting and modeling, performance measurement, operational and capital budgeting, and program evaluation also is provided. The relevance of cost accounting for program evaluation sometimes is not taught in courses on evaluation, which may help to explain why evaluation results often are ignored in the budget process.

The two course accounting sequence is designed to improve the quality of instruction and learning in the graduate-level survey courses in public financial management and budgeting required for all MPA students. At minimum, all students would take the nonprofit accounting course as a prerequisite for public financial management and budgeting. Required instruction in management control, and in accounting concepts and methods, teaches the framework and some of the techniques needed to understand financial management and budget functions. The need for sound accounting systems is understood by students as necessary to provide data for planning, budgeting, capital resource decision making, and program execution. Introduction to financial and management accounting, and to cost accounting as an elective, also establishes many of the skills needed to perform financial analysis—for example, for assessment of financial condition, budget preparation and execution, capital budgeting, cash flow, and investment.

Public Financial Management

The public financial management core course introduces students to the principal financial management functions of government and nonprofit organizations. The course begins with an explanation of the role of government in the economy (equity, efficiency, stability) and the use of fiscal, monetary, and the other policy instruments to achieve public policy objectives. This is followed by an analysis of government service production and distribution employing a production function model to illustrate relationships between resource inputs, production, outputs, and outcomes. This model introduces the concept of benefit/cost analysis to compare resource inputs with benefits received by citizens. It also introduces basic financial and microeconomic concepts such as discounted present value, public and private goods and costs, opportunity costs, externalities of production and consumption, economic rents, transaction costs, and so on, and highlights the importance of analyzing the distributional consequences of government financial and budgetary decisions. Examples of alternative tax rate burden distribution across different income segments are provided to illustrate regressivity, proportionality and progressivity, vertical/horizontal equity, and ability to pay. Efficiency/equity tradeoffs also are demonstrated through application of the production function/net benefit criterion approach for evaluating the outcomes of public taxing, spending, and service provision. Various public-sector input and output measurement methods are analyzed to indicate how work load, performance, net benefit, and other criteria are applied in budgeting, auditing, program evaluation and policy analysis. The usefulness of the net benefit criterion for assessing both short- and long-term public policy priorities may be illustrated through examples, for example, health and education cost and benefit distribution. The significance of distinguishing between public versus private costs and benefits also is explained in this initial microeconomic component of the course.

The second segment of the course introduces the basic financial management functions of government, including treasury and controllership, cash management and investment, debt management and municipal bonding, operations and capital budgeting, capital asset acquisition and inventory management, facilities operation and maintenance, and auditing. Also covered are financial aspects of personnel management, risk management and insurance, pension systems management, procurement contracting, and other related topics at the discretion of the instructor. The accounting system is explained within the context of this course as the central financial management information process that ties together all of the financial management functions of the organization.

The third component of the financial management course analyzes the principal sources of revenue for government. The levying of income, sales, property, and other taxes is explained. The objective of each type of tax is identified, and criteria for evaluating new or existing taxes and other sources of revenue are analyzed-efficiency, equity, yield, productivity, incidence, impact, visibility, political feasibility. These criteria are applied in examples to illustrate the economic effects of income, wealth, consumption, production, trade and other taxes, and other sources of public revenue generation. Concepts including revenue rights and competition, behavioral incentives/disincentives created through taxation and methods for evaluating tax capability and effort also are illustrated using examples from federal, state, and local government. In addition one session of this course is devoted to intergovernmental transfer payments and analysis of related issues such as revenue dependency, overlapping tax jurisdictions, and double taxation.

The fourth segment of the financial management course provides instruction in financial analysis concepts and techniques including present value, financial ratio analysis, unit revenue and cost analysis, breakeven pricing, rate of return, common size and variance analysis. Students will have been introduced to many of these techniques in earlier courses, which facilitates instruction on applications in public-sector financial management. Also included is instruction in methods for evaluating the financial condition of public organizations under the assumption that it is good practice to try to diagnose trends so that future problems may be anticipated and avoided.

The objectives of financial management achieved through budgeting are indicated at the conclusion of this course: capital asset acquisition management achieved through capital budgeting; operational planning and control are implemented through operational budgeting; management of liquid assets is carried out through cash budgeting, flow management, debt, and investment policy. This characterization provides the linkage between the financial management and the public budgeting core courses. Both the financial management and the budgeting courses that follow may incorporate presentations by practitioners to familiarize students with the issues faced by public agencies and to provide insight into some of the constraints posed in the working environment for example, conflict over program and spending priorities, political pressures, short time frames for action, and multiple clients.

Instruction in microcomputer spreadsheet and data base management applications is integrated into the public financial. management and budgeting courses. The use of microcomputers in these courses is facilitated through the assignment of cases to be completed using commonly available software (e.g., for spreadsheets, data base management, etc.), and the incorporation of workshops concentrating on specific types of financial and budgetary microcomputer applications, such as budget preparation, budget execution account monitoring, variance analysis, cost accounting, capital budget database preparation and analysis. Prerequisite introductory training in the use of microcomputers and software applications facilitates the laboratory component of instruction in these courses and accelerates student learning from case exercises.

Public Budgeting

The fifth course (fourth core course) in the curriculum is public budgeting. Budgeting is taught after management control, accounting, and financial management because it is an integrative functional means for achieving financial and management control, and because the performance of budgeting rests on accounting. Fundamentally, a budget is a compilation of accounts for purposes of planning, forecasting, decision, and execution. Budgets are the principal means of establishing parameters for programmatic and financial execution-that is, performance and control targets are negotiated, monitored, reported, and evaluated annually in the budget. The budgeting course includes the following elements: the objectives of budgeting, types of budgets and their purposes, budget cycle timing and participants, budget preparation techniques (adjusted base for cost/workload, new program, etc.), budget monitoring and control methods (amount, timing, location, volume, price/cost variance analysis), alternative approaches for budget formulation and analysis (performance, program, zero-base, target-level, etc.), the politics of the budgetary process (identifying the ploys and tactics of strategic representation), budgeting under resource uncertainty (cutback and budgeting restraint), relationships between budget reconciliation, auditing, accountability and management control, and the capital budget decision process.

The emphasis given to budgetary politics in this course can vary widely, based upon the expertise and inclination of the instructor. Given the fact that budgeting is intensively political and competitive, the political nature of budgeting in contrast to bureaucratic norms and preferences for a rational systems approach must be emphasized. Students should become fully aware of the triumph of substantive over procedural concerns in the annual budget decision process. The difficulty of meeting balanced budget requirements or reducing the federal deficit provides contemporary examples to illustrate this point.

Benefit/cost analysis of alternative capital project proposals is presented in this course with case examples to demonstrate technique and to contrast the application of rational versus political criteria in public decision making. This is enabled by the previous introduction to benefit/cost analysis in the nonprofit/cost accounting and financial management courses. Capital budgeting concepts and techniques also may be taught as a course separate from operational budgeting. Similarly, instruction in government contracting and contract management may be included in the budgeting course or taught in a separate elective course.

The unifying element of this course is a model of the budget process that articulates the components of budget preparation and execution. Preparation is explained to include executive policy formulation, definition of budget methodology or the rules of the game, preparation of estimates, executive and legislative negotiation, legislative authorization and appropriation targeting, appropriation decision making, and legislative/executive enactment. Budget execution in the model includes apportionment, allotment, allocation, spending, (preaudit, obligation, encumbrance, and disbursement), monitoring and control, audit, and evaluation. Differences between federal, state and local government cycles and practices are explained, with emphasis placed on the government most closely aligned with student employment opportunity. Thus, the introduction to budget systems and issues in municipal, state, federal, and other national governments and nonprofit organizations provided in this course will vary according to the focus of MPA program of which the financial management curriculum is a part. For example, special emphasis on comparative budgeting is valuable to demonstrate processes and techniques employed and lessons learned in other nations and political systems. Special problems in comparative national budgeting may be included in the budgeting core course taught as a separate elective where requisite faculty expertise is available to obtain value from the comparative approach.

Financial Management Information Systems

An elective course in financial information systems design, implementation, and evaluation is offered after budgeting to provide emphasis on computers in the curriculum in addition to the microcomputer instruction offered concurrently with two of the core courses. The purpose of this course is to teach methods for design and evaluation of computerized financial management systems, such as accounting, payroll, accounts receivable/payable, capital inventory management and control. Instruction is intended to give students a basic understanding of finance-related applications of microcomputers as well as mainframe systems, value-added networks, macrocomputers, and other sophisticated systems. A systems design component initiates the course to provide insight into the basic characteristics of systems per se and the application of systems analysis to financial management processes. This is followed by analysis of example systems in operation. Instruction in one or more programming languages is included in this course, and advanced material may be offered for students who desire to further develop this skill. The principal portion of the course is devoted to exercises in systems design, beginning with simple functions and proceeding to more complex systems. Students work with microcomputers and mainframe systems to become familiar with the opportunities and constraints in using different types of hardware and software. Use of a variety of tailored financial management software is included. The course differentiates between administrative and analytical software and provides the option for students to learn techniques useful for program and policy analysis as well as management control. A concluding segment provides instruction in criteria for assessing the adequacy of computerized financial management systems.

The rationale for teaching systems analysis, programming and computer applications after the core management control, accounting, financial management, and budgeting courses is twofold: to illustrate the financial and budgetary systems actually used in public organizations and to sensitize students to the importance of system design and implementation issues. In part, this course demonstrates the value of thinking about financial functions and systems in an integrated way, even if actual systems are not integrated. The integrated approach also helps to teach students about the degree of interdependence that is present between the various financial management functions of government. Furthermore, an understanding of functional and systems relationships provides a basis for subsequent instruction in cash management, investment, and debt management, each of which requires the integration of information from multiple financial management functional areas-for example, financial and managerial accounting to define relationships between inputs and results is needed to prepare and execute operating budgets.

Cash Management, Investment, And Debt Management

The financial management systems course is followed by an elective that covers cash management and investment, debt financing, and the dynamics of municipal bonding. The first segment of the course is devoted to cash flow forecasting and management. Instruction is provided in cash budgeting, working capital management, use of short, medium, and long-term investment instruments, mixed portfolio and "prudent person" investment practices for governments. The second segment of the course on debt policy covers the uses of various debt instruments, approaches to credit analysis, disclosure rules, liability and other debt issuance requirements, debt structuring, scheduling, and leveraging analysis of net and true interest costs, bond market procedures and terminology, bond preparation and sale methods, variables influencing debt issuance decisions, secondary market trading dynamics, municipal bond market behavior and performance. The course also introduces students to specific applications of debt policy in public enterprises, such as housing, hospitals, and utilities. Case examples in the uses and abuses of municipal bonds may be incorporated to demonstrate the advantages and risks associated with various debt strategies. The implications for cash and debt management policy for taxation, fee and service charge and other revenue-generation options are explored.

The final component of this course is devoted to fee, fine, service and regulatory policies and practices. Principles of public goods, excludability, and voluntariness are explained and related to average and marginal cost pricing. Price elasticity of demand, equity, and efficiency are presented as criteria for evaluating the objectives of pricing policy. Breakeven analysis for fee and service charge coverage analysis also is demonstrated. A review of regulatory policy objectives indicates the relationships between fines, penalties, and pricing policy in contemporary public organizations-for example, the principle that fines should equal or exceed compliance costs if they are to be effective may be introduced. Government experimentation with contracting-out and privatization as well as the theoretical foundations for such experimentation, may be presented in this course if not included previously in public budgeting or offered as a separate elective course.

Performance Auditing

The eighth and final course in the sequence is an elective in performance auditing to introduce the fundamentals of management audit theory and practice. Included in this course is a brief segment on financial auditing, although the overall focus is on how performance auditing is employed for management control to improve organizational effectiveness. Techniques of performance auditing are taught to provide skills needed by auditors as well as program analysts and evaluators. This course is offered last in the sequence because auditing is the final phase of the management control cycle; performance auditing evaluates both the financial and programmatic consequences of organizational actions. Instruction indicates how performance auditing renders judgments on the extent to which organizational objectives have been met and attempts to guide policymaking in pursuit of increased effectiveness and efficiency. Performance auditing provides the feedback link to future financial plans and budgets in the management control cycle.

CONCLUSIONS

The sequence and content of a public financial management curriculum offered within an MPA program outlined in this study demonstrates only one approach to implementation of the recommendations of the ASPA/ SBFM National Task Force report. Course sequencing and content are illustrative to suggest the need for continuing the dialogue initiated by the work of the National Task Force on public financial management curriculum reform.

The eight-course sequence follows the management control cycle for public organizations, with emphasis on financial systems as the principal means for implementing control objectives. This approach to public financial management curriculum design assumes that students will complete other courses complimentary to the financial management program including statistics, microand macroeconomics, public finance, policy analysis, program evaluation, and benefit/cost analysis in compliance with general public affairs program degree requirements. Other financial management related special-interest electives such as risk management, financial stress management, contracting-out and privatization, capital project planning and management, procurement contracting, purchasing and inventory control may be offered to enhance the curriculum so that it responds to the demands of students and the public-sector work environment. Professional development opportunities for in-service students also ought to be considered in curriculum design and selection of elective course offerings.

This approach to financial management curriculum design is more comprehensive than many public affairs programs offer at present. Where public affairs programs search for unique identity and comparative advantage, such an offering could provide strategic positioning benefits. However, as is the case with development of any specialized curricula, the benefits of investment to achieve market advantage and to increase academic reputation have to be weighed against opportunity costs. The National Task Force Report cites some of the difficulties involved in implementing its recommendations, including absence of faculty expertise and inability to hire new faculty. The approach outlined here may be contrasted with marginal adjustments to the public affairs curriculum to improve public financial management instruction that are more easily implemented-that is, the addition of one or two new financial management courses. Even where this is the case, a comprehensive financial management curriculum and course content model, provides an example of sequencing and topic coverage within such courses.

Those deliberating over the advisability and feasibility of modifying financial management instruction should recognize that comprehensive, change of the type indicated in this study moves the curricular focus of the public affairs program significantly in the direction of public financial management and away from public policy analysis. For a variety of reasons, a comprehensive public financial management curriculum may be more easily established in a generic school of management or in some schools of business than in many public affairs programs. This is because accounting and other financial management related courses typically are in management and business school curricula. However, existing in schools of management and business may not provide sufficient focus on the public sector to satisfy public affairs program requirements. Assessment of the feasibility of incorporating elements of the financial management curricula of schools of management and business public affairs programs is beyond the purpose and scope of this study. However, cooperative course offerings between business and public affairs programs are potentially advantageous to both curricula.

Further development of instruction in public financial management presents a challenge to public affairs faculty and administrators. If up-to-date and high-quality public financial management education is to be offered to students in the context of public affairs master's and doctoral degree programs, the addition of new courses and the modification of existing curricula appear to be necessary. The National Task Force report provided direction for reform and a stimulus to action. In consideration of these options, it should be emphasized that flexibility is needed in molding new courses into public affairs curricula so that innovation in public financial management instruction is compatible with faculty preferences, student demand, and the cultural characteristics of existing programs.

FLYING HOUR PROGRAM (FHP) CASH MANAGEMENT AT COMMANDER NAVAL AIR FORCES PACIFIC (CNAP)

INTRODUCTION

The Flying Hour Program (FHP) is the vehicle by which the Department of the Navy (DoN) budgets and allocates annual funding for the operation and maintenance of Navy and Marine Corps aircraft.[1] The FHP represented more than $3.2 billion of the Navy's FY2000 O&M, N appropriation.[2] Forty-eight percent of the FHP is allocated to the Commander Naval Air Forces Pacific (CNAP), and the majority of the remainder is allocated to the Commander Naval Air Forces Atlantic (CNAL). CNAP and CNAL are the two active duty Air Type Commanders (TYCOMS).

Despite the last four years of increased defense spending, the FHP, like many programs in DOD, has faced stringent budgets and limited resources, corresponding to an overall decline in dollars and tightening top line controls over the last decade. As a result, program managers have faced difficult decisions in budget execution, attempting to satisfy operational requirements with scarce dollars.

THE FHP CHAIN OF COMMAND

The dynamic environment of the FHP requires the participation of multiple Navy, Marine Corps, and DOD organizations. Two main functional chains of command exist to oversee the operation and financing of the FHP. The operational chain, (depicted in Figure 1 for the Pacific Fleet), gives direction for the daily mission tasking for all Navy and Marine Corps aircraft. This chain illustrates the flow of authority from the President to the squadron commander. Organizations within the operational chain provide input for consideration in budget formulation, but have a minimal role in formal budget development. The financial chain, depicted in Figure 2, illustrates the flow of the FHP budget process.

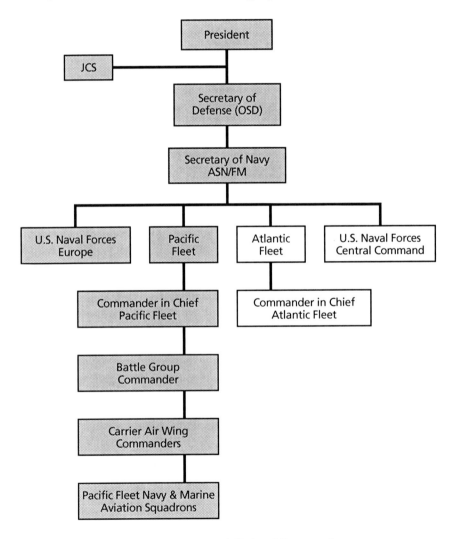

Figure 1.   Pacific Fleet FHP Operational Chain of Command.

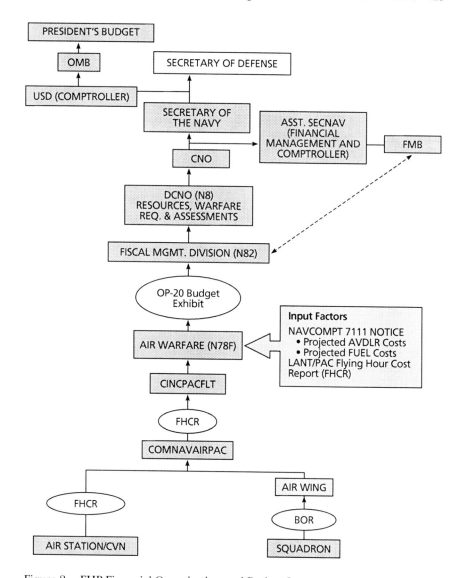

Figure 2.   FHP Financial Organization and Budget Inputs.

BUDGET FORMULATION

The primary FHP budget exhibit is the Operational Plan 20, (OP-20). The N-78 staff constructs the necessary FHP budget exhibits and works closely throughout the year with the Major Claimants such as Commander in Chief Pacific Fleet (CINCPACFLT) and Air Type Commanders (TYCOMs) such as

Commander Naval Air Forces Pacific (CNAP) in receiving the necessary budget inputs required for assembling and justifying the annual budget funding requirements. Figure 2 displays these budget inputs in relation to the financial organization. The three input mechanisms used at the squadron, air station, and N-78F levels are the Budget OPTAR Report (BOR), the Flight Hour Cost Report (FHCR), and the Operation Plan 20 FHP budget exhibit (Keating & Paulk, 1998, p. 29). The BOR and the FHCR are the primary financial management inputs used at CNAP to administer and track FHP obligations during the fiscal year. These reports collectively form the data used by N-78F to build new OP-20 budget exhibits.

Commander, Naval Air Forces Pacific plays an important role in FHP budget formulation by representing the flying hour users' needs and articulating the difficulties to the resource sponsor (N-78) in executing the FHP budget. The CNAP budget formulation role consists of two activities: (1) collecting and reporting FHP execution data and (2) developing FHP program and budget submissions (Keating & Paulk, 1998, p. 37).

BUDGET ALLOCATION

CNAP is the focal point for allocating, executing and monitoring flight hour funding for all Navy and Marine Corps Pacific fleet squadrons. Their primary goal and responsibility during allocation and execution is to achieve a specific level of readiness for each squadron within the constraints of the resources available (Assistant Chief of Naval Operations, 1996, p. 41).

The allocation of FHP funding begins at the start of the new fiscal year when FMB distributes quarterly allocations of the approved FHP funding to CNAP in the form of an Operating Budget (OB). The FHP OB, in theory, should provide the necessary dollars to execute CNAP's flying mission. With restricted DOD budgets and competing priorities, financial resources are scarce. Thus, the funds requested during budget formulation seldom actually match those required by CNAP to execute the FHP program. Therefore, CNAP's greatest challenge during allocation is to distribute these funds in such a way that will allow squadrons to achieve mission readiness while avoiding over obligation of FHP funds (Keating & Paulk, 1998, p. 41). CNAP's primary tool for distributing flight hour funds is through the Navy Operational Plan 20 (OP-20). The OP-20 serves as a budgeting formulation document and an execution-monitoring tool. During budgeting, the OP-20 displays funding requirements by aircraft type, model, series (T/M/S) and becomes the Navy's primary budget exhibit displaying the FHP funding requirements during submission and review to OSD and OMB.

By using the OP-20, the CNAP FHP manager and comptroller decide how to allocate flight hours to each squadron, air wing, and aircraft-owning activity, taking into account deployment schedules, and training requirements (Keating & Paulk, 1998, p. 42).

In distributing funds to squadrons and air stations, the OP-20 serves as a starting point. The Flying Hour Program Division (N01F3) and the Aviation Flight Hour Operations Office (N-3F) share the process of distributing FHP funds. The FHP manager (N01F3) is charged with the overall management of the program, but shares this responsibility with N-3F. N-3F, (also called the FHP Operations Officer—Ops-O), is responsible for ensuring squadrons are allocated the proper number of flight hours and associated funding levels required to meet CNO's readiness goals for aircraft (Commander Naval Air Forces Pacific, 1998). Primary Mission Readiness (PMR) serves as a subjective means to distribute a limited number of flight hour funds among the various activities. PMR is the number of flight hours required to complete all events scheduled on the Training & Readiness Matrix. Completing all events is known as 100% PMR. PMR is currently maintained at a Navy wide rate of 83% plus 2% of the flying hours-per-formed in aircraft simulators (Keating & Paulk, 1998, p. 43).

At CNAP, the Ops O primarily relies on the OP-20 and the 83% PMR goal to distribute flight hours by T/M/S. The OP-20 assists in the allocation of funds to the fleet as it is separated into three schedules to reflect different mission areas. Each T/M/S is funded to a slightly different level of hours and dollar amounts because of differences in operating expenses (e.g., jets versus helicopters). These schedules serve as a rough guideline for flight hour OPTAR distribution throughout the fleet. Schedules are introduced as follows (Assistant Chief of Naval Operations, 1996):

Schedule	Mission/Definition
A	TACAIR/ASW—Carrier air wings, Marine air wings, land and sea-based units committed to combat operations funded at 83% PMR. This category constitutes the bulk of the Navy/Marine Corps aviation warfighting capability, which primarily consists of those squadrons capable of executing the "joint strike" and "crisis response" missions in support of the National Military Strategy. (1A1A fund code)
B	FLEET AIR TRAINING (FAT)—This category (also referred to as Fleet Replacement Squadrons (FRS)), consists of squadrons that train pilots and navigators prior to joining TACAIR/ASW and Fleet Air Support units. These squadrons are dedicated to training fleet aircrews in each particular type aircraft and funded at 100% student throughput. (1A2A fund code)
C	FLEET AIR SUPPORT (FAS)—The primary mission of these squadrons is to provide direct and indirect support (including logistics) to Navy and Marine Corps fleet operating units and shore installations. Their funding is based on Naval Center for Cost Analyses (NCCA) methodologies and historical execution. Common mission examples include Carrier-on-Board Delivery, and Search and Recovery. (1A1A fund code).

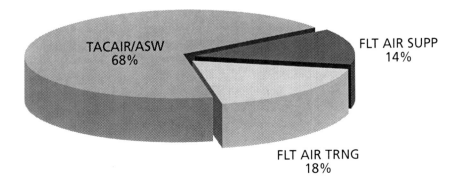

Figure 3.   FHP schedule funding percentages. *Source:* Assistant Chief of Naval Operations (1998).

The percentage of FHP resources spent for squadrons within the above schedules is indicated in Figure 3.

In conjunction with the OP-20, final distribution of funding to fleet squadrons is calculated by matching squadron flying "activity levels" with the CNO PMR goal of 83%. An activity level indicates a phase of employment for a squadron during its 18-month "turnaround deployment cycle." A turnaround cycle is the eighteen-month period used for scheduling aircraft deployments, along with all the requisite aircraft and air wing training in preparation for deployment. Flight hour requirements vary at each stage of the turnaround cycle. Air wings are typically funded at the levels shown below:

Month 1:	Personnel turnover and leave	40% PMR
Months 2–6:	Turnaround training	65% PER
Months 7–10:	Turnaround training	75% PMR
Months 11–16:	Pre-deployment training	95% PMR
Month 17:	Pre-deployment Stand down	50% PMR
Deployment Month 1:		70% PMR
Deployment Months 2–5:		115% PMR
Deployment Month 6:		60% PMR

Using the 83% PMR goal as guidance, the CNAP Ops-O uses the OP-20 schedule and builds quarterly master flight hour execution plans for each air wing once CINCPACFLT passes the "controls" (fiscal FHP dollar limits) to CNAP. The objective is to attain an overall PMR goal of 83% while ensuring squadrons receive necessary funding to fly enough flight hours to meet training requirements. The level of funding and flight hours required varies from the 83% PMR baseline depending on squadron location within the turnaround cycle. In the aggregate, an 83% PMR level is achieved. In addition to achieving the 83% PMR goal, the Ops-O and FHP mangers must avoid any over obligation of FHP funds and a resulting 1517 Anti-deficiency Act violation (Keating & Paulk, 1998, p. 45).

BUDGET EXECUTION

Navy Operations and Maintenance, (O&M, N) funding for the FHP is made available annually but is provided to the fleet quarterly. Beginning with the new fiscal year on October 1, each Navy and Marine squadron and their supporting air station or ship, if deployed, receives one quarter's worth of flight operation funding from CNAP. These quarterly funds are called Operational Target Functional Categories (OFCs) or commonly known as Operating Targets (OPTARS). An OPTAR represents the anticipated funding level necessary to support the costs of a squadron's flight operations. Receipt of the OPTAR gives the squadron authorization to place obligations against CNAP's FHP funds up to the amount of the issued OPTAR grant (Keating & Paulk, 1998, p. 32).

CNAP's monitoring role in FHP execution is to track and review squadron and air station obligations. CNAP does this through the FHCR and BOR costing information reports. These reports serve to:

- Prevent over expenditure of allocated funds
- Ensure funds are used for approved purposes only
- Compare squadron, air wing and air station readiness training and support activities to current on-hand FHP funds
- Identify excess funds for redistribution to other units
- Measure ship/station/squadron budget execution performance
- Support and provide justification for subsequent fiscal year budget inputs and decisions
- Prepare required FHP management control reports (Keating & Paulk, 1998, p. 46).

Overseeing the distribution of flight hour funds within CINPACFLT requires a tremendous management effort between the squadrons, air stations, air wing commanders, and the resource sponsor. At any given time, FHP managers are monitoring the execution of five air wings, a dozen air stations, and more than 100 squadrons. The final objective is to spread the limited FHP funding across all activities while achieving mission readiness goals and to ensure the proper execution of all allocated funds by the end of the fiscal year (Keating & Paulk, 1998, p. 47).

Budget execution is ultimately where the FHP budget is validated to assess whether sufficient funds have been forecasted and allocated to achieve the flying hour requirements of CNAP. Because of overall federal budget constraints, competing priorities and limited resources, the final version of the OP-20 often contains less funding than the originally budgeted OP-20. The hope and expectation during the execution year is that the actual FHP cost data are relatively consistent with the budget estimates. However, in recent years, execution costs for CNAP's FHP have exceeded the budgeted estimates. When FMB passes the "controls" (fiscal FHP dollar limits) to CINCPACFLT, there are fewer resources available than necessary to fully execute the FHP. CINCPACFLT passes additional controls to CNAP reflecting managerial decisions (withholds) that may reprogram FHP funds for other priorities.

The most influential factor creating FHP funding problems is the fact that there are limited resources to fund any program among competing priorities within the DoN. A constrained fiscal environment and other spending priorities often drive unpopular funding decisions. When this occurs, the onus is on CNAP FHP managers and comptrollers to embark upon "creative financing" to try to achieve aviation readiness goals without committing an Anti-deficiency Act violation.

TRENDS IN CNAP ANNUAL FHP EXECUTION

The author conducted personal interviews with past and present staff members at CNAP Headquarters in San Diego, California in order to gather trends in FHP budget execution over the past three years. The following pages represent his findings.

Beginning of the Fiscal Year

CNAP FHP managers start each fiscal year recognizing that there are insufficient funds to continue operations through the end of the year. CNAP continuously updates CINCPACFLT on their money position. At the start of the fiscal year, CINCPACFLT's execution philosophy and direction to CNAP is to fly the requirement, making necessary expenditures in order to properly execute the program. As the year continues, the reality at CNAP is that they must fly to the dollars. Table 1 is the initial balance sheet for CNAP's FY 1998 FHP and is indicative of the three years analyzed.

CNAP normally requests a higher percentage of annual funds for the first quarter of the fiscal year in order to "buy back" the previous year's bow wave. (Bow waves are discussed later.) For example, CNAP requested 28% of the total FHP funds for FY 01 for the first quarter. CNAP is required to provide justification up the chain of command for requesting quarterly

Table 1.   CNAP Initial FY 98 FHP Balance Sheet

Shortfalls	
Delta (OP-20 vs Controls)	$ (116,000,000)
Under Pricing and Bow Wave	$ (89,000,000)
Unfilled Customer Order Buy Back	$ (12,000,000)
Critical Unfunded Requirements	$ (16,000,000)
Increased Repairables Cost	$ (14,000,000)
Reprogramming	$ (24,000,000)
Total	$ (271,000,000)
Assets	
Contingency dollars	$ 40,000,000
Maintenance efficiency	$ 30,000,000
USN/USMC reimbursables	$ 10,000,000
USN/USMC supply credits	$ 10,000,000
USMC hours asset	$ 18,000,000
Total	$ 108,000,000
FHP Delta	$ (163,000,000)

Source: Commander Naval Air Forces Pacific (1998)

funds in excess of 25% of annual funding. When CNAP managers determine that there are insufficient funds to continue through the end of a particular quarter, they may request that CINCPACFLT advance money from a later quarter into the current quarter. CINCPACFLT is the custodian for numerous operating funds, including those for the Pacific fleet surface and submarine communities, and may or may not have resources available to advance to CNAP for the FHP. CNAP managers prefer not to request advances from CINCPACFLT unless absolutely unavoidable (Personal interview, March 2001).

Reprogramming

During the execution of FHP funds, several opportunities exist to shift or reprogram FHP dollars. This occurs because of changing priorities, and insufficient funding levels for other programs. Reprogramming is designed to give operational and financial commanders increased flexibility to meet unforeseen program changes that may occur during budget execution. With approval from the chain of command, CNAP FHP managers can reprogram up to $15 million between fund codes (Department of Defense, 2000, p. 64). They shift money within the FHP from an under-executed account (if one exists) to an over-executed account. In the second quarter of FY 01, CNAP shifted money from TACAIR/ASW (1A1A fund code) to the smaller FAT (1A2A fund code) in order to close out quarterly budgets in the black. When CNAP managers shift resources between fund codes, often money is moved from 1A1A to 1A2A. The priority resides with the smaller FRS account that provides funding for training replacement pilots and other aircrew (Personal interview, March 2001).

CNAP managers routinely reprogram money from the FHP to the smaller Flying Other (FO) account that has experienced under-funding the past several years. Even though detrimental from a cash management perspective, augmenting some of these programs out of the current year FHP budget is essential. For example, if missile range and/or temporary assignment of duty (TAD) funding is inadequate, squadrons may not be able to achieve the required training because they can't fully utilize the facilities and pay the travel expenses for people, regardless of the available flight hours. The support programs are integral to achieving the readiness milestones necessary to deploy a combat capable force.

Quarterly Shortfalls

CNAP has problems each quarter with requirements exceeding available cash. As the funds provider to operating units, they do not want to order squadrons to stop flying operations because of a cash flow problem. The distribution of funding on a quarterly basis causes CNAP to experience timing issues for incurring liabilities. The problem is similar to a bank obtaining coverage by the federal reserve. The bank knows the money is there, but has not yet received it. As available resources are spent toward the end of a quarter, CNAP managers know that the new quarter's resources will come, but cash has not yet been distributed by CINCPACFLT.

Execution Philosophy

During the first seven months of FY01, CNAP managers' estimates for the current year FHP funding shortfall have ranged from $235 to $325 million. The entire shortfall does not manifest itself all in the fourth quarter; rather, it works its way through the year. The CNO directs CINCPACFLT to fly 83% PMR, and CNAP must determine how to accomplish this aviation readiness goal. They monitor overall daily spending rates and consider timing of employment of the aircraft carriers in the deployment cycle. CNAP managers must make decisions such as how low to deplete flying hours of the two Air Wings at home. Because of funding shortfalls, in a worst-case scenario, they may have to temporarily halt flying operations of squadrons returning from deployment. Part of the job of CNAP managers is to ensure that all of the squadrons among the TACAIR, helicopter, patrol, and other aviation communities equally "share the pain" of under-funding. With the limited funds available and number of reporting units, trying to properly allocate resources to the squadrons throughout the year becomes a huge cash flow juggling act (personal interview, March 2001).

If CNAP managers communicate an impending funding shortfall to the fleet, units may constrain themselves because of money. CNAP managers promote prudent program execution yet avoid constraining fleet flying. The signals that CNAP managers send during execution are very important. Limiting fleet operations because of money shortfalls would artificially reduce the FHP, ultimately misrepresenting its true cash requirements. This would be detrimental because the starting point in budget formulation for future years is what is spent in the current year.

Challenges with Reporting Units

Once CNAP managers distribute quarterly funding to the fleet, managing flying hour execution rates and maintenance expenditures is the responsibility of individual squadrons, air stations, and other reporting units. Although managers at CNAP direct fleet units to fly the requirements and not to be constrained by available dollars, some Commanding Officers may view requesting additional funds as a poor reflection on their command. Therefore, command influence at the unit level plays a role in execution. Commanding Officers may attempt to stretch available dollars with various management techniques. Canceling requisitions for aircraft parts, rescheduling training events, or delaying needed aircraft maintenance are methods to temporarily defer costs. With more than one hundred different reporting units, there are several different levels of management controlling the execution process and there are different styles within the various units.

Additional challenges with which CNAP FHP managers must contend include accuracy and timeliness in reporting by units. For example, reporting errors in a unit's 7B (fuel) OPTAR may occur because of calculations with fuel chits, causing unexpected overages or shortages in OFC-01 accounts. CNAP must be extremely careful about overspending their accounts. Because of a lag in reporting obligations, not all costs are captured by the accounting system in the quarter in which they occur. Often bills exist for which CNAP is liable, yet CNAP may be unaware of their existence. CNAP must routinely manage the risk of Anti-deficiency Act violations because requirements often exceed final monetary authority.

Conclusion of Fiscal Year

As CNAP managers continue to monitor daily FHP expenditure rates throughout the year, available cash dwindles. They have advanced money as far forward as possible and can now project a date that they will have to completely stop all fleet operations because all money will be expended. This date is usually in early to mid fourth quarter. To continue operations, managers must rely on funding relief to overcome shortfalls.

As shortfalls are communicated up the chain of command, CNAP money managers monitor progress on potential sources of funding relief to know if and when to order all fleet units to stop spending and cease operations. CNAP managers describe the process as trying to determine "when and how hard to slam on the brakes" (Commander Naval Air Forces, 1998). They do not know if funding relief will be forthcoming, how much it will be, nor when it will occur.

Funding Relief

One form of funding relief comes from the distribution of "contingency funds." Contingency funds are appropriated by Congress to offset costs of ongoing "known" operations. An example of known contingency funds were those used to fund Operation Southern Watch (OSW) in Iraq in FY98. These funds came from the Overseas Contingency Operations Transfer Fund (OCOTF). Once appropriated by Congress and released by OSD, these funds are held by FMB and provided only when fleet operations in direct support of contingencies exceed the appropriated FHP budget. "Unknown" contingency funds are appropriated through emergency supplemental bills to cover unforeseen contingencies. An example of unknown contingency funds were the funds appropriated in July 1998 to cover the unplanned costs of deploying a second aircraft carrier to the Persian Gulf.

Additional sources of funding relief may come from a CNO Reserve (withhold at the CNO level), reprogramming from other accounts within the DOD appropriation (for example from procurement accounts), or Defense supplemental appropriations from Congress.

If units within CNAP are flying high sortie rates in support of contingencies during the first quarter of the fiscal year, they may expend cash faster than is available. This is another case in which CNAP will request to move money forward. CNAP managers describe this as "covering contingencies out-of-hide." They are loaning themselves their own money to pay the cost of contingencies until reimbursed later in the fiscal year. CNAP managers continually attempt to reconcile timing issues associated with the expenditure and receipt of cash.

The Navy midyear review process affords CNAP managers another opportunity to communicate shortfalls up the chain of command. Following midyear review, the critical question becomes "Will we get the funding relief requested in the midyear review process from a Defense Supplemental appropriation or some other mechanism toward the end of the fiscal year?" When CNAP does receive funding relief, but the amount received is insufficient to meet requirements, they then scramble to figure out how to make it through the end of the year. For example, they conduct "what if" drills of shutting down Air Wings for 30 days to 60 days to determine how much they could avoid spending.

Withholds

The FHP is the largest financial account that CNAP manages and has been subject to withholds to fix other funding shortfalls. CNAP has no control over these types of "reprioritizations" imposed by higher levels in the chain of command. These actions affect not only the FHP budget, but other OM&N accounts as well. Budget managers do not know what will be the final withhold or tax that will be levied against their programs, but monitor discussions in the summer review process. By the time the fiscal year starts and the budget has been received, managers concern themselves with execution, and cannot really influence decisions to tax their program.

Over the past several years, CINCPACFLT has withheld money from the FHP account to fund enhanced fleet computer operability with initiatives such as the Navy-Marine Corps Intranet (NMCI), Y2K improvements, and Information Technology for the 21st Century (IT-21) (personal interview, January 2001).

Unanticipated Expenses

Another challenge in executing the FHP is the annual occurrence of unexpected expenditures. These expenditures are often significant and can cause major fiscal difficulties for CNAP FHP managers. These unanticipated expenses are referred to as "emergent unfundeds." Emergent unfundeds generally arise because of unforeseen maintenance costs associated with reliability problems with aircraft components. The fleet issues maintenance bulletins because of a mishap or inspection that uncovers a defect that may ground an entire aircraft type until the problem is corrected.

The FHP is not resourced to fund these life-cycle costs that require engineering investigations and testing. Often, however, FHP funds are used to pay for repairs to aircraft that have been grounded or "red-striped" when NAVAIR does not have procurement (APN-5) funds available.

Marine Corps AV-8B and H-53 aircraft have recently experienced numerous failures, which have resulted in grounding of these airframes. Normal operating costs of these two aircraft comprise approximately half of the Marine Corps portion of the FHP. Because of their recent groundings, the Marines under-executed their portion of the FHP budget for first quarter FY01 (personal interview, March 2001).

ANNUAL COST DEFERMENT METHODS

Bow-Waving

The primary annual financing mechanism that CNAP uses to sustain flying operations through the fiscal year is called "bow-waving." Bow-waving refers to deferring the cost of something from the current fiscal year to the next fiscal year. CNAP uses this technique with Aviation Depot Level Repair parts (AVDLRs) in order to keep aircraft operating. When a Ready for Issue (RFI) repair part is taken from the "shelf" the bad or broken part is inducted into the depot facility for repair if the item cannot be fixed at the Aviation Intermediate Maintenance activity (AIMD). To prevent the charge in the current fiscal year, the AIMDs will retain the AVDLRs until the next fiscal year. This cash flow technique enables fleet units to continue flying when the budget would have been exhausted if the AVDLRs were processed. However, the practice of bow-waving ensures further under-funding in the future because the costs of the bow-wave are not part of OP-20 pricing. Table 2 shows the cost of AVDLRs that were bow-waved in the past four fiscal years.

Table 2.   Bow-Waved Amounts [Ref. 6]

Fiscal Year	Amount
97	$65M
98	$26M
99	$55.5M
00	0

Source: Personal interview (March 2001)

Unfilled Customer Orders (UCOs)

Another cash flow transaction CNAP has used to get through the execution year in is Unfilled Customer Orders (UCOs). UCOs are a cash flow generating strategy in which fleet operating units administratively cancel or de-obligate outstanding requisitions for AVDLRs to recover the cash as a means to pay for more urgent requirements. This strategy is a mechanism used by CNAP to prevent over-obligation of budgeted FHP funds. Under the agreement between CNAP and Navy Inventory Control Point (NAV-ICP), all requisitions cancelled must be reordered within 45 days after the new fiscal year (Keating & Paulk, 1998, p. 181).

FUNDING CYCLE PROBLEMS: THE BATHTUB EFFECT

As CNAP managers have struggled to maintain the viability of FHP budgets, they have been forced to reduce funding allotted to squadrons in the Inter-Deployment Training Cycle (IDTC). The resultant reduction of flying hours and PMR for squadrons has created what CNAP managers refer to as the bathtub effect (Figure 4). The height of operating tempo occurs during deployment for Naval forces. As units return to the United States from overseas deployments, some crews rotate and new replacement personnel arrive, there is an expected decrease in the level of flying from the high tempo of deployment. Within the first couple of months upon returning, leave, training and rotations occur. Readiness levels decrease as crews

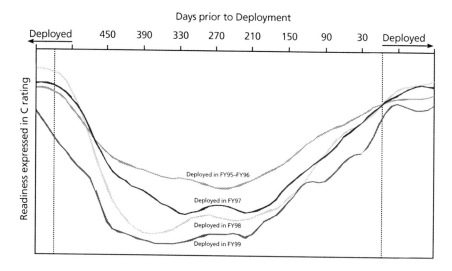

Figure 4.   Bathtub effect.

are dismantled and the process of training for the next deployment begins (personal interview, January 2001).

To stay safe and proficient however, flying still occurs but at reduced levels from deployment. As funding levels have been reduced in recent years, the easiest target for reduction of flying has become the "home guard" squadrons. The trend in recent years is to reduce IDTC squadrons to lower levels of PMR.

Although difficult to quantify for the entire force, CNAP managers reported aggregate PMR execution rates of 57–60% for carrier aviation squadrons from the month of return from deployment through the tenth month prior to deployment for fiscal years 1998 to 2000. For FY01, funding for this same time period in the IDTC has been reduced to 53% PMR (personal interview, January 2001).

As the depth of the bathtub increases, proficiency atrophies as pilots fly fewer hours per month. The real concern of planners is that there is a steeper ramp going on deployment coming out of IDTC. As aircrews are faced with increasing intensity and more challenging flying during deployment, their skills may not match the level of flying required because of the reduction in flying hours throughout the IDTC.

SUMMARY

Table 3 summarizes key final amounts for the fiscal years that have been researched. This table is not intended to serve as a balance sheet, but reflects some of the important amounts identified. Numbers are approximate and reflect information provided to the author from multiple sources.

Table 3.   Summary of Final Key Amounts for FY98, 99, and 00 (Millions of dollars).

	FY 98	FY 99	FY 00
Initial Controls from CINCPACFLT	$ 1,380	$ 1,290	$ 1,289
CINCPACFLT Withholds (Y2K, IT-21, others	$ (27)	$ (53)	$ (27)
CNAP reprogramming to Underfunded Programs (Staff OPTAR, Ranges, TAD, Simulators)	$ (37)	$ (30)	$ (21)
Contingency Funds	$ 84	$ 87	$ 65
Reprogramming in, CNO Reserve, Supplementals	$ 25	$ 68	$ 63
Total Funds Spent on FHP	$ 1,388	$ 1,343	$ 1,393
Previous year's bow wave	$ 65	$ 26	$ 56
FHP Funds Spent on Critical Unfundeds (Aircraft Life Cycle Costs)	$ 16	$ 53	$ 32
PMR achieved	79.4	80.0	76.6

CONCLUSIONS

Recognizing that there are insufficient funds to properly execute the annual FHP budget, CNAP managers initially request a higher percentage of annual funding for the first quarter in CINCPACFLT's phasing of funding. As expenditures outstrip resources in different fund codes, reprogramming money and requesting that CINCPACFLT advance funds from future quarters enables fiscally balancing each account. CNAP managers reduce operating tempo for units in the Inter-Deployment Training Cycle (IDTC) and reduce expenses on the margins by leading initiatives to cut maintenance and supply costs.

CNAP managers use cost deferment methods in order to make it through the year avoiding Anti-deficiency violations. These procedures include bow waving AVDLRs to future fiscal years and using Unfilled Customer Orders (UCOs). Throughout the process, CNAP managers monitor expenditure rates and continually communicate shortfalls. By articulating their fiscal position up the chain of command, the hope is that funding relief that will be provided toward the end of the year.

Each year the POM process produces the OP-20 budgeting document that attempts to match resources to requirements and is used as the initial starting point to determine the FHP budget. In budget execution many things happen to the dollars that were originally in the OP-20 budget. When the dollars available to execute the FHP reach the managers at CNAP, some of the money that was originally in the budget is being used for other programs.

The overall budgeting system does not recognize valid bills from many different programs and fund them; therefore the FHP (CNAP's only real source of discretionary money) is raided every year. The process forces CNAP managers to creatively finance throughout the year and hope for relief at the end of the year. The resultant dollar amount to execute the FHP constitutes an overly restrictive control on CNAP managers. It adds transaction costs to CNAP managers in the form of continually trying to communicate shortfalls, second guessing true Fleet execution, and inventing methods of creative financing, including the risk of violating the Anti-deficiency Act. The challenges of budget execution documented in this research are difficult enough without the additional restrictions of excessive control placed upon CNAP's FHP managers.

FHP budget development and execution trends continue in FY 01. CNAP managers estimate a $235 million shortfall and hope to receive a Defense Supplemental Appropriation late in the summer FY01 (personal interview, April 2001). As in the three years covered in this research, large funding shortfalls frustrate FHP managers' efforts in developing a coherent plan to execute the program.

Instead of providing budget relief at the end of the year, proper initial funding of all programs within Naval Aviation, or use of some alternative method of funding flying hours would alleviate the uncertainties and system stress throughout the year and especially in third and fourth quarter execution. With such substantial reform, CNAP managers will be able to focus on properly supporting fleet requirements, while eliminating the need of creative and risky financing. Until restrictive controls are removed, CNAP managers will not meet readiness requirements, they will have to consider shutting down non-deployed squadrons for extended periods of time, and they will risk Anti-deficiency Act violations.

NOTES

1. This case study was written by Lt. Commander Ernie Philips as an essay derived from his Master's degree thesis on the execution of the Flight Hour Program budget.

2. "Highlights of the Department of the Navy FY 2000 Budget," [http://navweb.secnav.navy.mil/pubbud/01pres/highbook/01pb_highlights.pdf] .

REFERENCES

Assistant Chief of Naval Operations for Air Warfare. (1996 Draft). N-88 "Flying Hour Program (FHP) Desktop Procedures Guide."

Assistant Chief of Naval Operations for Air Warfare Naval Aviation. (1998). "Flying Hour Program Brief." Washington, DC.

Commander Naval Air Forces Pacific Flying Hour Program Brief for VADM Bowman, March 5, 1998.

Department of Defense Financial Management Regulation, DoD 7000.14-R (2000, August), Vol. 3, Ch. 6, p. 6–4.

Keating, P.J., & Paulk, D.A. (1998, December). *Examination of the Flying Hour Program (FHP) Budgeting Process and an Analysis of Commander Naval Air Forces Pacific (CNAP) FHP Underfunding.* Master's Thesis, Naval Postgraduate School, Monterey, CA.

Personal interview with Flying Hour Program staff member, Commander Naval Air Force Pacific, San Diego, CA, April 27, 2001.

Personal interview with Flying Hour Program staff member, Commander Naval Air Force Pacific, San Diego, CA, March 28–30, 2001.

Personal interview with Flying Hour Program staff member, Commander Naval Air Force Pacific, San Diego, CA, January 17–18, 2001.

APPENDIX C

CFO ACT IMPLEMENTATION:

A CASE STUDY OF THE
SPECIAL WARFARE COMMAND

INTRODUCTION:
THE CFO ACT AND IMPLEMENTATION ISSUES

The Chief Financial Officer's Act of 1990 (CFO) was implemented to create a structure and systems that would improve financial management practice and support resource decision making toward a more responsible government and a better-informed public. The legislation addressed three problem areas: organizational short-term focus and fragmentation; inadequate internal controls and accounting systems; and a total lack of audited financial statements.

Financial decision making had been split between the Office of Management and Budget, the General Services Administration, and the Treasury. A Chief Financial Officer of the United States would provide centralized financial management leadership. It was decided this position should reside in the OMB because this "budget power center" was best suited to establish government-wide financial reform policies.

Managing the cost of government operations was made more difficult by control weaknesses and a lack of comprehensive financial information. The adoption of Generally Accepted Accounting Principles (GAAP) used by businesses would move the government from cash budgeting and accounting to capital budgeting and accrual accounting. This would recognize assets such as buildings or equipment as capital items with specific values and rates of depreciation. Thus, the value of an asset over its entire life could be assessed. Budget manipulation would be unnecessary because all liabilities would appear on the balance sheet.

Such financial statements could then be audited, ensuring discipline in financial management, providing an analytic tool to understand the government's condition and operations, and highlighting the adequacy of agency conduct and practice.

Thus, the CFO Act not only created a CFO for the whole government, but an additional CFO in all major departments and agencies, as well as a CFO Council to assist in implementation. Agencies were required to submit proposals for consolidating financial management functions, particularly accounting and budgeting, under their CFO, with five year plans describing the implementation of this consolidation; audited financial statements and management reports were to be done annually. Additionally, Chief Financial Officers were to approve and manage financial system design and enhancement projects; oversee recruitment and training of agency financial personnel; implement asset management systems; and monitor agency budget execution.

Additional legislation and governing bodies were created to enable and enhance implementation. The Federal Accounting Standards Advisory Board (FASAB) was established by the comptroller general, the secretary of the Treasury, and the director of OMB to develop cost and financial accounting standards specifically for the federal government. The Government Performance and Results Act (GPRA) of 1993 emphasizes strategic planning, performance measurement, and customer satisfaction. The Government Management Reform Act (GMRA) of 1994 extended the auditing requirement to all types of accounts within five months of the close of the fiscal year. It also established the time line for the first government-wide audit in FY97.

Significant progress has been made since that first audit was prepared. Of 24 agencies required to prepare financial statements, 21 are expected to receive an unqualified opinion for FY99. Twenty-two agencies have successfully produced accountability reports for FY99. More reliable financial information has improved the evaluation of federal programs and activities. The Health Care Financing Administration has reduced improper payments every year since 1996 as a result of an extensive audit analysis done by the Department of Health and Human Services Inspector General (OMB, 1999, p. 3).

To help agencies share lessons learned, the Joint Financial Management Improvement Program (JFMIP) Program Management Office (PMO) was established in November 1998. The JFMIP PMO serves as an information clearinghouse for federal financial systems, developing requirements and testing vehicles, addressing integration issues, and facilitating communication with the private sector. JFMIP began testing vendor core financial software in June 1999 to qualify it for use in the federal government in FY00, to be supplied by the Government Service Agency (GSA) (OMB, 1999, pp. 5–6).

Recruiting, training and retaining qualified personnel to use these and other financial management systems is another key priority of the CFO Council. Training guidelines and recruitment strategies have been issued. Core competencies for financial management positions have been developed, and a pilot program using standard position descriptions for accountants has begun. The Federal Training Technology Initiative will be used to develop training programs with outside facilitators (OMB, 1999, p. 7).

Other priorities in which the CFO Council has made significant progress are: improving the management of receivables by expanding the Treasury Offset Program and Agency Debt Referral; using electronic commerce by increasing the usage of government purchase cards, Electronic Funds Transfer, and the Financial Electronic Data Exchange, which helps the Veterans Administration collect insurance payments and the Department of Education collect student loan payments. Internet Credit Card Collections will expand to from five to thirteen agencies to collect fees, donations, fines and other payments. The Electronic Federal Tax Payment System will allow the IRS to deduct payments from individual bank accounts. Administration of federal grant programs will improve by reducing the cash draw-down systems in use to three by October 2003. Standardization of the indirect cost rate calculation, which determines what percentage of a federal grant may be used for facilities and administrative costs, will help streamline grant application and reporting processes (OMB, 1999, pp. 8–12).

For all the government-wide success of the CFO Council in implementing the CFO Act and subsequent legislation, however, there are several obstacles to obtaining an unqualified audit opinion on the government-wide financial statements. All agencies need to eliminate intragovernmental transactions. The cost of loans receivable and loan guarantee programs need to be properly reported. The full extent of improper payments needs to be assessed, and the discrepancies between agency records and Treasury records of disbursements need to be resolved. A more effective process to reconcile the change in net position with the budget surplus or deficit needs to be established (OMB, 1999, p. 4).

A significant problem area in obtaining an unqualified audit opinion is the Department of Defense (DOD). The Federal Financial Management Status Report and Five Year Plan reports, "DOD is making progress in meeting the audited financial statement requirements of the CFO Act. However, significant and longstanding systems deficiencies preclude DOD from projecting an unqualified consolidated audited financial statement until after 2000." Coupled with the challenge of eliminating intragovernmental transactions, the "magnitude" of DOD problems makes the goal of an unqualified government-wide audit opinion "daunting." Specific issues include: understating of environmental and disposal liabilities because no estimate was reported for some major weapons systems and some nuclear weapons are inadequately documented. Health benefits, accounts payable, and other liabilities are not supported by auditable systems and data. Property, plant, equipment (PP&E), and inventory data cannot be audited to demonstrate the dollar value of assets supporting DOD operations (OMB, 1999, p. 4). In Congressional testimony in May 2000, the General Accounting Office noted that many of DOD's fixes would result in a one-time year-end number for financial statement purposes but would not "produce the timely and reliable financial and performance information DOD needs to manage its operations every day" (GAO, 2000, p. 1).

CFO ACT IMPLEMENTATION AT
NAVAL SPECIAL WARFARE COMMAND

One command is making great effort to comply with CFO Act requirements. The Naval Special Warfare Command (NAVSPECWAR) in Coronado, California, is the Navy's component to the United States Special Operations Command (SOCOM). Responsible for the "...administration, training, maintenance, support and readiness of all United States-based active and reserve Naval Special Warfare forces," NAVSPECWAR develops strategy, operations, and tactics to carry out assigned missions to support Theater Commanders in Chief (CINCs). Though their operational chain-of-command is clear, their financial management personnel serve two masters: the Navy and the joint command of SOCOM. This presents unique challenges to their ability to comply with the CFO Act, primarily centered around their relationships with DOD through the Defense Finance and Accounting Service (DFAS); with the Navy and SOCOM as their superiors with differing systems; and with various entities all struggling to resolve the PP&E and inventory issues that plague DOD.

CFO IMPLEMENTATION BY THE DEFENSE FINANCE AND
ACCOUNTING SERVICE

DFAS was established in January 1991 as the sole finance and accounting entity for DOD to "provide effective and efficient financial information, accounting, and payment services" (DFAS, 2000, p. 1–4). Since each service and defense agency had their own systems and business practices, DFAS's priority has been consolidation and integration of operations locations from 338 to 25, and of installation level finance and accounting systems from 324 to 83 in January 2000, with a goal of 30 or fewer by 2005 (DFAS, 2000, p. 1–2).

The DFAS Corporate Database was established to store and maintain all shared financial data for on-line transaction processing. The DFAS Corporate Warehouse supports reporting, analytical processing and archival functions in a central information repository. Yet many systems cannot share data. Some systems create incomplete or inaccurate reports because of the incompatibility with other systems and a lack of standardization. Interfaces among systems range from manual data entry from hard-copy to real-time electronic interchange. Thus, transactions are slow and prone to errors, creating problem disbursements, degraded data, multiple data entry, duplicate system interfaces, and an inability to trace transactions to source data. These limitations preclude validation of disbursements with the corresponding obligations prior to disbursing funds. Thus, DFAS must choose between making potentially invalid payments or paying late penalties while taking the time it needs to establish validation. (DFAS, 2000, p. 2.3).

NAVSPECWAR has found this makes it impossible for a command to validate DFAS data as well. Reports are generated without input from the field and with fiscal years lumped together. DFAS would need to provide a detailed crosswalk from their accounting reports and a backup on their data sources to assist command validation, yet this has never been done. However, NAVSPECWAR has yet to see any impact on DFAS or the command if the reports are incorrect (Dissing, 2000).

Thus, when DFAS surveyed commands about a proposed change to the DOD Financial Management Regulation (DODFMR) to enable DFAS to automatically obligate funds for transactions up to $2500, NAVSPECWAR was not in favor of it. Volume 3, Chapter 8 of the DODFMR establishes standards for recording commitments and obligations. Price Waterhouse Coopers, the DFAS contractor, has proposed several changes on the premise that a number of unrecorded obligations exist in the accounting system and that the time it takes to record them is too great. They suggest that if DFAS identifies an incurred obligation that has not been recorded in the accounting records, DFAS will immediately record the obligation if it is less than $2500. If it is greater than $2500, DFAS will provide documentation to the DOD component fund manager and allow 10 calendar days for the fund manager to record the obligation or demonstrate that it was already done. DFAS vows to contact the fund manager immediately and initiate research if by recording the obligation it results in an apparent Anti-deficiency Act violation. The change proposal also states that if the fund manager identifies that DFAS has recorded a duplicate obligation, DFAS will reverse it upon receiving adequate documentation (Dissing, 2000).

NAVSPECWAR disagrees with these premises and proposed changes, because most commands use systems that interface obligation data into the accounting system, eliminating unrecorded or incorrectly recorded obligations. They feel that most problem disbursements are created not by missing obligations but by erroneous or duplicate payments posting against a valid line of accounting or invoices with inaccurate data, such as citing a document number that is different from the obligating document.

Allowing DFAS to obligate funds to pay an invoice presents several difficulties. The Suspended Transaction Listing would no longer exist. This mechanism provided visibility of problems and allowed fund holders to validate transactions, preventing erroneous transactions from impacting the funds available balance while allowing payments to be processed. If DFAS obligates funds, invoices would find matching obligating documents but would not be validated. Since DFAS is not within NAVSPECWAR's funding chain, it should not have obligation authority over funds for which it does not have Anti-deficiency Act responsibilities. It calls into question who would be held responsible for violations. These changes appear to make DFAS "look good on paper at everyone else's expense" without solving any problems (Dissing, 2000).

DFAS has some sense of the difficulties involved, since its strategic plan covers nearly a ten-year period to achieve what they call the Objective CFO-compliant Environment (OCE) that will also satisfy the requirements of the Federal Financial Management Improvement Act and OMB Circulars A-123 (Management Accountability and Control), A-127 (Financial Management Systems), and A-130 (Management of Federal Information Resources). The Near-Term (FY99–FY00) phase focuses on eliminating redundant systems; establishing target architecture framework while continuing integration of legacy financial systems; and initiating the reengineering of selected financial systems into the OCE. The Mid-Term (FY01–FY04) phase will complete the elimination of redundant systems and integration of finance and accounting systems, accelerating the completion of the target architecture framework; and continuing reengineering of selected systems into the OCE. The Long-Term (FY05–FY08) phase completes the development of the DFAS Corporate Information Infrastructure (DCII) and continues the integration of selected financial systems into the OCE, a process that will continue past FY08 (DFAS, 2000, pp. 4.2–4.3).

It appears that CFO Act compliance for DFAS will not occur anytime soon. DFAS is holding military services and DOD agencies accountable for their feeder systems, which provide 80 percent of the data used by DFAS systems. "Achieving the OCE—to include the production of auditable financial statements—is critically dependent on the ability of feeder systems to produce high quality data and execute CFO-compliant processes"

(DFAS, 2000, p. 5.5). Feeder systems must migrate to CFO-compliant environments in concert with the migration of DFAS so that the systems will be compatible and exchange data in standard formats. "Massive collaborative efforts among stakeholders" will be required (DFAS, 2000, p. 5.5).

CFO ACT IMPLEMENTATION IN SPECIAL OPERATIONS COMMAND AND THE NAVY

Collaboration is the hallmark of the United States Special Operations Command (USSOCOM), created in 1986, which incorporates the Joint Special Operations Command (JSOC), United States Army Special Operations Command (USASOC), the Air Force Special Operations Command (AFSOC) and NAVSPECWAR to, "...provide special operations forces to the National Command Authorities, Regional Combatant Commanders, and American ambassadors and their country teams for successful conduct of worldwide special operations, civil affairs, and psychological operations during both peace and war" (Kingston, 1999, p. 2). USSOCOM develops joint Special Operations Forces (SOF) doctrine, tactics, and procedures; conducts training with SOF-specialized instruction to ensure joint interoperability; and ensures professional development and readiness of all joint SOF personnel (Kingston, 1999, p. 3).

USSOCOM also manages the program and budget of Major Force Program (MFP) 11, which contains seven elements for operational activities, force enhancements, training, general support, advanced SOF RDT&E, planning and design, and headquarters management. SOF-peculiar items can be standard items used by other DOD forces and modified by SOF; items initially designed for or used by SOF but adopted for use by other forces; and items deemed by the CINC as critically urgent for immediate mission accomplishment (Kingston, 1999, pp. 3–6).

DOD has decreed that USSOCOM produce CFO financial statements, even though USSOCOM must act as translator among Army, Air Force, and Navy financial systems since it does not have one of its own, nor does it have a staff and infrastructure to support CFO compliance efforts. The FY99 reports, made without additional input from the service commands, are now being audited. As the services have also produced reports, SOF assets may be double-counted; neither the Army nor the Navy has the capability to segregate SOF data, although that capability is required by DOD regulations. The Air Force has maintained a separate SOF budgeting process for years and has successfully received budget increases for their support of SOF (Dissing, 2000).

NAVSPECWAR has already detected significant errors in the parts of the report they have seen. USSOCOM's total cost of ownership programs produced inaccurate financial data. The ship inventory did not use DOD category definitions and placed all of NAVSPECWAR's craft in the wrong categories. The Navy MFP 11 report includes several commands in addition to NAVSPECWAR, such as Naval Sea Systems Command, Special Operations Command Pacific, USASOC, and Naval Air Systems Command. These cross a variety of DFAS headquarters and financial systems, resulting in incorrect or incomplete data collection. NAVSPECWAR can help improve the accuracy of the MFP 11 reports with the help of DFAS Indianapolis, but there are too many elements they do not control to be able to correct the entire report.

Although MFP 11 funds 100% of NAVSPECWAR activities, since 1995 they have been doing CFO Act reports through the Navy. (The Navy provides limited support in the form of chemical/biological gear and radios, but it is not listed in the NAVSPECWAR budget.) For FY99 NAVSPECWAR strictly followed Navy guidelines and only reported information the Navy did not already have. This included: an inventory of ships and craft, since the Navy has no register of these vessels except for Patrol Coastals; military construction in progress—funded by USSOCOM it does not enter the Navy database until completed and registered with Naval Facilities Engineering Command (NAVFAC); and Civil Engineering Support Equipment (vehicles), because it could not be verified that NAVFAC listed them in their database although they issued the licenses. They did not report: ammunition already recorded by the Navy; Plant Property Class 3 and 4 awaiting implementation of the Defense Plant Accounting System; and Land and Facilities Class 1 and 2, owned and reported by the Navy, yet without distinguishing it as SOF.

This multitude of reporting systems has caused the Navy its own problems with CFO Act compliance. For FY99 the Naval Audit Service was unable to express an opinion on the Department of the Navy Principal Statements. The Statements were not provided in a timely manner to enable the necessary audit work and the Management Representation Letter was missing. The following systems deficiencies were noted: the Department of the Navy does not have transaction-driven standard general ledger accounting systems to accurately report the value of assets and liabilities; accounting systems do not have sufficient audit trails to enable transaction level verification; and financial and non-financial feeder systems do not collect and record data on an accrual basis—financial data is based on budgetary information and adjusted (Bragg, 2000, p. 1).

In addition, internal controls "did not provide reasonable assurance that resources were properly managed and accounted for, that the Department of the Navy complied with applicable laws and regulations, and that the FY1999 Department of the Navy General Fund financial statements contained no material misstatements" (Bragg, 2000, p. 2). In fact, the Navy was found out of compliance with the Statement of Federal Financial Accounting Standards No. 6, the Federal Managers' Financial Integrity Act of 1982; the Government Performance and Results Act of 1993, OMB Bulletin No. 97-01 as amended, and the CFO Act (Bragg, 2000, p. 2).

At a presentation to the American Society of Military Comptrollers' Professional Development Institute in May 2000, the Office of Financial Operations of the Assistant Secretary of the Navy (Financial Management and Comptroller) outlined the issues, strategies, and requirements for gaining compliance. They noted that resources required to make the legislative changes are often in short supply; that personnel are transaction rather than analysis oriented; the existence of the "use it or lose it" mentality instead of examining the bottom-line; and an ineffective relationship with DFAS. Yet they used the DFAS method of strategic planning for a three-phased approach. The Near-Term Action Plan provides general and specific steps to alleviate current audit issues and "ensure all commands/ activities are managing accounting and finance information and processes effectively and efficiently" (OFO, 2000, p. 30). The Short-Term Action Plan outlines the Navy Working Groups and initiatives for achieving Under Secretary of Defense (Comptroller) Implementation Strategies for Property, Plant and Equipment; Inventory and Related Property; Liabilities (Environmental Restoration, Hazardous Waste Disposal); and Human Resources. The Long-Term Action Plan addresses "critical, overarching organizational, system and process issues:" refining and articulating a unified vision of Navy Financial Management; cooperation between financial and functional areas; refining business processes; monitoring policy execution; improving the financial statement production process; reviewing the mix of personnel resources; and feeder system issues of compliance, redundancies, and interfaces.

UNIQUE NATURE OF PLANT, PROPERTY, AND EQUIPMENT IN CFO ACT IMPLEMENTATION

The Undersecretary of Defense (Comptroller) (USD(C)) Implementation Strategy for Plant, Property, and Equipment outlines methods for achieving unqualified opinions on the Department's financial statements. Issued in 1998, in a series of memorandums, time lines of accomplishment and monthly reporting requirements are established. Unless a DOD component has a fully operational property accountability system that meets CFO requirements, including the capability to maintain historical cost data and calculate depreciation, implementation of such a system must be expedited (USD(C), 1998, p.1).

For property acquired prior to FY1999, if an asset is fully depreciated based on its initial acquisition or transfer date and useful life, its cost will be reported with an offsetting amount as accumulated depreciation. Assets that are not fully depreciated must be evaluated by a USD(C) Comptroller to determine carrying value, accumulated depreciation and book value. Newly acquired assets will be capitalized at acquisition cost, and departments will establish procedures to identify and report assets with capital leases in accordance with Standard Federal Financial Accounting Standard No. 6 (USD(C), 1998, p. 1).

Verification of property accountability records and/or systems will ensure that all property, plant, and equipment are properly recorded. Data fields of installation-level PP&E databases must be reconciled with headquarters and/or centralized databases to ensure reliability of data (USD(C), 1998, p. 2).

The system that DOD ultimately chose for department-wide use is the Defense Plant Accounting System, originally developed by the Army. It has not yet been installed for NAVSPECWAR, so definition issues of PP&E are still prominent. Boston Whalers and dive boats could be classified as support craft or General PP&E. Combat Rubber Raiding Craft are viewed as consumables, purchased from GSA, but some may view them as boats (Dissing, 2000).

Many discussions have ensued between the DOD Inspector General (IG) conducting USSOCOM's audit and NAVSPECWAR over the classification of boats and which command will report which data. SOCOM apparently chose a threshold of $100,000 above which to report watercraft as ships. This dollar figure is briefly mentioned in the USD(C) memorandums as a topic for further discussion amongst OMB, GAO, and DODIG, but is not yet listed in any other written guidance. NAVSPECWAR maintains that SOCOM's database is incomplete and does not recognize the specific definition of commissioned ships. They have 13 ships and everything else is a boat. DODIG maintains that the DODFMR does not include a category for boats in the National Defense PP&E category, despite Navy trying to add one; the DOD agency-wide report merges boats into an "Other Ships" category. NAVSPECWAR states that the $100,000 threshold will not accurately represent their PP&E because entire types of boats, used for National Defense, will be eliminated (Dissing, 2000).

Dialogue is also ongoing between NAVSPECWAR and NAVFAC over who should report CESE equipment. NAVFAC believes they have no reporting requirement as the Naval Comptroller Manual only requires activity-level, not claimant level reporting. NAVSPECWAR maintains that not reporting it is in violation of the CFO Act, but is concerned that both entities are reporting the same data: NAVFAC because they are unable to split the registered vehicles out from the rest of the motorpool, and

NAVSPECWAR because they want to ensure it is done. The Navy must decide whose responsibility this requirement will be (Dissing, 2000).

This is but a symptom of the larger ills between NAVFAC and NAVSPECWAR. NAVFAC receives more than $100,000 annually for CESE support and management, yet the only service provided is Navy license plates. Although vehicles are bought via NAVFAC channels, program requirements are managed by NAVSPECWAR headquarters staff, and component commands maintain them. This is highly inefficient and expensive funds management, yet Navy accounting systems are targeted to give useful data to service providers, not customers (Dissing, 2000).

NAVSEA also provides support and management, but NAVSPECWAR is unsure of where the money goes. NAVSEA is currently asking for more than $600,000 in prior year bills for overhaul contracts, but cannot provide any documentation as to when or what overhauls were done. Overhead fees are paid to manage the contracts but the managers cannot provide basic data. In another case, NAVSEA is requesting $140,000 to write a maintenance manual for the Ford trucks used to haul NAVSPECWAR's boats in and out of the water. This manual would replace the standard owners' manuals that come with the trucks. Money from one fiscal year requirement is routinely applied to other fiscal year requirements, which may not necessarily be those of NAVSPECWAR. Yet if they protest, NAVSEA can refuse to certify their watercraft. NAVSPECWAR feels it is being held hostage by the Navy's requirements to use services it does not need.

LESSONS LEARNED

A high level member of the Comptroller staff at NAVSPECWAR offered the following view on compliance, "I really think that if we were on our own we could produce a compliant statement. We are small enough to get our hands around the information. But we are not independent." Herein lies the key to the successful implementation of the CFO Act—commands, reporting entities, OMB, GAO, and Congress must all work together to achieve compliance.

NAVSPECWAR is rewriting their Memorandum of Agreement with the Navy to resolve duplicative reporting issues and definitions. They are working closely with the DODIG during USSOCOM's audit to help both parties understand their unique requirements. They are negotiating with DFAS Indianapolis to clear up some of the anomalies in the MFP 11 reports. They are raising the flag against inefficiencies and old-school support and management through outside bodies such as NAVFAC and NAVSEA.

The new Chief of Naval Operations, ADM Vern Clark outlined his "Framework for Action" to include manpower, current readiness, future readiness, quality of service, and a new Navy-wide command realignment. Vice Chief of Naval Operations ADM Donald Pilling will establish the office of naval war fighting requirements to parallel the resource office of N8. This will give fleet commanders a "louder voice in the budget process" (Defense Daily, 2000, p. 6).

The Under Secretary of Defense (Comptroller) William J. Lynn, is asking for help: "We, frankly, are interested in hiring 'Big Six' accounting firms to help us with our financial systems. Efforts to reform the process are harmed by the political process. The length of time needed to change the system is longer than any one administration. If the subsequent administration puts the reform on the backburner, as has happened in the past, the system will accrue more inaccurate financial data" (Mulholland, 2000).

Mr. Lynn's enthusiasm was probably motivated by the Congressional testimony by GAO in July 2000, noting that no major part of DOD has yet been able to pass an independent audit because of "pervasive weaknesses in DOD's financial management systems, operations and controls." DOD continues to be considered a high-risk area vulnerable to fraud, waste, abuse and mismanagement whose efforts to improve its efficiency of operations are severely hampered by its lack of control. Establishing an integrated financial system is key to overcoming unreliable cost and budget information used to measure performance and reduce costs (GAO, 2000, p. 1).

Certainly, OMB is anxious to have the Department of Defense on board. It will soon be the only federal department unable to produce CFO-compliant financial statements, continuing to put the rest of the government on hold from achieving government-wide unqualified audit results.

An extraordinary degree of cooperation between the military services and defense agencies is required. Stovepipes and traditional parochialism will have to be abandoned in favor of standardized, uniform processes for financial management easily understood and adhered to by all. If not, as one defense official has said, using the Revolution in Business Affairs to pay for the Revolution in Military Affairs will be a non-starter.

ACKNOWLEDGMENT

This case study was written by Lt. Martin Sable, U.S. Navy and edited by L.R. Jones for this volume.

REFERENCES

Assistant Secretary of the Navy (Financial Management and Comptroller). 1994. NCB-31 Memorandum on Assignment of Subheads for Fiscal Year 1995 in Defense Agency Appropriations. ASNFM: September 13.

Assistant Secretary of the Navy (Financial Management and Comptroller). 1999. "Memorandum FMO-123, Budget and Accounting Classification Code Structure and Mapping to Defense Data Dictionary System." ASNFM: January 5.

Assistant Secretary of the Navy (Financial Management and Comptroller). 1999. "Memorandum on Property, Plant, and Equipment Accountability." ASNFM: July 13.

Assistant Secretary of the Navy (Financial Management and Comptroller). 2001. "Memorandum: Department of the Navy Financial and Feeder Systems Compliance Process." ANSFM: February 14.

Bragg, N. 2000. "Audit for CFO Compliance." Naval Audit Service, Department of the Navy, Washington, D.C.

Defense Daily. 2000. "Framework for Action" Washington, D.C.: Department of Defense.

Defense Finance and Accounting Service. 2000. "Financial Systems Strategic Plans: Foundation for the Future." DFAS: January. http://www.dfas.mil/library/dassp.pdf

Defense Finance and Accounting Service. No Date. "Standard Accounting and Reporting System Field Level (STARS-FL) Online User's Manual." DFAS, Cleveland.

Department of Defense. 1996. "Regulation 7000.14-R." DoD Financial Management Regulation, Vol. 6, Reporting and Policy Procedures. DOD: February.

Department of the Navy. 20001. "Memorandum on Department of the Navy Future Years Defense Program Improvement Project: Program Element Restructure." DON: June 29.

Department of the Navy. No Date. Memorandum: NAVSO P-1000 074202—Activity Group Coding Structure Criteria for Operations and Maintenance. DON.

Department of Systems Management. 1995. "Practical Comptrollership Course Manual." Naval Postgraduate School. NPS/SM: Monterey, CA. July.

Dissing, P. 2000. "Personal Memorandum." Coronado, CA: Special Warfare Command.

Federal Accounting Standards Advisory Board. 1997. "Statement of Federal Financial Accounting Standards (SFFAS) No. 6, Accounting for Property, Plant, and Equipment." FASAB: September 30.

General Accounting Office. 2000. "Department of Defense: Progress in Financial Management Reform." T-AIMD/NSIAD-00-163. GAO: May 9.

General Accounting Office. 2000. "Implications of Financial Management Issues." GAO/T-AIMD/NSIAD-00-264 Department of Defense. GAO: July 20.

Hleba, T. 2000. "Topics for the DoD Financial Manager." Practical Financial Management: A Handbook of Practical Financial Management. Naval Postgraduate School, Department of Systems Management.

Inspector General, Department of Defense. 2000. "U.S. Special Operations Command's Reporting of Real Property Assets on the FY 00 DoD Agency-Wide Financial Statements." Project # 1FH-0044.001, Draft Report. DoDIG: April 27.

Joint Financial Management Improvement Program. 2001. "Core Financial System Requirements." (Exposure Draft), JMFIP: June.

Kingston, J. 1999. "The United States Special Operations Command Mission." Naval Postgraduate School, Department of Systems Management, Master's of Science in Management Degree Thesis.

Jones, L.R. and J.L. McCaffery. 1992. "Financial Management Reform in the Federal Government." Naval Postgraduate School, Department of Administrative Science. Technical Report NPS-AS-93-002. NPS/AS: June.

Jones, L.R. and J.L. McCaffery. 1992. "Federal Financial Management Reform and the Chief Financial Officer's Act." Public Budgeting and Finance 12/4 (Winter): 75–86.

Jones, L.R. and J.L. McCaffery. 1993. "Implementation of the CFO Act." Public Budgeting and Finance. 13/1 (Spring): 68–76.

Maher, M. 1997. Cost Accounting: Creating Value for Management. Fifth edition. Chicago: McGraw-Hill.

Mulholland, P. 2000. "Implementing the CFO Act." Washington, D.C.: Defense Daily.

Nemfakos, Charles P. 2000. "Message from the Senior Civilian Official for the Office of the Assistant Secretary of the Navy (Financial Management & Comptroller)." Department of the Navy Future Years Defense Plan Improvement Project on Program Element Restructure. DON.

Office of Financial Operations (OFO). 2000. "Presentation to the ASMC/PDI National Conference." Assistant Secretary of the Navy (Financial Management and Comptroller), Washington, D.C.: ASNFM, May.

Office of Management and Budget. 1999. "Federal Financial Management Status Report and Five Year Plan." OMB: June 30. http://www.whitehouse.gov/omb/financial

Office of the Under Secretary of Defense (Comptroller). 2001. "Program Budget Decision (PBD) 818." USD/C: June 11.

Office of the Under Secretary of Defense (Comptroller). 2001. Department of Defense Financial Management Improvement Plan. January. http://www.dtic.mil/comptroller/OOFMIP

Office of the Under Secretary of Defense (Comptroller). 2001. "Summary of Financial management Reforms." September. http://www.dtic.mil/comptroller/sumfinman.htm

Office of the Under Secretary of Defense (Comptroller). 1998. "Implementation Strategy for Plant, Property, and Equipment." Washington, D.C.: OUSD(C).

Public Law 101-576. 1990. "Chief Financial Officer's Act of 1990." 101st Congress. November 15.

Shields, James L. 1992. "Department of Defense Implementation of the Chief Financial Officer Act." Naval Postgraduate School, Department of Administrative Science, Master's of Science in Management Degree Thesis.

Sabel, M. 2001. "Interview with Naval Special Warfare Command Personnel." Coronado, CA: June.

Stickney, C.P., and R.L. Weil. 1995. Financial Accounting. An Introduction of Concepts, Methods, and Uses, Ninth edition. Chicago: McGraw-Hill.

United States Special Operations Command. No Date. "Capabilities Based Priorities List (CBPL)—Priority Ranked/Rated listing of All USSOCOM Programs." USSOCOM.

BIBLIOGRAPHY

Abney, G., & Lauth, T. (1989, Summer). The executive budget in the states: Normative idea and empirical observation. *Policy Studies Journal, 17,* 829–840.

Air Combat Command (ACC). (1994). Government Performance and Results Act Performance Plans Fiscal Year 1995, HQ, ACC.

Albritton, R.B., & Dran, E.M. (1987). Balanced budgets and state surpluses: The politics of budgeting in Illinois. *Public Administration Review, 47,*143–152.

Analytical Perspectives, Budget of the United States (1997).

Analytical Perspectives, Budget of the United States (1996).

Anthony, R. (1985, November-December). Games government accountants play. *Harvard Business Review,* 161–170.

Anthony, R.N., & Herzlinger, R.E. (1975). *Management control in nonprofit organizations.* Homewood, IL: R.D. Irwin.

Anthony, R., & Young, D. (1984). *Managerial control in non-profit organizations.* Homewood, IL: Irwin.

Appleby, P. (1980). The role of the budget division. Reprinted in A. Schick (Ed.), *Perspectives on budgeting.* Washington, DC: ASPA.

Appleby, P. (1957, Summer). The role of the budget division. *Public Administration Review, 17,* 156–158.

Archer, S.H., Choate, G.M., & Racette, G. (1979). *Financial management: An introduction.* New York: Wiley.

Army Audit Agency (AAA). (1995). *Annual performance plan fiscal year 1995.* Washington, DC: Department of the Army, Office of the Auditor General.

Army Research Laboratory (ARL). (1994). *FY95 performance plan.*: U.S. Army Research Laboratory.

Arnold, D. (1979). *Congress and the bureaucracy.* New Haven, CT: Yale University Press.

Assistant Chief of Naval Operations for Air Warfare. (1996 Draft). N-88 Flying Hour Program (FHP) Desktop Procedures Guide.

Assistant Chief of Naval Operations for Air Warfare Naval Aviation. (1998). Flying Hour Program Brief. Washington, DC.

Associated Press. (1997, January 15). Clinton budget to seek money for welfare: Pentagon spending will be targeted. *Washington Times,* p. 5.

Aucoin, P. (1995). *The new public management: Canada in comparative perspective.* Montreal: Institute for Research in Public Policy.

Axelrod, D. (1988). *Budgeting for modern government.* St. Martin's Press.

Axelrod, R. (1975, March). The place of policy analysis in political science: Five perspectives. *American Journal of Political Science, 6*(1), 418–436.

Bailey, J.H., & O'Connor R.J. (1975). Operationalizing incrementalism: Measuring the muddles. *Public Administration Review, 35,* 60–66.

Bailey, M. (1967). Decentralization through internal prices. In S. Enke (Ed.), *Defense management* (pp. 337–352). Englewood Cliffs, NJ: Prentice-Hall.

Barton, D. (1982). Regulating a monopolist with unknown costs. *Econometrical, 50.*

Barzelay, M., with Armajani, B.J. (1992). *Breaking through bureaucracy: A new vision for managing in government.* Berkeley: University of California Press.

Beckner, N.V. (1960). Government efficiency and the military: Buyer-seller relationship. *Journal of Political Economy, 68.*

Behn, R. (1996). Public management: Should it strive to be art, science, or engineering. *Journal of Public Administration Research and Theory, 6*(1), 91–193.

Behn, R.D. (1995). The big questions of public management. *Public Administration Review, 55*(4), 313–324.

Behn, R.D. (1980). Leadership for cutback management: The use of corporate strategy. *Public Administration Review, 40*(6), 613–620.

Berner, K., & Daggett, S. (1993). *A defense budget primer.* Washington, DC: Congressional Research Service.

Bennett, J., & DiLorenzo, T. (1983). Public employee labor unions and the privatization of public services. *Journal of Labor Research, 4,* 43.

Bennett, J., & Johnson, M. (1980). *Better government at half the price: Private production of public services.* Caroline House.

Bennett, J., & Johnson, M. (1979). Public v. private provision of collective goods and services. *Public Choice, 34,* 55–63.

Berman, L. (1979). *The office of management and the budget and the presidency, 1921–1979.* Princeton, NJ: Princeton University Press.

Biller, R.P. (1980). Leadership tactics for retrenchment. *Public Administration Review, 40,* 604–608.

Black, E.L., & Walker, K.B. (1997). *Reengineering the business core curriculum: Aligning business schools with business for improved performance.* Fayetteville: University of Arkansas, Department of Accounting, College of Business Administration.

Blankart, C.B. (1979). Bureaucratic problems in public choice: Why do public goods still remain public? In R. Roskamp (Ed.), *Public choice and public finance* (pp. 155–167). Cujas.

Blechman, B., Gramlick, E., & Hartman, R. (1975). *Setting national priorities: The 1976 budget* (pp. 193–207). Washington, DC: The Brookings Institute.

Block, P. (1995, Fall). Rediscovering service: Weaning higher education from its factory mentality. *The Educational Record, 76*(4), 6–13.

Bolles, A.S. (1896/1969). *The financial history of the United States from 1774 to 1789.* New York: D. Appleton.

Borins, S.F. (1995, Spring). The new public management is here to stay. *Canadian Public Administration,* 122–132.

Borins, S.F. (1994, October). *Government in transition: A new paradigm in public administration.* A Report on the Inaugural Conference of the Commonwealth Association for Public Administration and Management, CAPAM, Toronto, Canada.

Bower, J.L., & Christenson, C.J. (1978). *Public management: Text and cases.* Homewood, IL: R.D. Irwin.

Bowsher, C.A. (1985, Summer). Governmental financial management at the crossroads: The choice is between reactive and proactive financial management. *Public Budgeting & Finance, 5*(2), pp. 9–22.

Breton, A., & Wintrobe, R. (1975). The equilibrium size of a budget maximizing bureau. *Journal of Political Economy, 83,* 195–207.

Browne, V.J. (1949). *The control of the public budget.* Washington, DC: Public Affairs Press.

Bruggeman, W. (1995, September). The impact of technological change on management accounting. *Management Accounting Research, 6*(3), 241–252.

Brundage, P. (1970). *The bureau of the budget.* New York: Praeger.

Budget Concepts. (1996). Washington, D.C: USGPO.

Budget of the United States Government, 1976, p. 49.

Bunce, P., Fraser, R., & Woodcock, L. (1995, September). Advanced budgeting: A journey to advanced management systems. *Management Accounting Research, 6*(3), 253–265.

Burkhead, J. (1956/1959). *Government budgeting.* New York: John Wiley and Sons.

Caiden, N. (1991, Spring). Do politicians listen to experts. *Public Budgeting and Finance, 11*(1), 41–49.

Caiden, N. (1983, Winter). Guidelines to federal budget reform. *Public Budgeting and Finance, 3*(4), 4–22.

Caiden, N. (1982, November/December). The myth of the annual budget. *Public Administration Review, 42,* 516–523.

Caiden, N., & Wildavsky, A. (1974). *Planning and budgeting in poor countries.* New York: Wiley.

Caldwell, L.K. (1944, Spring). Alexander Hamilton: Advocate of executive leadership. *Public Administration Review, 4.* [Reprinted in J.W. Fesler (1982), *American public administration: Patterns of the past* (pp. 71–89). Washington, DC: ASPA]

Chandler, A. (1962). *Strategy and structure: Chapters in the history of industrial enterprise.* Cambridge, MA: MIT Press.

Cheung, S.N.S. (1983). The contractual nature of the firm. *Journal of Law and Economics, 25.*

Cheung, S.N.S. (1973, April). The fable of the bees. *Journal of Law & Economics, 16,* 11–33.

Citizen's guide to the federal budget. (1995). Fiscal Year 1996. Historical Budget Summary. Washington, DC: U.S. Government Printing Office.

Clynch, E., & Lauth, T. (Eds.). (1991). Introduction. *Governors, legislatures, and budgets: Diversity across the American states.* New York: Greenwood Press.

Coase, R. (1937). The nature of the firm. *Economica, 4.*

Cogan, J.F., Muris, T.J., & Schick, A. (1994). *The budget puzzle.* Stanford, CA: Stanford University Press.

Cohen, E.A., & Gooch, J. (1990). *Military misfortune: The anatomy of failure in war.* New York: The Free Press.

Cohen, S., & Eimicke, W. (1995). *The new effective public manager: Achieving success in a changing government.* San Francisco: Jossey-Bass.

Commander Naval Air Forces Pacific Flying Hour Program Brief for VADM Bowman, March 5, 1998.

Comptroller General of the United States. (1981). *Funding gaps jeopardize federal government operations.* Washington, DC: General Accounting Office.

Congressional Quarterly Almanac. (1982) pp. 258–261.

Cothran, D. (1981). Program flexibility and budget growth. *Western Political Quarterly, 34,* 593–610.

Curro, M., & Yocom, C. (1996, August). *A decade of change: Federal budget practices in the 1990's.* Paper presented at the Conference on Applied Public Finance, Willamette University, Salem, OR.

Davis J.W., & Ripley, R.B. (1967, November). The bureau of the budget and executive branch agencies: Notes on their interaction. *Journal of Politics, 29,* 749–769.

Defense Commissary Agency (DeCA). (1994). *Annual performance plan.* HQ, DeCA.

Defense Daily. (1997). DOD launches acquisition reform week, seeks to further cut costs. March 17, p. 408.

Defense Commissary Agency (DeCA), *Annual performance plan,* HQ, DeCA (1994).

Defense Logistics Agency (DLA), *Performance plan fiscal year 1995,* HQ, DLA (1994).

Defense Logistics Agency (DLA), *Performance plan fiscal year 1994,* HQ, DLA (1994).

Defense Logistics Agency (DLA). (1994b). *The DLA corporate plan.* HQ, DLA.

Demski, J., & Feltham, G. (1967). *Cost determination.* Ames: Iowa State University Press.

Department of Defense Financial Management Regulation, DoD 7000.14-R (2000, August), Vol. 3, Ch. 6, p. 6–4.

Derthick, M. (1975). *Uncontrollable spending for the social services.* Washington, DC: The Brookings Institution.

Dewey, D.R. (1968). *Financial history of the United States.* New York: Longmans, Green.

Dollenmayer, J. (1990, Winter). Landmarks in federal financial management. *Government Accountants Journal,* p. 2

Domenici, P. (1996, December 16). Make it a two year budget. *Washington Post National Weekly Edition,* p. 22.

Draper, F., & Pitsvada, T. (1981). Limitations in federal budget execution. *Government Accountants Journal, 30,* 3.

Drucker, P. (1982). The deadly sins in public administration. In F.S. Lane (Ed.), *Current issues in public administration* (2nd ed.). New York: St. Martin's Press.

Drucker, P. (1974). *Management: Tasks, responsibilities, practices.* New York, Harper & Row.

Drucker, P. (1953). *The practice of management.* New York: Harper & Brothers.

Duncombe, S., & Kinney, R. (1987, Spring). Agency budget success: How it is defined by agency officials in five western states. *Public Budgeting and Finance, 7,* 24–37.

Dunleavy, P., & Hood, C. (1994, July-September). From old public administration to new public management. *Public Money & Management, 1(3),* 9–16.

Eghtedari, A, & Sherwood, F. (1960). Performance budgeting in Los Angeles. *Public Administration Review, 20,* 63–85.

Euske, K. (1984). *Management control planning, control, measurement, and evaluation.* Reading, MA: Addison-Wesley.

Euske, N.A., & Euske, K.J. (1993). Institutional theory: Employing the other side of rationality in nonprofit organizations. *British Journal of Management.*

Evans, P.B., & Wurster, T.S. (1997, September-October). Strategy and the new economics of information. *Harvard Business Review,* 71–82.

Executive Office of the President, Office of Management and Budget (OMB). (1994). *Preparation and submission of budget estimates,* Circular A-11, Director, OMB.

Feldman, M., & March, J. (1981, June). Information in organizations as signal and symbol. *Administrative Sciences Quarterly,* 171–186.

Fenno, R. (1966). *The power of the purse.* Boston: Little, Brown.

Ferejohn, J. (1974). *Pork barrel politics.* Stanford, CA: Stanford University Press.

Fiorina, M. (1977). *Congress: Keystone of the Washington establishment.* New Haven, CT: Yale University Press.

Fischer, G.W., & Kamlet, M.S. (1984). Explaining presidential priorities: The competing aspiration levels model of macrobudgetary decision making. *American Political Science Review, 78,* 356–371.

Fisher, L. (1975). *Presidential spending power.* Princeton, NJ: Princeton University Press.

Fountain, J. (1994). Comment: Disciplining public management research. *Journal of Policy Analysis and Management, 13*(2), 269–277.

Fox, R. (1974). *Arming America: How the U.S. buys weapons.* Cambridge, MA: Harvard University Press.

Franklin, A.L. (1995, October). *Managing for results in Arizona state government: Arizona budget reform implementation.* Paper presented at the National Conference of the Association for Budgeting and Financial Management, Washington, DC.

Frant, H. (1996a). High-powered and low-powered incentives in the public sector. *Journal of Public Administration Research & Theory, 6*(3), 365–381.

Frant, H. (1996b). *Politics and effectiveness in the design of public organizations.* Unpublished manuscript, School of Public Administration and Policy, University of Arizona.

Frant, H. (1993). Rules and governance in the public sector: The case of civil service. *American Journal of Political Science, 37*(4), 990–1007.

Gaebler, T., & Osborne, D. (1993). *Reinventing government.* New York: Penguin Books, 1993.

Gallo, C.L. (1995). *DLA planning, programming, budgeting, and execution (PPBE) schedule.* Executive Director, Strategic Programming & Contingency Operations, HQ, DLA.

Garson, G.D., & Overman, E.S. (1983). *Public management research in the United States.* New York: Praeger.

Gates, B.L. (1980). *Social program administration: The implementation of social policy.* Englewood Cliffs, NJ : Prentice-Hall.

Gist, J. (1977, May). Increment and base in the congressional appropriation process. *American Journal of Political Science, 21,* 341–354.

Godek, P.A. (2000, December). *Emergency supplemental appropriations: A Department of Defense perspective.* Master's Thesis. Naval Postgraduate School, Monterey, CA.

Goldberg, V. (1976). Regulation and administered contracts. *Bell Journal of Economics, 7,* 426–428.

Gore, A. (1995). *Common sense government: Works better & costs less.* Third Report of the National Performance Review. Washington, DC: U.S. Government Printing Office.

Gore, A. (1993). *From red tape to results: Creating a government that works better and costs less.* Report of the National Performance Review. New York: Times Books/Random House.

Gosling, J. (1987, Spring). The state budget office and policy making. *Public Budgeting and Finance, 7,* 51–56.

Greider, W. (1981, December). The education of David Stockman. *The Atlantic Monthly.*

Grizzle, G. (1986). Does budget format really govern the actions of budgetmakers? *Public Budgeting and Finance, 6,* 60–70.

Gross, B. (1969). The new systems budgeting. *Public Administration Review, 29,* 113–137.

Gulick, L.H., & Urwick, L. (Eds.). (1937). *Papers on the science of administration.* New York: Institute of Public Administration, Columbia University.

Hamilton, A. (1961). *The federalist papers.* [See the version edited by J.E. Cooke, *The federalist.* Middletown, CT: Wesleyan University Press, 1961].

Hammer, M. (1990, July-August). Reengineering work: Don't automate, obliterate. *Harvard Business Review,* 104–112.

Hamre, J.J. (1995). *DoD corporate level performance goals and measures under GPRA-action memorandum.* Under Secretary of Defense, Comptroller.

Hamre, J.J. (1994, Winter). The future of financial management: Focus on performance. *Armed Forces Comptroller.*

Hanke, S. (1985). Privatization: Theory, evidence, implementation. In Harris (Ed.), *Control of federal spending.* Academy of Political Science.

Hanke, S. (1983). Land policy. In R. Howill (Ed.), *Agenda 83* (p. 65). Washington, DC: Heritage Foundation.

Hanke, S. (1982). The privatization debate. *Cato Journal, 656.*

Hargrove, E.C., & Glidewell, J.C. (Eds.). (1990). *Impossible jobs in public management.* Lawrence: University Press of Kansas.

Heckathorn, D.D., & Maser, S.M. (1987, Spring). Bargaining and the sources of transaction costs: The case of government regulation. *Journal of Law, Economics and Organization, 3*(1), 69–98.

Heclo, H. (1984). Executive budget making. In G.B. Mills & J. Palmer (Eds.), *Federal budget policy in the 1980s.* Washington, DC: The Urban Institute Press.

Heclo, H. (1975, Winter). OMB and the presidency: The problem of neutral competence. *Public Interest, 38,* 80–98.

Herzlinger, R.E., & Nitterhouse, D. (1994). *Financial accounting and managerial control for nonprofit organizations.* Cincinnati, OH: South-Western Pub.

Hinricks, H., & Taylor, G. (Eds.). (1969). *Program budgeting and benefit-cost analysis.* Pacific Palisades, CA: Goodyear.

Hodsoll, F. (1992, Winter). Facing the facts of the CFO Act. *Public Budgeting and Finance, 12*(4), 72–74.

Hofsted, G.H. (1967). *The game of budget control.* Van Gorcum.

Holstrom, B. (1979). Moral hazard and observability. *Bell Journal of Economics, 10.*

Hood, C. (1991, Spring). A public management for all seasons. *Public Administration, 69*(1), 3–20.

Hyde, A. (1978). A review of the theory of budget reform. In A. Hyde & J. Shafitz (Eds.), *Government budgeting* (pp. 71–77). Oak Park, IL: Moore.

Johnson, C., Jones, L.R., and Thompson, F. (1997). Management and control of budget execution. In J. Rabin and R. Golembiewski, (Eds.) *Handbook of public budgeting,* 2nd edition, New York: Marcel Dekker.

Johnson, B.E. (1984). From analyst to negotiator: The OMB's new role. *Journal of Policy Analysis and Management, 3*(4), 501–515.

Jones, L.R. (1993, Spring). Counterpoint essay: Nine reasons why the CFO Act may not achieve its objective. *Public Budgeting and Finance, 13*(1), 87–94.

Jones, L.R. (1986). Budget deficits and restraint management in western provincial governments. *American Review of Canadian Studies, 16,* 279–291.

Jones, L.R., & Bixler, G.C. (1992). *Mission financing to realign national defense.* Greenwich, CT: JAI Press.

Jones, L.R., and Euske, K. (1991). Strategic misrepresentations in budgeting. *Journal of Public Administration Research and Theory, 3*(4), 28–45.

Jones, L.R., Guthrie, J., and Steare, P. (Eds.) (2001). *Learning from public international public management experience. Vols. A & B.* New York: JAI–Elsevier Press

Jones, L.R., & McCaffery, J. (1993, Spring). Implementation of the CFO Act. *Public Budgeting and Finance, 13*(1), 68–76 .

Jones, L.R., & McCaffery, J. (1992, Winter). Federal financial management reform and the Chief Financial Officer's Act. *Public Budgeting and Finance, 12*(4), 75–86.

Jones, L.R., & McCaffery, J. (1989). *Government response to financial constraints.* Westport, CT: Greenwood.

Jones, L.R., and Thompson, F. (1999). *Public management: Institutional renewal for the twenty-first century.* New York: JAI–Elsevier Press.

Jones, L.R., & Thompson, F. (1994). *Reinventing the Pentagon.* San Francisco: Jossey-Bass.

Jones, L.R., & Thompson, F. (1986, Spring). Reform of budget execution control. *Public Budgeting and Finance, 6*(1), 33–49.

Joyce, P. (1993a, July). *Using performance measures in the federal budget process.* Washington, DC: Congressional Budget Office.

Joyce, P. (1993b, Fall). The reiterative nature of budget reform: Is there anything new in federal budgeting? *Public Budgeting and Finance, 13*(3), 45.

Joyce, P.G. (1993c, Winter). Using performance measures for federal budgeting: Proposals and prospects. *Public Budgeting and Finance, 13*(4), 3–17.

Joyce, P.G. (1996, Summer). Jesse Burkhead and the multiple uses of federal budgets: A contemporary perspective." *Public Budgeting and Finance, 16*(2), 70–75.

Jun, J.S. (1976). Management by objectives in the public sector. *Public Administration Review, 36,* 1–45.

Juran, J.M. (1944). *Bureaucracy, a challenge to better management: A constructive analysis of management effectiveness in the federal government.* New York: Harper & Brothers.

Kamlet, M.S., & Mowery, D.C. (1980). The budgetary base in federal resource allocation. *American Journal of Political Science, 74,* 804–821.

Kaplan, R.S. (1991, Autumn). The topic of quality in business school education and research. *Selections, 13*–21.

Kearns, P.S. (1994). State budget periodicity: An analysis of the determinants and the effect on state spending. *Journal of Policy Analysis and Management, 13,* 331–362.

Keating, P.J., & Paulk, D.A. (1998, December). *Examination of the Flying Hour Program (FHP) Budgeting Process and an Analysis of Commander Naval Air Forces Pacific (CNAP) FHP Underfunding.* Master's Thesis, Naval Postgraduate School, Monterey, CA.

Kelly, J., & Wanna, J. (2001). Are Wildowsky's guardians and spenders still relevant? In L.R. Jones, J. Guthrie, and P. Steare (Eds.), *Learning from international management reform* (pp. 589–614). New York: JAI–Elsevier Press.

Kemp, K.A. (1984). Accidents, scandals, and political support for regulatory agencies. *Journal of Politics, 46,* 401–427.

Killeen, A. (1990, Summer). A successful budget process. *Public Budgeting and Finance, 10,* 110–114.

Kotler, P. (1975). *Marketing for nonprofit organizations.* Englewood Cliffs, NJ: Prentice-Hall.

Kotler, P., & Andreasen, A.R. (1987). *Strategic marketing for nonprofit organizations.* Englewood Cliffs, NJ: Prentice-Hall.

Kozar, M.J. (1993). *An analysis of obligation patterns for the Department of Defense operations and maintenance appropriations.* Master's Thesis, Naval Postgraduate School, Monterey, CA.

Kozar, M., & McCaffery, J. (1994, October). DOD O&M obligation patterns: Some reflections and issues. *Navy Comptroller, 5*(1), 2–13.

Labaree, L.W. (1958). *Royal government in America: A study of the British colonial system before 1783.* New Haven, CT: Yale University Press.

Lan, Z., & Rosenbloom, D. (1992, November-December). Public administration in transition? *Public Administration Review, 52*(6), 535–537.

Landau, M. (1977, May). The proper domain of policy analysis. *American Journal of Political Science, 21*(2), 418–425.

Lapsley, I. (1994, September-December). Responsibility accounting revived? Market reforms and budgetary control. Management Accounting Research, 5(3,4), 337–352.

Larkey, P. (1979). *Evaluating public programs: The impact of general revenue sharing on municipal government.* Princeton, NJ: Princeton University Press.

Lauth, T.P. (1987). Exploring the budgetary base in Georgia. *Public Budgeting and Finance, 7,* 72–82.

Lee, R.D. (1991, May-June). Developments in state budgeting: Trends of two decades. *Public Adminstration Review, 51,* 254–262.

Lee, R.D., & Johnson, R. (1983). *Public budgeting systems.* Baltimore, MD: University Park Press.

Lehan, E.A. (1981). *Simplified government budgeting.* Chicago: Municipal Finance Officers Association of America.

LeLoup, L.T. (1978). The myth of incrementalism: Analytical choices in budgetary theory. *Polity, 10,* 488–509.

LeLoup, L.T., & Moreland, W.B. (1980). Agency strategies and executive review: The hidden politics of budgeting. In A. Schick (Ed.), *Perspectives on budgeting* (pp. 180–192). Washington, DC: American Society for Public Administration.

LeLoup, L.T., & Moreland, W.B. (1978). Agency strategies and executive review: The hidden politics of budgeting. *Public Administration Review, 38,* 232–239.

Levine, C. (1985). Where policy comes from: Ideas, innovations, and agenda choices. *Public Administration Review, 45,* 255–258.

Levine, C. (1978). Organizational decline and cutback management. *Public Administration Review, 38,* 316–324.

Levy, F. (1979, Summer). On understanding Proposition 13. *The Public Interest, 56,* 66–89.

Lewis, G.B. (1984). Municipal expenditures through thick and thin. *Publius, 14,* 31–40.

Lewis, C.W., & Logalbo, A.T. (1980). Cutback principles and practices: A checklist for managers. *Public Administration Review, 40,* 184–188.

Lovelock, C.H., & Weinberg, C.B. (1989). *Public & nonprofit marketing.* Redwood City, CA: Scientific Press.

Lynch, T. (1995). *Public budgeting in America.* Englewood Cliffs, NJ: PrenticeHall.

Lynn, L.E. (1996). *Public management as art, science, and profession.* Chatham NJ: Chatham House.

Lynn, L.E., Jr. (1994, Spring). Public management research: The triumph of art over science. *Journal of Policy Analysis and Management, 13,* 231–259.

Maroni, A. (1996, Fall). DoD implementation of the Government Performance and Results Act (GPRA). *Armed Forces Comptroller,* pp. 23–26.

Masujima, T., & O'uchi, M. (Eds.). (1993). *The management and reform of Japanese government.* Tokyo: The Institute of Administrative Management.

Mautz, R.K. (1991). Generally accepted accounting principles. *Public Budgeting and Finance, 11*(4), 3–11.

McAndrew, C.R. (1990, Winter). Strengthening controls for better government. *Association of Government Accountants Journal,* pp. 27–40.

McCaffery, J.L. (1987a). Budgetmaster: A budgeting practicuum 1987. Pacific Grove, CA: McCaffery.

McCaffery, J. (1987b). The development of public budgeting in the United States. In R.C. Chandler (Ed.), *A centennial history of the American administrative state* (pp. 345–379). New York: Macmillan and Co.

McCaffery, J., & Mutty, J. (1999). The hidden process in budgeting: Budget execution. *Journal of Public Budgeting, Accounting, and Financial Management, 11,* 233–275.

McCaffery, J., & Wolfgang, D. (1998). Performance budgeting with Donald Wolfgang. In J. Shafritz (Ed.), *International encyclopedia of public policy and administration.* Boulder, CO: Westview Press, 1623–1629.

McCaffery, J., & Wolfgang, D. (1995, October). *From performance measurement to performance budgeting.* Paper presented at the National Conference of the Association for Budgeting and Financial Management, Washington, DC.

McTighe, J. (1979). Management strategies to deal with shrinking resources. *Public Administration Review, 39,* 86–90.

Merewitz, L., & Sosnick, S.H. (1972). *The budget's new clothes.* Chicago: Markham.

Meyers, R. (1995, October). *Is there a key to the normative budgeting lock?* Paper presented at the National Conference of the Association for Budgeting and Financial Management, Washington, DC.

Meyers, R. (1994). *Strategic budgeting.* Ann Arbor: University of Michigan Press.

Meyers, R. (1990, April 9). *Strategic budgeting in the federal government.* Paper delivered at the Annual Conference of the American Society for Public Administration, Los Angeles, CA.

Meyerson, R.B. (1979). Incentives compatibility and the bargaining problem. *Econometrica, 47.*

Mikesell, J. (1986). *Fiscal administration.* Chicago: Dorsey Press.

Milgrom, P., & Roberts, J. (1992). *Economics, organization, and management.* Englewood Cliffs, NJ: Prentice-Hall.

Miller, G.J. (1992). *Managerial dilemmas: The political economy of hierarchy.* Cambridge: Cambridge University Press.

Miller, J.C. (1959). *Alexander Hamilton: Portrait in paradox.* NY: Harper.

Mirlees, J. (1976). The optimal structure of incentives and authority within an organization. *Bell Journal of Economics, 7.*

Mitnick, B. (1977). The theory of agency: The policing "paradox" and regulatory behavior. *Public Choice, 30.*

Moore, M.H. (1995). *Creating public value: Strategic management in government.* Cambridge, MA: Harvard University Press.

Morgan, J. (1949). Bilateral monopoly and the competitive output. *Quarterly Journal of Economics, 63.*

Mosher, F.C. (1954). *Program budgeting: Theory and practice.* New York: Public Administration Service.

Muris, T.J. (1994). The uses and abuses of budget baselines. In J.F. Cogan, T.J. Muris, & A. Schick (Eds.), *The budget puzzle* (pp. 41–78). Stanford, CA.: Stanford University Press.

Natchez, P.B., & Bupp, I.C. (1973). Policy and priority in the budgetary process. *American Political Science Review, 67,* 951–963.

New Zealand Treasury. (1987). *Report on management reforms* (p. 21).Wellington: New Zealand Treasury.

Novick, D. (Ed.). (1969). *Program budgeting.* New York: Holt.

OECD. (1995). *Budgeting for results: Perspectives on public expenditure management.* Paris: Organisation for Economic Co-operation and Development.

Office of the Auditor General of Canada. (1995). *Toward better governance: Public service reform in New Zealand and its relevance to Canada.* Ottawa: Author.

Osborne, D., & Gaebler, T. (1992). *Reinventing government: How the entrepreneurial spirit is transforming the public sector from schoolhouse to statehouse, city hall to the Pentagon.* Reading, MA: Addison Wesley.

Otley, D. (1994). Management control in contemporary organizations: Towards a wider framework. *Management Accounting.*

P.L. 103–62, Government Performance and Results Act of 1993. (1993).103d Congress.

Pearson, N.M. (1943). The budget bureau: From routine business to general staff. *Public Administration Review, 3,* 126.

Peck, M., & Scherer, F. (1962). *The weapons acquisition process: An economic analysis.* Cambridge, MA: Harvard Business School.

Peckman, J.A. (Ed.). (1983). *Setting national priorities: The 1984 budget.* Washington, DC: The Brookings Institution.

Perry, W.J., Secretary of Defense. (1996, March). *Annual report to the President and Congress.* Washington, DC: U.S. Government Printing Office.

Personal interview with Flying Hour Program staff member, Commander Naval Air Force Pacific, San Diego, CA, April 27, 2001.

Personal interview with Flying Hour Program staff member, Commander Naval Air Force Pacific, San Diego, CA, March 28–30, 2001.

Personal interview with Flying Hour Program staff member, Commander Naval Air Force Pacific, San Diego, CA, January 17–18, 2001.

Pfeffer, J., & Salancik, G. (1974). Organizational decision making as a political process: The case of a university budget. *Administrative Sciences Quarterly, 19,* 135–151.

Pfiffner, J. (1991). OMB: Professionalism, politicization, and the presidency. In C. Campbell & M. Wyszomirski (Eds.), *Executive leadership in Anglo-American systems* (pp. 195–225).

Pierce, L.C. (1971). *The politics of fiscal policy formation.* Pacific Palisades, CA: Goodyear.

Pitsvada, B.T. (1983). Flexibility in federal budget execution. *Public Budgeting and Finance, 3*(2), 83–101.

Poole, R. (1982). Air traffic control: The private sector option. *Heritage Foundation, Backgrounds, 216.*

Poole, R. (1980). *Cutting back city hall.*: University Books.

Poole, R. (1976, May). Fighting fires for profit. *Reason.*

Powell, F.W. (1939). *Control of federal expenditures.* Washington, DC: The Brookings Institution.

Powers, K.A., & Thompson, F. (1994). Managing coprovision: Using expectancy theory to overcome the free-rider problem. *Journal of Public Administration Research and Theory, 4*(2), 179–196.

Pressman, J.L., & Wildowsky, A. (1973). *Implementation.* Berkeley, CA: The University of California Press.

Pyhrr, P.A. (1977). The zero-base approach to government budgeting. *Public Administration Review, 37,* 1–8.

Quinn, J.B. (1992). Intelligent enterprise: A knowledge and service based paradigm for industry. New York: Free Press.

Reschenthaler, G.B., & Thompson, F. (1996). The information revolution and the new public management. *Journal of Public Administration Research and Theory, 6*(1), 125–144.

Rhodes R.A.W. (1991, Spring). The new public management. *Public Administration, 69*(1), entire issue.

Rickards, R.C. (1990, Summer). Budget presentations in Texas. *Public Budgeting and Finance, 10*(2), 72–87.

Riso, G. (1988). Role of the federal chief financial officer. *Public Budgeting and Finance, 8*(3), 55–62.

Rivlin, A.M. (1995, Summer). Linking resources to results: Management and budgeting in a time of resource constraints. *The Public Manager*, p. 3.

Rodriguez, J. (1996, Winter). Connecting resources with results. *Budget and Finance*, pp. 2–4.

Rogers, J., & Brown, M. (1999). Preparing agency budgets. In R. Meyers (Ed.), *Handbook of government budgeting* (pp. 441–469). San Francisco: Jossey-Bass.

Rose, J.H. (1911a). *William Pitt and national revival*. London: G. Bell and Sons.

Rose, J.H. (1911b). *William Pitt and the great war*. London: G. Bell and Sons.

Rose, J.H. (1912). *Pitt and Napoleon*. London: G. Bell and Sons.

Rose, R. (1977). Implementation and evaporation: The record of MBO. *Public Administration Review, 37*, 64–71.

Rose, R. (1976). *Managing presidential objectives*. New York: Free Press.

Rosenberg, N., & Birdsall, L.E. (1986). *How the west grew rich: The economic transformation of the industrial world*. New York: Basic Books.

Rosenbloom, D.H. (1993, November-December). Have an administrative Rx? Don't forget the politics! *Public Administration Review, 53*, 503–507.

Rubin, I.S. (1993, September/October). Who invented budgeting in the United States? *Public Administration Review, 53*(5), 438–444.

Rubin, I.S. (1985). *Shrinking the federal government: The effect of cutbacks on five federal agencies*. New York: Longman.

Rubin, I., & Stein, L. (1990, July-August). Budget reform in St. Louis: Why does budgeting change? *Public Administration Review, 50*, 421–425.

Savas, E.S. (1977). Policy analysis for local government. *Policy Analysis, 3*, 49–77.

Schedler, K. (1995). *Ansatze einer Wirkungsorientirten Verwaltungsfuhrung: Von der Idee des New Public Managements (NPM) zum konkreten Gestaltungsmodell*. Bern: Verlag Paul Haupt.

Scherer, F. (1964). *The weapons acquisition process: Economic incentives*. Cambridge, MA: Harvard Business School.

Schick, A. (1994). *The federal budget*. Washington, DC: The Brookings Institution.

Schick, A. (1990). *The capacity to budget*. Washington, DC: The Urban Institution.

Schick, A. (1988). Micro-budgetary adaptations to fiscal stress in industrialized democracies. *Public Administration Review, 48*, 523–533.

Schick, A. (1982a). *Reconciliation and the congressional budget process*. Washington, DC: American Enterprise Institute.

Schick, A. (1982b). Contemporary problems in financial control. In F. Lane (Ed.), *Current issues in public administration* (2d ed., pp. 361–371). New York: St. Martin's Press.

Schick, A. (1980a). *Zero-base budgeting*. Washington, DC: National Association of State Budget Officers.

Schick, A. (1980b). *Congress and money: Budgeting, spending and taxing*. Washington, DC: Urban Institute.

Schick, A. (1978). The road from ZBB. *Public Administration Review, 30*, 177–180.

Schick, A. (1973). A death in the bureaucracy: The demise of federal PPB. *Public Administration Review, 33*, 146–156.

Schick, A. (1970, Summer). The budget bureau that was: Thoughts on the rise, decline and future of a presidential agency. *Law and Contemporary Problems, 35*, 519–539.

Schick, A. (1966, December). The road to PPB: The stages of budget reform. *Public Administration Review, 26,* 243–258.

Schick, A. (1964). Control patterns in state budget executions. *Public Administration Review, 24,* 97–106.

Schick, A., Keith, R., & Davis, E. (1991). *Manual on the federal budget process.* Washington, DC: Congressional Research Service.

Schlesinger, J. (2001, August 15). The enforcer: Bush budget director jousts with congress, and big fight is likely. *The Wall Street Journal,* pp. 1, 7.

Schwartz, H. (1994, July). Small states in big trouble. *World Politics, 46*(4), 527–555.

Seckler-Hudson, C. (1978). Performance budgeting in Government. In A. Hyde & J. Shafritz (Eds.), *Government budgeting* (pp. 80–93). Oak Park, IL: Moore Publishers.

Seiko, D.T. (1940). *The federal financial system.* Washington, DC: The Brookings Institution.

Sharkansky, I. (1969). *The politics of taxing and spending.* New York: Bobbs Merril.

Sharkansky, I. (1968). Agency requests, gubernatorial support and budget success in state legislatures. *American Political Science Review, 62,* 1220–1231.

Shepsle, K., & Weingast, B. (1981). Political preferences for the pork barrel. *American Journal of Political Science, 25.*

Shewhart, W.A., & Deming, W.E. (1945). *Statistical method from the viewpoint of quality control.* Washington, DC: The Graduate School, The U.S. Department of Agriculture.

Shubik, M., & Stark, R. (Eds.). (1983). *Auctions, bidding, and contracting.* New York: New York University Press.

Shycoff, D.B. (1992). *Performance budgeting memorandum.* Washington, DC: Comptroller of The Department of Defense.

Sigelman, L. (1986). The bureaucrat as budget maximizer: An assumption examined. *Public Budgeting and Finance, 6,* 50–59.

Simon, H. et al. (1954). *Centralization vs. Decentralization in organizing the controller's department.* New York: The Controllership Foundation.

Simons, R. (1995). *Levers of control: How managers use innovative control systems to drive strategic renewal.* Boston: Harvard Business School Press.

Skinner, B.F. (1978). *Reflections on behaviorism and society.* Englewood Cliffs, NJ: Prentice-Hall.

Smith, G.D. (1941). The bureau of the budget. *Public Administration Review, 1,* 106.

Smith, R.G. (1983, May). Feet to the fire. *Reason,* 23–29.

Smithies, A. (1955). *The budgetary process in the United States.*

Sokolow, A.D., & Honadle, B.W. (1984, September/October). How rural local governments budget: The alternatives to executive preparation. *Public Administration Review, 44,* 373–383.

Staats, E. (1981). Financial management improvements: An agenda for federal managers. *Public Budgeting and Finance, 1*(1), 44.

Stanbury, W.T., & Thompson, F. (1995, September/October). Toward a political economy of government waste. *Public Administration Review, 55*(5), 418–427.

Stark, R. (1983). On cost analysis for engineered construction. In R. Englebrecht-Wiggins, M. Shubik, & R. Stark (Eds.), *Auctions, Bidding, and contracting.* New York: New York University Press.

Stark, R., & Varley, T. (1983). Bidding, estimating, and engineered construction contracting. In R. Englebrecht-Wiggins, M. Shubik, & R. Stark (Eds.), *Auctions, bidding, and contracting* (pp. 121–135). New York: New York University Press.

Statutes at Large. (1789, September 29). U.S. Congress, Chapter XXIII, p. 95.

Steinberg, H.I. (1996, March). The CFO Act: A look at federal accountability. *Government Accounting*, p. 57.

Steinhoff, J., Skelly, J., & Narang, J. (1990, Winter). Modernizing systems and practices. *Association of Government Accountants Journal*, pp. 48–56.

Straussman, J.D. (1986). Courts and public purse strings: Have portraits of budgeting missed something? *Public Administration Review, 46*, 345–351.

Taft, W.H., President of the United States. (1912, January 27). *Message on economy and efficiency in the government service.* H. Doc 458 62–2.

Thompson, F. (1984). How to stay within the budget using per-unit prices. *Journal of Policy Analysis and Management, 4*(1).

Thompson, F. (1981). Utility maximizing behavior in organized anarchies. *Public Choice, 36.*

Thompson, F. (1997). The new public management. *Journal of Policy Analysis and Management, 16*(1), 165–176.

Thompson, F., & Fiske, G. (1978). One more solution to the problem of higher education finance. *Policy Analysis, 3*(4).

Thompson, F., & Jones, L.R. (1986, Spring). Controllership in the public sector. *Journal of Policy Analysis and Management, 5*(3), 74–76.

Thompson, F., & Zumeta, W. (1981). Controls and controls: A reexamination of control patterns in budget execution. *Policy Sciences 13*, 25–50.

Thompson, J. (1967). *Organizations in action.* New York: McGraw Hill.

Thomson, M.A. (1938). *A constitutional history of England* (Vol. IV). London: Methuen & Co.

Thurmaier, K. (1998). Budget analyst. In J. Shafritz (Ed.), *International encyclopedia of public policy and administration* (pp. 233–240). Boulder, CO: Westview Press.

Thurmaier, K. (1997). Decisive decisionmaking in the executive budget process: Analyzing the political and economic propensities of central budget bureau analysts. *Public Administration Review.*

Thurmaier, K. (1995). Decisive decisionmaking in the executive budget process. *Public Administration Review, 55*(5), 429–438.

Thurmaier, K. (1992). Budgetary decisionmaking in central budget bureaus: An experiment. *Journal of Public Administration Research and Theory, 2*(4), 463–487.

Tomkin, S.L. (1983). OMB budget examiner's influence. *The Bureaucrat, 12*, 43–47.

Trebilcock, M.J. (1994). *The prospects for reinventing government.* Toronto: C.D. Howe Institute.

Tucker, H.J. (1982). Incremental budgeting: Myth or model? *Western Political Quarterly, 35*, 327–338.

Tyszkiewicz, M., & Daggett, S. (1998, December 8). *A Defense budget primer.* CRS Report for Congress.

U.S. Bureau of Census. (1994). *Census of governments, Vol. I: Government organization.* Washington, DC: U.S. Department of Commerce, Bureau of the Census.

U.S. Army Corps of Engineers. (1994). *Performance plan for fiscal year 1995.* Washington, DC: U.S. Army Corps of Engineers.

U.S. Office of Management and Budget. (2000, October 2). Mission Statement, Strategic Plan, FY 2001–2005.

U.S. Senate, Subcommittee on Intergovernmental Relations. (1977). *Compendium of materials on zero-base budgeting in the states.* Washington, DC: U.S. Government Printing Office.

Verville, A.-L. (1995, Fall). What business needs from higher education? *The Educational Record, 76*(4), 46–50.

Vining, A.R., & Weimer, D. (1990, March-April). Government supply and government production failure: A framework based on contestability. *Journal of Public Policy, 10*, 54–90.

Wanat, J. (1975). Bureaucratic politics in the budget formulation arena. *Administration and Society, 7*, 191–212.

Weicker, J. (1980). *Housing.* Washington, DC: American Enterprise Institute.

Weimer, D.L., & Vining, A.R. (1992). *Policy analysis: Concepts and practice* (2nd ed.). Englewood Cliffs, NJ: Prentice-Hall.

Weiss, J. (1982, Fall). Coping with complexity: An experimental study of public policy decision-making. *Journal of Policy Analysis and Management, 2*, 65–82.

White, B. (1999). Examining budgets for chief executives. In R. Meyers (Ed.), *Handbook of government budgeting* (pp. 462–484). San Francisco: Jossey-Bass.

White, J. (1985). Much ado about everything: Making sense of federal budgeting. *Public Administration Review, 45*, 623–630.

White, J., & Wildavsky, A. (1990). *The deficit and the public interest.* Berkeley: The University of California Press.

White, L.D. (1958). *The Republican Era.* New York: Macmillan.

White, L.D. (!954). *The Jacksonians.* New York: Macmillan.

White, L.D. (1951). *The Jeffersonians.* New York: Macmillan.

White, L.D. (1948). *The Federalists.* New York: Macmillan.

Wholey, J., & Hatry, H. (1992). The case for performance monitoring. *Public Administration Review, 52*(6), 604–610.

Wildavsky, A. (1992). *The new politics of the budgetary process* (2nd ed.). New York: Harper Collins Publishers.

Wildavsky, A. (1988). *The new politics of the budgetary process.* Boston: Little, Brown and Co.

Wildavsky, A. (1985). The logic of public sector growth. In J.E. Lane (Ed.), *State and market* (pp. 231–270). London: Sage Publications, Ltd.

Wildavsky, A. (1984a). On the balance of budgetary cultures. In R. Chandler (Ed.), *A history of American public administration* (pp. 379–382). New York: John Wiley.

Wildavsky, A. (1984b). *The politics of the budgetary process* (4th ed.). Boston: Little, Brown and Co.

Wildavsky, A. (1980). *How to limit government spending.* Los Angeles/Berkeley: University of California Press.

Wildavsky, A. (1979). *The politics of the budgetary process* (3rd ed.). Boston: Little, Brown.

Wildavsky, A. (1976, January). Principles for a graduate school of public policy. *The Journal of Urban Analysis, 3*(1), 127–152.

Wildavsky, A. (1975). *Budgeting: A comparative theory of the budgetary process.* Boston: Little, Brown and Co.

Wildavsky, A. (1974). *The politics of the budgetary process* (2nd ed.). Boston: Little, Brown.

Wildavsky, A. (1964). *The politics of the budgetary process.* Boston: Little, Brown.

Wildavsky, A. (1961). Political implications of budget reform. *Public Administration Review, 21,* 183–190.

Wildavsky, A., & Hammann, A. (1956). Comprehensive versus incremental budgeting in the Department of Agriculture. *Administrative Sciences Quarterly, 10,* 321–346.

Williamson, O. (1975). *Markets and hierarchies.* New York: Free Press.

Williamson, O. (1964). *The economics of discretionary behavior.* Englewood Cliffs, NJ: Prentice-Hall.

Willoughby, K. (1993). Decision making orientations of state government budget analysts: Rationalists or incrementalists? *Public Budgeting and Financial Management, 5*(1), 67–74.

Wilmerding, Jr., L. (1943). *The spending power: A history of the efforts of Congress to control expenditures.* New Haven, CT: Yale University Press.

Wolfgang, D. (1994, June). *Performance measurement and The Government Performance and Results Act of 1993.* Master's Thesis. Naval Postgraduate School, Monterey, CA.

Womack, J.P., Jones, D.T., & Roos, D. (1990). *The machine that changed the world: Based on the Massachusetts Institute of Technology 5-million dollar 5-year study on the future of the automobile.* New York: Rawson Associates.

World Bank. (1995). *Bureaucrats in business: The economics and politics of government ownership.* New York: Oxford University Press.

Zimmerman, J. (1977). The municipal accounting maze: An analysis of political incentives. *Journal of Accounting Research, 21,* 107–144.

Zody, R. (1998a). Budget ethics. In J. Shafritz (Ed.), *International encyclopedia of public policy and administration* (pp. 251–252). Boulder, CO: Westview Press.

Zody, R.E. (1998b). Budget tools, commonsense. In J. Shafritz (Ed.), *International encyclopedia of public policy and administration* (pp. 290–294). Boulder, Co: Westview Press.

Zuboff, S. (1988). *In the age of the smart machine: The future of work and power.* New York: Basic Books.